Hot Topics in Emergency Radiology

Editors

JENNIFER W. UYEDA
SCOTT D. STEENBURG

RADIOLOGIC CLINICS OF NORTH AMERICA

www.radiologic.theclinics.com

Consulting Editor
FRANK H. MILLER

January 2023 • Volume 61 • Number 1

ELSEVIER

1600 John F. Kennedy Boulevard • Suite 1800 • Philadelphia, Pennsylvania, 19103-2899

http://www.theclinics.com

RADIOLOGIC CLINICS OF NORTH AMERICA Volume 61, Number 1
January 2023 ISSN 0033-8389, ISBN 13: 978-0-323-98753-0

Editor: John Vassallo (j.vassallo@elsevier.com)
Developmental Editor: Karen Solomon

Radiologic Clinics of North America (ISSN 0033-8389) is published bimonthly by Elsevier Inc., 360 Park Avenue South, New York, NY 10010-1710. Months of issue are January, March, May, July, September, and November. Periodicals postage paid at New York, NY and additional mailing offices. Subscription prices are USD 544 per year for US individuals, USD 1007 per year for US institutions, USD 100 per year for US students and residents, USD 643 per year for Canadian individuals, USD 1415 per year for Canadian institutions, USD 739 per year for international individuals, USD 1415 per year for international institutions, USD 100 per year for Canadian students/residents, and USD 315 per year for international students/residents. To receive student and resident rate, orders must be accompanied by name of affiliated institution, date of term and the signature of program/residency coordinatior on institution letterhead. Orders will be billed at individual rate until proof of status is received. Foreign air speed delivery is included in all *Clinics* subscription prices. All prices are subject to change without notice. **POSTMASTER:** Send address changes to *Radiologic Clinics of North America*, Elsevier Health Sciences Division, Subscription Customer Service, 3251 Riverport Lane, Maryland Heights, MO63043. **Customer Service: Telephone: 1-800-654-2452** (U.S. and Canada); **1-314-447-8871** (outside U.S. and Canada). **Fax: 1-314-447-8029. E-mail: journalscustomerservice-usa@elsevier.com (for print support); journalsonlinesupport-usa@elsevier.com (for online support).**

Reprints. For copies of 100 or more of articles in this publication, please contact the Commercial Reprints Department, Elsevier Inc., 360 Park Avenue South, New York, New York 10010-1710. Tel.: +1-212-633-3874; Fax: +1-212-633-3820; E-mail: reprints@elsevier.com.

Radiologic Clinics of North America also published in Greek Paschalidis Medical Publications, Athens, Greece.

Radiologic Clinics of North America is covered in *MEDLINE/PubMed (Index Medicus), EMBASE/Excerpta Medica, Current Contents/Life Sciences, Current Contents/Clinical Medicine, RSNA Index to Imaging Literature, BIOSIS, Science Citation Index,* and *ISI/BIOMED.*

Contributors

CONSULTING EDITOR

FRANK H. MILLER, MD, FACR, FSAR, FSABI
Lee F. Rogers, MD, Professor of Medical
Education; Chief, Body Imaging Section;
Medical Director, MRI; Professor, Department
of Radiology, Northwestern Memorial Hospital,
Northwestern University Feinberg School of
Medicine, Chicago, Illinois, USA

EDITORS

JENNIFER W. UYEDA, MD
Assistant Professor, Department of Radiology,
Emergency Radiology, Brigham and Women's
Hospital, Boston, Massachusetts, USA

SCOTT D. STEENBURG, MD, FASER
Assistant Professor, Department of Radiology
and Imaging Sciences, Indiana University
School of Medicine, Indiana University Health,
Indianapolis, Indiana, USA

AUTHORS

**FERCO H. BERGER, MD, EDER, FASER,
FESER**
Associate Professor, Deputy-Chief
(Operations) and Head, Division of Emergency
and Trauma Radiology, Sunnybrook Health
Sciences Centre, University of Toronto,
Department of Medical Imaging, Toronto,
Ontario, Canada

MARC A. CAMACHO, MD, MS, FACR
Assistant Professor, Chief, RAF Watch/Acute
Care Radiology Division, Head, Acute Care
Radiology Section, Department of Radiology,
University of South Florida Morsani College of
Medicine, Florida State University College of
Medicine, Radiology Partners, Radiology
Associates of Florida, Tampa General Hospital,
Tampa, Florida, USA

MAURICIO CASTILLO, MD, FACR
Professor, Department of Radiology, Division
of Neuroradiology, University of North Carolina
School of Medicine, Chapel Hill, North
Carolina, USA

SACHIV CHAKRAVARTI, BS
Johns Hopkins University, Baltimore,
Maryland, USA

AISARA CHANSAKUL, MPH
Research Associate, Weill Cornell Medical
Center, New York, New York, USA

SUZANNE T. CHONG, MD, MS, FASER
Professor of Radiology, Emergency Radiology
Division, Indiana University School of
Medicine, Indiana University Health,
Department of Radiology and Imaging
Sciences, IUH University Hospital,
Indianapolis, Indiana, USA

NOAH DITKOFSKY, MD, FRCPC
Division of Emergency, Trauma and Acute Care
Radiology, St. Michael's Hospital, Toronto,
Ontario, Canada

JEFFREY W. DUNKLE, MD, FACR
Assistant Professor, Vice Chair of Clinical
Affairs, Indiana University School of Medicine,
Indiana University Health, Department of

Radiology and Imaging Sciences, IUH University Hospital, Indianapolis, Indiana, USA

YIGAL FRANK, MD
Division of Emergency, Trauma and Acute Care Radiology, St. Michael's Hospital, Toronto, Ontario, Canada

DANIEL D. FRIEDMAN, MD
Mallinckrodt Institute of Radiology, Washington University School of Medicine, St Louis, Missouri, USA

TAREK N. HANNA, MD
Department of Radiology and Imaging Sciences, Emory University School of Medicine, Atlanta, Georgia, USA

JAMLIK-OMARI JOHNSON, MD, FASER
Chief of Radiology, Emory University School of Medicine, Professor, Department of Radiology and Imaging, Atlanta, Georgia, USA

SURAJ KAPOOR, MD
Mallinckrodt Institute of Radiology, Washington University School of Medicine, St Louis, Missouri, USA

VENKAT KATABATHINA, MD
Professor of Radiology, UT Health San Antonio, San Antonio, Texas, USA

ABHISHEK KERALIYA, MD
Brigham and Women's Hospital, Emergency Radiology, Boston, Massachusetts, USA

LOKESH KHANNA, MD
Assistant Professor of Radiology, UT Health San Antonio, San Antonio, Texas, USA

BHARTI KHURANA, MD
Department of Radiology, Trauma Imaging Research and Innovation Center, Brigham and Women's Hospital, Harvard Medical School, Boston, Massachusetts, USA

MARA KUNST, MD
Assistant Professor, Department of Radiology, Lahey Hospital and Medical Center, Tufts University School of Medicine, Boston, Massachusetts, USA

M. STEPHEN LEDBETTER, MD, MPH, FASER
Assistant Professor, Medical Director, Enterprise Medical Imaging Informatics, Department of Radiology, Brigham and Women's Hospital, Mass General Brigham, Harvard Medical School, Boston, Massachusetts, USA

MIHAN LEE, MD, PhD
Resident, Weill Cornell Medical Center, New York, New York, USA

SHOBHIT MATHUR, MD
Division of Emergency, Trauma and Acute Care Radiology, St. Michael's Hospital, Toronto, Ontario, Canada

VINCENT M. MELLNICK, MD, FSAR
Abdominal Imaging Division, Mallinckrodt Institute of Radiology, Washington University School of Medicine, St Louis, Missouri, USA

CHRISTINE "COOKY" MENIAS, MD
Professor, Department of Radiology, Mayo Clinic, Scottsdale, Arizona, USA

ROBERT MORELAND, MD, FRCPC
Division of Emergency, Trauma and Acute Care Radiology, St. Michael's Hospital, Toronto, Ontario, Canada

RAWAN ABU MUGHLI, MD
Assistant Professor, Division of Emergency and Trauma Radiology, Sunnybrook Health Sciences Centre, University of Toronto, Department of Medical Imaging, Toronto, Ontario, Canada

FELIPE MUNERA, MD
Department of Radiology, Jackson Memorial Hospital, University of Miami Miller School of Medicine, Department of Radiology, Ryder Trauma Center, Miami, Florida, USA

JAYKUMAR RAGHAVAN NAIR, MD
Division of Emergency, Trauma and Acute Care Radiology, St. Michael's Hospital, Toronto, Ontario, Canada

BIPIN NANDA, MD
Division of Emergency, Trauma and Acute Care Radiology, St. Michael's Hospital, Toronto, Ontario, Canada

SAVVAS NICOLAOU, MD, FASER
Professor of Radiology, Head and Medical Director, Department of Radiology, Vancouver General Hospital, University of British Columbia, Vancouver, British Columbia, Canada

DEVANG ODEDRA, MD, MASC, FRCPC
Department of Medical Imaging, North York General Hospital, Toronto, Ontario, Canada

FABIO M. PAES, MD, MBA
Department of Radiology, Jackson Memorial Hospital, University of Miami Miller School of Medicine, Department of Radiology, Ryder Trauma Center, Miami, Florida, USA

MICHAEL N. PATLAS, MD, FRCPC, FASER, FCAR, FSAR
Division of Emergency/Trauma Radiology, Department of Radiology, McMaster University, Hamilton General Hospital, Hamilton, Ontario, Canada

PAULO PUAC-POLANCO, MD, MSc
Assistant Professor, Department of Radiology, McMaster University, St. Joseph's Healthcare, Juravinski Innovation Tower, Hamilton, Ontario, Canada

MOHAMED Z. RAJPUT, MD
Mallinckrodt Institute of Radiology, Washington University School of Medicine, St Louis, Missouri, USA

ANTHONY ROSEN, MD
Associate Professor, Weill Cornell Medical Center, New York, New York, USA

JESSICA A. ROTMAN, MD
Attending and Assistant Professor, Unity Health Toronto, Division of Emergency, Trauma and Acute Care Radiology, St. Michael's Hospital, Toronto, Ontario, Canada

JEAN SEBASTIEN ROWE, MD
Department of Radiology and Imaging Sciences, Emory University School of Medicine, Atlanta, Georgia, USA

NINAD SALASTEKAR, MBBS, MPH
Department of Radiology and Imaging Sciences, Emory University School of Medicine, Atlanta, Georgia, USA

AARON D. SODICKSON, MD, PhD
Associate Professor, Medical Director of Enterprise Emergency Radiology, Department of Radiology, Brigham and Women's Hospital, Mass General Brigham, Harvard Medical School, Wayland, Massachusetts, USA

ARAVIND SOMASUNDARAM, MD
Department of Radiology and Imaging Sciences, Emory University School of Medicine, Atlanta, Georgia, USA

ANDRES SU, MD
Department of Radiology and Imaging Sciences, Emory University School of Medicine, Atlanta, Georgia, USA

ANJI TANG, MD
Department of Radiology, Brigham and Women's Hospital, Trauma Imaging Research and Innovation Center, Brigham and Women's Hospital, Harvard Medical School, Boston, Massachusetts, USA

CARLOS TORRES, MD, FRCPC
Professor, Department of Radiology, Radiation Oncology and Medical Physics, University of Ottawa, Ottawa, Ontario, Canada

JENNIFER W. UYEDA, MD
Assistant Professor, Department of Radiology, Emergency Radiology, Brigham and Women's Hospital, Boston, Massachusetts, USA

DANIEL VARGAS, MD
Assistant Professor of Radiology, UT Health San Antonio, San Antonio, Texas, USA

ANDREW WONG, MD, PhD
Department of Radiology, Trauma Imaging Research and Innovation Center, Brigham and Women's Hospital, Harvard Medical School, Boston, Massachusetts, USA

PHILLIP K. WONG, MD
Department of Radiology and Imaging Sciences, Emory University School of Medicine, Atlanta, Georgia, USA

JEREMY R. WORTMAN, MD
Assistant Professor, Department of Radiology,
Lahey Hospital and Medical Center, Tufts
University School of Medicine, Boston,
Massachusetts, USA

ALEC J. WRIGHT, MD
Mallinckrodt Institute of Radiology,
Washington University School of Medicine, St
Louis, Missouri, USA

HEI SHUN YU, MD
Brigham and Women's Hospital, Emergency
Radiology, Boston, Massachusetts, USA

CARLOS ZAMORA, MD, PhD
Associate Professor, Division Head of
Neuroradiology, Department of Radiology,
University of North Carolina School of
Medicine, Chapel Hill, North Carolina,
USA

Contents

> Multi-energy computed tomography is a technology that is being increasingly used in the emergency room (ER) setting and has many applications that can impact patient care, including virtual monoenergetic imaging and material-specific imaging. It is important for radiologists to understand this technology, and how it can be optimally used in the ER setting.

> Computed tomography (CT) plays an important role in trauma because imaging findings directly impact management. Advances in CT technology, specifically multienergy CT, have allowed for simultaneous acquisition of images at low and high kilovolt peaks. This technique allows for differentiation of materials given that materials have different absorption behaviors. Various multienergy CT postprocessing applications are helpful in the setting of trauma, including bone subtraction, virtual monoenergetic imaging, iodine-selective imaging, and virtual noncontrast imaging. These techniques have been applied from head to toe and have been used to improve image quality and increase conspicuity of injuries, which increases diagnostic confidence.

> Historically, computed tomography of the abdomen and pelvis had been performed routinely with enteric contrast to help improve diagnostic accuracy. However, the utility of enteric contrast has been called into question recently, particularly in the high-patient-volume setting of the emergency department. This article reviews the role of enteric contrast in the emergency setting. Particular emphasis is given to specific clinical scenarios in which enteric contrast provides value. These include the identification of abdominal postsurgical complications such as anastomotic leaks and fistulas, detection of penetrating bowel injuries, evaluation of acute appendicitis, and assessment of small-bowel obstructions.

> Intimate partner violence (IPV) is a major public health problem with adverse health and mental consequences. Patient- and clinician-related barriers to screening include underreporting, misattribution of IPV to other causes, and patients not seeking help or facing social stigmas and discrimination. Radiology may help overcome these barriers through objective imaging evaluation, noting mismatches between image findings and provided clinical history. Recognizing injury patterns specific to IPV on imaging aids early identification and intervention even when the patient is not forthcoming. This article examines the ways radiologists have adapted to meet an ever-increasing demand for diagnosis and reporting of IPV.

Elder abuse, defined as "harm inflicted on an older person in a relationship where there is an expectation of trust, and/or when the person is targeted based on age or disability," can be challenging for clinicians to identify. Radiologists can help raise appropriate suspicion for elder abuse based on a patient's imaging. This article reviews common distributions and radiographic patterns of injury sustained in physical elder abuse. It also discusses limitations and unique challenges to the radiologic assessment of elder abuse, including issues of communication with frontline providers, and broad overlap in the appearance of abusive and accidental injuries in the setting of old age and deconditioning.

Patients with head and neck cancers are susceptible to emergencies related to tumor infiltration, systemic disorders, or treatment. Computed tomography plays a major role in imaging assessment and MRI provides further characterization. Hematologic disorders may lead to hemorrhage, thrombosis, or ischemia. Patients are susceptible to metabolic derangements that are often not recognized. Complications in the neck are threatening due to compromise of vascular structures and airway.

Oncology patients can present with acute, life-threatening conditions that may arise either due to underlying malignancy or secondary to cancer therapy. Select oncologic emergencies show characteristic imaging findings on radiographs, ultrasound, computed tomography, and MRI that helps in timely diagnosis. Radiologists need to be aware of typical imaging findings in such patients in an emergency setting and should be able to guide the clinicians for proper patient management. Appropriate knowledge of the treatment and its timing is pivotal in diagnosing treatment-related complications.

Establishing an emergency radiology division in a practice that has long-standing patterns of operational routines comes with both challenges and opportunities. In this article, considerations around scheduling and staffing, compensation, and equity and parity are provided with supporting literature references. Furthermore, a panel of experts having established, grown and managed emergency radiology divisions in North America and Europe share their experiences through a question and answer format.

Understanding the pathophysiology of a disease allows physicians to make a diagnosis, alter its natural course, and develop and implement appropriate preventative and management strategies. With ballistic injuries, an understanding of how the mechanism of injury translates to the injuries observed makes it possible to make sense of what can, at times be a complex imaging appearance and mitigate against the long-term complications of gunshot wounds. In this article, the authors describe the different types of ballistic projectiles, their mechanism of injury as well as the injury patterns they cause. In addition, both lead arthropathy and MR imaging safety in patients with retained ballistic debris are discussed.

Imaging of Trauma in Pregnancy 129

Devang Odedra, Vincent M. Mellnick, and Michael N. Patlas

A pregnant patient with acute trauma is not commonly encountered by clinicians and radiologists. A multidisciplinary approach is key. Although radiography and ultrasound examination are frequently used modalities in the setting of maternal–fetal trauma, the fear of radiation should not preclude from carrying out a thorough diagnostic workup of the patient with a computed tomography scan. MRI mainly serves as a problem solving and follow-up modality. After stabilizing the mother, fetal wellbeing should be assessed with external fetal monitoring and a dedicated obstetric ultrasound examination. Radiologists should be familiar with the sonographic and computed tomography findings of catastrophic entities.

Computer Tomography Angiography of Peripheral Vascular Injuries 141

Fabio M. Paes and Felipe Munera

Peripheral vascular injuries are a rare finding in the setting of trauma but an important source of morbidity and mortality when present. Fast and accurate diagnosis followed by rapid repair of vascular injuries are important for achieving the best clinical outcomes. The advancements in computer tomography (CT) and decades of experience in vascular imaging have allowed radiologists to become important contributors for the diagnosis and characterization of peripheral vascular injury. We review the epidemiology of peripheral vascular injuries, indications for imaging, ways to optimize CT technique, imaging findings, and common challenges for accurate diagnosis of such injuries.

Imaging of Soft Tissue Infections 151

Ninad Salastekar, Andres Su, Jean Sebastien Rowe, Aravind Somasundaram, Phillip K. Wong, and Tarek N. Hanna

Although superficial infections can often be diagnosed and managed clinically, physical examination may lack sensitivity and specificity, and imaging is often required to evaluate the depth of involvement and identify complications. Depending on the area of involvement, radiography, ultrasound, CT, MR imaging, or a combination of imaging modalities may be required. Soft tissue infections can be nonnecrotizing or necrotizing, with the later having a morbid and rapid course. Infectious tenosynovitis most commonly affects the flexor tendon sheaths of the hand, characterized by thickened and enhancing synovium with fluid-filled tendon sheaths.

PROGRAM OBJECTIVE

The objective of the *Radiologic Clinics of North America* is to keep practicing radiologists and radiology residents up to date with current clinical practice in radiology by providing timely articles reviewing the state of the art in patient care.

TARGET AUDIENCE

Practicing radiologists, radiology residents, and other healthcare professionals who provide patient care utilizing radiologic findings.

LEARNING OBJECTIVES

Upon completion of this activity, participants will be able to:

1. Describe the difficulties and complications that radiologists may face when providing care in the emergency room.
2. Discuss the significance of using a multidisciplinary approach when using imaging techniques in the emergency room setting to assess, diagnose, and treat illnesses and traumatic injuries, particularly in special patient populations.
3. Recognize imaging methods, such as multi-energy CT enteric contrast, as valuable tools for identifying, diagnosing, evaluating, and guiding treatment for the variety of medical conditions, injuries, and trauma seen in emergency rooms.

ACCREDITATION

The Elsevier Office of Continuing Medical Education (EOCME) is accredited by the Accreditation Council for Continuing Medical Education (ACCME) to provide continuing medical education for physicians.

The EOCME designates this journal-based CME activity for a maximum of 12 *AMA PRA Category 1 Credit*(s)™. Physicians should claim only the credit commensurate with the extent of their participation in the activity.

All other healthcare professionals requesting continuing education credit for this enduring material will be issued a certificate of participation.

DISCLOSURE OF CONFLICTS OF INTEREST

The EOCME assesses conflict of interest with its instructors, faculty, planners, and other individuals who are in a position to control the content of CME activities. All relevant conflicts of interest that are identified are thoroughly vetted by EOCME for fair balance, scientific objectivity, and patient care recommendations. EOCME is committed to providing its learners with CME activities that promote improvements or quality in healthcare and not a specific proprietary business or a commercial interest.

The planning committee, staff, authors, and editors listed below have identified no financial relationships or relationships to products or devices they or their spouse/life partner have with commercial interest related to the content of this CME activity:

Rawan Abu Mughli, MD; Ferco H. Berger, MD, EDER; Marc A. Camacho, MD, MS, FACR; Mauricio Castillo, MD, FACR; Sachiv Chakravarti; Aisara Chansakul; Suzanne T. Chong, MD, MS; Noah Ditkofsky, MD, FRCPC; Jeffrey W. Dunkle, MD; Yigal Frank, MD; Daniel D. Friedman, MD; Tarek N. Hanna, MD; Jamlik-Omari Johnson, MD; Suraj Kapoor, MD; Venkat Katabathina, MD; Abhishek Keraliya, MD; Lokesh Khanna, MD; Bharti Khurana, MD; Mara Kunst, MD; Pradeep Kuttysankaran; M. Stephen Ledbetter, MD, MPH; Mihan Lee, MD, PhD; Shobhit Mathur, MD; Vincent M. Mellnick, MD; Christine Menias, MD; Robert Moreland, MD, FRCPC; Felipe Munera, MD; Jaykumar Raghavan Nair, MD; Bipin Nanda, MD; Savvas Nicolaou, MD; Devang Odedra, MD, MASc; Fabio M. Paes, MD, MBA; Michael N. Patlas, MD; Paulo Puac-Polanco, MD, MSc; Mohamed Z. Rajput, MD; Anthony Rosen, MD; Jessica A. Rotman, MD; Jean Sebastien Rowe, MD; Ninad Salastekar, MBBS, MPH; Aaron D. Sodickson, MD, PhD; Aravind Somasundaram, MD; Scott D. Steenburg, MD, FASER; Andres Su, MD; Anji Tang, MD; Doreen Thomas-Payne, MSN, BSN, RN, PMHNP-BC; Carlos Torres, MD, FRCPC; Jennifer W. Uyeda, MD; Daniel Vargas, MD; Andrew Wong, MD/PhD; Phillip K. Wong, MD; Alec J. Wright, MD; Hei Shun Yu, MD; Carlos Zamora, MD, PhD

The planning committee, staff, authors, and editors listed below have identified financial relationships or relationships to products or devices they or their spouse/life partner have with commercial interest related to the content of this CME activity:

Jeremy R. Wortman, MD: *Cosultant*: United Imaging Intelligence

UNAPPROVED/OFF-LABEL USE DISCLOSURE

The EOCME requires CME faculty to disclose to the participants:

1. When products or procedures being discussed are off-label, unlabelled, experimental, and/or investigational (not US Food and Drug Administration [FDA] approved); and
2. Any limitations on the information presented, such as data that are preliminary or that represent ongoing research, interim analyses, and/or unsupported opinions. Faculty may discuss information about pharmaceutical agents that is outside of FDA-approved labelling. This information is intended solely for CME and is not intended to promote off-label use of these medications. If you have any questions, contact the medical affairs department of the manufacturer for the most recent prescribing information.

TO ENROLL

To enroll in the *Radiologic Clinics of North America* Continuing Medical Education program, call customer service at 1-800-654-2452 or sign up online at http://www.theclinics.com/home/cme. The CME program is available to subscribers for an additional annual fee of USD 356.00.

METHOD OF PARTICIPATION

In order to claim credit, participants must complete the following:

1. Complete enrolment as indicated above.
2. Read the activity.
3. Complete the CME Test and Evaluation. Participants must achieve a score of 70% on the test. All CME Tests and Evaluations must be completed online.

CME INQUIRIES/SPECIAL NEEDS

For all CME inquiries or special needs, please contact elsevierCME@elsevier.com.

RADIOLOGIC CLINICS OF NORTH AMERICA

SERIES OF RELATED INTEREST

Advances in Clinical Radiology
Available at: https://www.advancesinclinicalradiology.com/
Magnetic Resonance Imaging Clinics
Available at: https://www.mri.theclinics.com/
Neuroimaging Clinics
Available at: www.neuroimaging.theclinics.com
PET Clinics
Available at: www.pet.theclinics.com

THE CLINICS ARE AVAILABLE ONLINE!
Access your subscription at:
www.theclinics.com

Preface
Hot Topics in Emergency Radiology

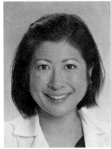
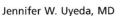
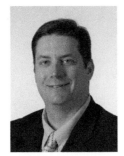

Jennifer W. Uyeda, MD   Scott D. Steenburg, MD, FASER

Editors

When we were approached by Elsevier to guest edit an issue on Emergency Radiology, our thoughts immediately went to the 2019 *Radiologic Clinics of North America* issue titled "Trauma and Emergency Radiology," edited by Stephan W. Anderson, MD from Boston University. Our goal with this current issue was to include topics that are unique and timely but without substantial overlap with the 2019 issue, which is no small feat given the breadth and high quality of material included in the outstanding 2019 issue.

In this issue, we believe that we have assembled an excellent group of highly regarded, leading experts focusing on high-yield and timely topics that are relevant to the practicing emergency radiologist. Herein, we include topics and areas of emerging research that may be new to some radiologists. Topics include multienergy CT in the setting of trauma, the use of enteric contrast in the Emergency Department, intimate partner violence and elder abuse, a head-to-toe review of oncologic emergencies, a panel discussion focused on the challenges of starting an emergency radiology division, wound ballistics for the emergency radiologist, imaging of traumatized pregnant patient, imaging of peripheral vascular trauma, and a multimodality imaging review of soft tissue infections. We certainly hope you enjoy and benefit from this unique collection.

We want to sincerely thank and congratulate the contributing authors for sharing their valuable time and expertise. Last, we would like to thank the staff at Elsevier for their assistance, guidance, and flexibility throughout the development of this issue.

Jennifer W. Uyeda, MD
Department of Radiology
Brigham and Women's Hospital
75 Francis Street
Boston, MA 02115, USA

Scott D. Steenburg, MD, FASER
Department of Radiology and
Imaging Sciences
Indiana University School of Medicine and
Indiana University Health
550 North University Boulevard, Room 0663
Indianapolis, IN 46202, USA

E-mail addresses:
juyeda@bwh.harvard.edu (J.W. Uyeda)
ssteenbu@iuhealth.org (S.D. Steenburg)

Radiol Clin N Am 61 (2023) xv
https://doi.org/10.1016/j.rcl.2022.09.004
0033-8389/23/© 2022 Published by Elsevier Inc.

Multi-Energy CT Applications
Problem-Solving in Emergency Radiology

Jeremy R. Wortman, MD[a,b,*], Mara Kunst, MD[a,b]

KEYWORDS

• Dual-energy computed tomography (CT) • Multi-energy CT • Emergency radiology • Spectral CT

KEY POINTS

- Multi-energy computed tomography (MECT) is a technology that is being increasingly used in the emergency department setting.
- There are many MECT applications that can impact patient care in the emergency room (ER) setting, and it is important for radiologists to be aware of how MECT can be optimally used in ER patients.
- Virtual monoenergetic imaging at low energy allows for increased iodine conspicuity, which can improve image quality of contrast-enhanced CT studies and improve detection of pathology.
- Iodine-selective imaging allows for iodine quantification and subtraction, which has many applications in ER patients.

Abbreviations	
FDA	food and drug administration
tPA	tissue plasminogen activator
rCBF	relative cerebral blood flow
DWI	diffusion weighted imaging
DSA	digital subtraction angiography
US	ultrasound
MRA	magnetic resonance angiography
IV	intravenous
SNR	signal to noise ratio
CNR	contrast to noise ratio
ROI	region of interest

INTRODUCTION

Multi-energy computed tomography (MECT), also referred to as dual-energy CT or spectral CT, is an imaging technology that has the potential to improve diagnosis and impact patient care. With an increasing number of emergency departments using MECT scanners, it is important for radiologists to know how this technology can be used

[a] Department of Radiology, Lahey Hospital and Medical Center, 41 Mall Road, Burlington, MA 01805, USA;
[b] Tufts University School of Medicine, 145 Harrison Avenue, Boston, MA 02111, USA
* Corresponding author. Department of Radiology, Lahey Hospital and Medical Center, 41 Mall Road, Burlington, MA 01805.
E-mail address: jeremy.wortman@lahey.org

Radiol Clin N Am 61 (2023) 1–21
https://doi.org/10.1016/j.rcl.2022.08.004
0033-8389/23/© 2022 Elsevier Inc. All rights reserved.

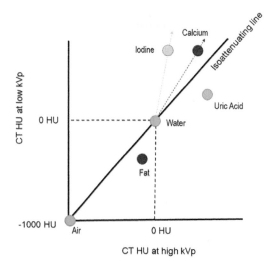

Fig. 1. HU values of different materials are displayed at low kVp (*y* axis) and high kVp (*x* axis). Water and air are calibrated at 0 and -1000, respectively, at both low and high kVp. Fat and uric acid demonstrate lower photon absorption as kVp decreases. Conversely, iodine and calcium show increased photon absorption as kVp decreases.

in the emergency room (ER) setting. In this article, the authors review the various MECT applications that can be optimally used for problem-solving in emergency radiology, focusing on evaluation of the nontraumatic ER patient.

MULTI-ENERGY COMPUTED TOMOGRAPHY OVERVIEW, PHYSICS, AND TECHNICAL PRINCIPLES

On conventional single-energy CT (SECT), imaging is performed with a single polyenergetic energy spectrum, usually ranging from 80 to 140 kVp. With MECT, CT data are acquired using two different energy levels: low energy (generally 70–100 kVp) and high energy (140–150 kVp). By imaging with two energy spectra, MECT allows some materials to be differentiated based on their chemical compositions. In order for materials to be differentiated, they must demonstrate differences in x-ray absorption behavior as a function of kilovolt peak. These differences are referred to as the *dual-energy ratio* or *CT number ratio* of materials, which is defined as the ratio of the attenuation (in Hounsfield units [HU]) of the material at low kVp to the attenuation of the material at high kVp. Some materials, such as iodine and calcium, show increased x-ray absorption and thus increased HU as kVp decreases; other materials, such as uric acid and fat, show increased x-ray absorption and increased HU as kVp increases. With MECT, these types of materials

can be isolated within images and can be quantified (**Fig. 1**).

POST-PROCESSING TOOLS

In this section, the authors review the most common post-processing applications used for problem-solving in emergency radiology. In the remainder of this article, the authors review the literature and show examples of how these applications can be used in emergency radiology.

Material-Specific Imaging

Materials that are isolated and quantified using MECT can be displayed visually with the use of *material-specific imaging*. Among these images, the most common are material-specific imaging of iodine, uric acid, and calcium.

Because of the ubiquitous use of iodine in CT imaging, material-specific imaging of iodine is one of the most common MECT post-processing techniques (**Fig. 2**). Iodine-selective images can demonstrate iodine content visually, either in gray scale or in color. Color-coded "iodine overlay" images have the advantage of demonstrating iodine content superimposed on an image with more anatomic detail, usually a virtual noncontrast (VNC) image. Although iodine concentration (in mg/mL of iodine) can be measured directly from iodine selective images, this cannot be performed in the Picture Archive and Communication System (PACS) and requires use of a vendor post-processing software package.

Conversely, if iodine is subtracted from images, this creates a VNC image. Attenuation measurements from VNC images have been shown to be accurate and comparable to true non-contrast (TNC) images in a variety of clinical settings. Unlike iodine maps and overlay images, attenuation (HU) on VNC images can be measured directly in PACS without using a post-processing software package, allowing them to be easily incorporated into clinical workflow.

Several other material-specific imaging applications are available with MECT. Material-specific imaging of uric acid allows uric acid content can be displayed in gray scale or with color-coded images, which can be used to distinguish uric acid from calcium-based stones and to image patients with gout to assess disease burden. Material-specific imaging of calcium can be used to create virtual non-calcium (VNCa) images, which subtract trabecular bone, help visualize bone marrow edema, and improve detection of marrow replacing lesions such as lytic metastases.

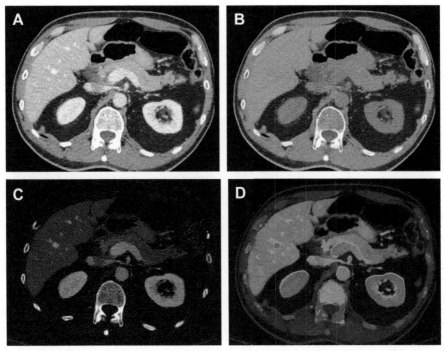

Fig. 2. Example of iodine-selective imaging. From a conventional image (*A*), iodine can be subtracted from the image creating a virtual non-contrast (VNC) image (*B*). Iodine content can be imaged in gray scale with an iodine no water image (*C*). Iodine can be imaged in color with an iodine overlay image (*D*).

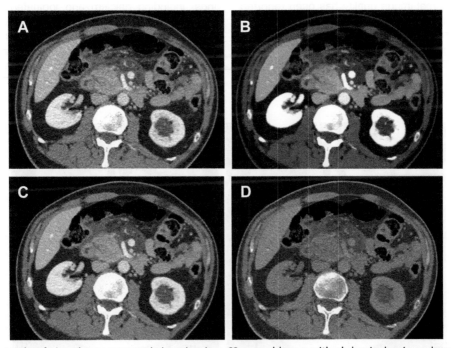

Fig. 3. Example of virtual monoenergetic imaging in a 62-year-old man with abdominal pain and pancreatitis. Compared with conventional images (*A*), iodine content is more conspicuous on 40 keV images (*B*); 70 keV images (*C*) are similar in appearance to conventional images. On high-keV images at 170 keV (*D*), iodine enhancement decreases.

Virtual Monoenergetic Images

With MECT, virtual monoenergetic images (VMI) are post-processed, simulated images that display the scan as if it had been performed at a single-energy level (kiloelectron volt [keV]). These simulated, monoenergetic images can range from low energy (around 40 keV) to high energy (around 200 keV) (**Fig. 3**). At low keV, iodine content will be accentuated; at high keV, iodine will be less conspicuous, and metallic beam hardening artifact will be reduced.

CLINICAL APPLICATIONS
Applications in Emergency Neuroradiology

Brain parenchyma
Technique and image quality Head CT image quality relies on maximizing grey-white matter differentiation, defining the bone/brain interface while minimizing beam-hardening artifacts. Although mean CT values of specific anatomic structures can vary by keV, conventional CT imaging is best simulated by combining low- (80 kVp) and high (140 kVp)-energy CT data, with a reported optimal ratio of 0.6.[1] Optimal keV selection for VMI will vary based on scanner generation, manufacturer, and reconstruction algorithm but can also be individualized to highlight pathology based on lesion type and location. In the supratentorial brain parenchyma, optimal image quality has been reported as 65 keV in adults and 60 to 65 keV in children.[2–4] In the posterior fossa, where beam-hardening artifact may limit lesion detection, higher keV imaging (80–100 keV) has shown some benefit but must be balanced with image noise and soft tissue contrast[5] for individual lesion detection. As in other

body parts, high-energy monoenergetic images are useful in decreasing beam-hardening artifacts from dental hardware and metallic intracranial devices (**Fig. 4**).

Pathology
Hemorrhage and mimics Evaluation for intracranial hemorrhage (ICH) is the most common indication for emergent head CT evaluation. As such, it has laid the groundwork for several FDA-approved artificial intelligence (AI) algorithms that are trained to detect hyperdense findings in specific anatomic locations and flag them as potential hemorrhage on a radiology worklist. For ICH detection, monoenergetic keV selection depends on the hemorrhage density and location, with at least one report citing best delineation of hemorrhage in gray matter at 120 keV and white matter at 40 keV.[6] In the age of AI, low-keV monoenergetic imaging may also aid in the detection of sometimes subtle isodense subdural hematomas by emphasizing differential attenuation of blood products in the hemorrhage itself and by accentuating the margins of the displaced brain parenchyma (**Fig. 5**).

Beyond detection, MECT has a well-documented role in the characterization of ICH and distinction from mimics. Using material decomposition, hemorrhage can reliably be distinguished from other hyperdense intracranial findings, including calcium and iodinated contrast. Through VNCa and VNC techniques, MECT allows point-of-care problem-solving without having to rely on MR imaging, which may be contraindicated, not available or introduce significant delays that may be detrimental to the patient presenting with a neurologic emergency.

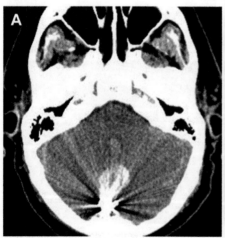 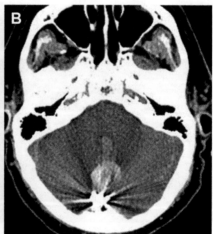

Fig. 4. Embolization material partially obscures the adjacent parenchymal hematoma in this patient with a ruptured arteriovenous malformation on conventional image (A). Beam-hardening artifact is reduced at 170 keV (B), at a cost of increased noise and decreased soft tissue contrast of the adjacent cerebellum.

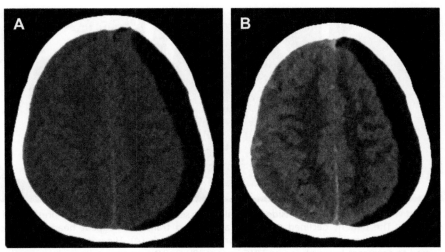

Fig. 5. A left-sided hypodense chronic subdural hematoma is clearly visible on both images. A more subtle iso-dense right acute subdural hematoma is difficult to visualize on the conventional image (A) and was not detected by an AI detection algorithm. On a 50-keV monoenergetic image (B), the right subdural hematoma is more conspicuous due to increased highlighted internal heterogeneity of blood products and enhanced visualization of displaced gray matter.

One area that has shown promise in MECT is distinguishing hemorrhage from calcium. Although most calcifications can be readily distinguished from hemorrhage, occasionally a small hyperdense focus will be indeterminate on SECT. Traditionally, these would be further characterized by MR imaging; alternatively, some institutions will follow these with serial CT to monitor for change in size. By using VNCa and calcium overlay images, these lesions can be characterized with greater diagnostic accuracy and diagnostic confidence.[7] When combined with other features, including the location, appearance, and associated findings, accuracy in distinguishing calcium from hemorrhage was been reported as high as 100% in small lesions.[8] In addition, bone removal with MECT calcium subtraction can be used in emergency neuroradiology; this technique may allow for improved visualization of small acute subdural hematomas or hemorrhagic contusions adjacent to the skull base.[9]

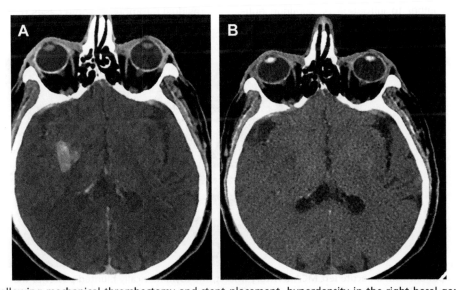

Fig. 6. Following mechanical thrombectomy and stent placement, hyperdensity in the right basal ganglia was present on SECT (A). The patient was re-scanned with MECT, and a VNC image (B) revealed contrast staining rather than hemorrhage, allowing the patient to receive the anticoagulation needed to maintain the patency of the stent.

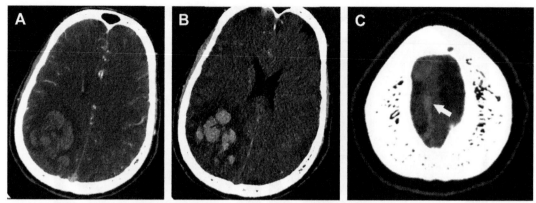

Fig. 7. In a patient who presented to an outside hospital with a seizure, a head CT was interpreted as displaying a right parietal mass. The patient declined neurologically during transfer. A repeat head CT was performed following a contrast-enhanced CT of the chest, abdomen, and pelvis (*A*). Hyperdensity in the right parietal lobe is confirmed to represent hemorrhage on VNC images (*B*). On VNC images, a hyperdense cortical vein can also be seen (*C, white arrow*).

Distinguishing hemorrhage from contrast Distinguishing iodinated contrast from hemorrhage was among the first described clinical advantages of MECT in neuroradiology[10] and has found important clinical relevance in the assessment of the acute stroke patient following reperfusion therapy. Contrast staining following intra-arterial thrombolysis or mechanical thrombectomy can linger in the cerebral parenchyma for 24 to 48 hours, overlapping with the time window for postprocedural hemorrhage or hemorrhagic transformation.[11] VNC images are able to safely and reliably distinguish contrast from hemorrhage,[12] a role of critical importance when deciding whether to introduce or continue antiplatelet or anticoagulant medication (**Fig. 6**).

In the ER setting, it is not uncommon for a noncontrast head CT to be performed following previous contrast administration. On these examinations, hyperdense, extra-axial collections may represent acute subdural hematomas or iodine leakage into a chronic subdural effusion/hygroma. MECT and VNC images can also help to distinguish these,[13] thereby avoiding the need for follow-up imaging and allowing more timely administration of anticoagulant medication.

In addition to eliminating the contribution of contrast to the attenuation of the cerebral parenchyma, contrast is also virtually removed from the vessels with VNC images, revealing underlying or residual thrombus in some cases (**Fig. 7**).

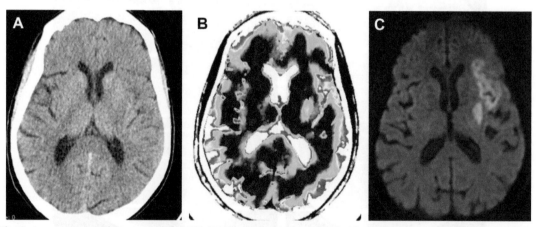

Fig. 8. In a patient with an acute left MCA territory infarct, the asymmetrically blunted posterior margin of the left lentiform nucleus is difficult to appreciate on CT using standard brain windows (*A*). Use of MECT reconstructed images to accentuate water or edema in gray and white matter (*B*), the infarct in the left lentiform nucleus and insula is clearly visualized. The corresponding MR imaging diffusion-weighted image (*C*) confirms this finding. MCA, middle cerebral artery.

Ischemia In the setting of acute stroke, head CT is obtained to exclude hemorrhage before tPA administration and also to assess for early ischemic changes. CT findings of early ischemia can be extremely subtle, particularly in the first 6 hours, when response to tPA or mechanical thrombectomy is highest. Nonetheless, these findings have significant prognostic implications, as large, completed infarcts are at increased risk for hemorrhagic transformation following thrombolytic therapy.[14,15] Although MR imaging is considered the gold standard for imaging cerebral infarcts, CT correlates have long been sought after to avoid the limitations and time delays inherent to MR imaging. For many years, CT perfusion imaging has filled this role, with validated software packages demonstrating accurate identification of completed infarction through a calculated decreased CBF relative to normal brain tissue (rCBF) less than 30%.[16] However, this technique uses an additional contrast bolus and a large amount of radiation to achieve this goal.

By using material decomposition to separate brain parenchyma into gray matter, white matter, and water, MECT reconstructed images are able to accentuate differences in fractional lipid content in gray and white matter, improving depiction of water, and therefore edema without additional contrast or radiation. These "X maps"[17,18] have shown increased sensitivity and accuracy for early stroke detection correlating with DWI in early studies (Fig. 8).

Similarly, modified VNC images that separate air, water, and iodine result in a uniform density background image, against which there is improved edema visualization,[19] allowing for more accurate detection of edema and end-infarct volume as compared with conventional CT images (Fig. 9).

Cerebral Vasculature

Technique and image quality
CT angiography (CTA) is the preferred noninvasive screening examination for evaluation of the head and neck vessels. The examination is quite technique-dependent, however, and can be limited by a suboptimal contrast bolus injection or timing, as well as beam-hardening artifacts commonly arising from dental or procedural hardware, adjacent venous contrast bolus, or patient's shoulders. Low-energy VMI can accentuate contrast in vessels, though at the expense of increased image noise. By using additional techniques to reduce noise, 40 keV images have been shown to demonstrate the optimal image quality on CTA examinations.[20] This technique can be used to decrease radiation dose or contrast amount in select patients.[21]

CTAs are also frequently recommended following endovascular aneurysm treatment, where accentuated intravascular contrast needs to be closely balanced with artifact reduction to evaluate vessels immediately adjacent to clip and coils. In these cases, monoenergetic images from 40 to 70 keV combined with metal artifact reduction software produced the best image quality.[22]

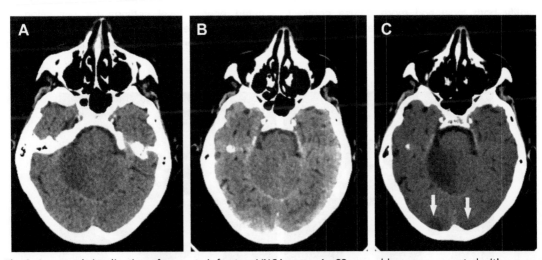

Fig. 9. Improved visualization of an acute infarct on VNC images. An 82-year-old woman presented with syncope and was found to have a basilar thrombus. A large area of completed acute infarction in the right superior cerebellar artery territory is only faintly visible on the conventional images (A) and is not well visualized on 50 keV images (B). The infarct is clearly visualized on VNC images (C), which also improves visualization of infarcts in both occipital poles (white arrows in C).

Pathology

Stenosis assessment With its superior image quality and its visualization of intraluminal contents, DSA is the gold standard for estimating percent vessel stenosis before surgery or stenting. Nonetheless, CTA is frequently used as a noninvasive substitute and has shown strong correlation to DSA imaging.[23] The difficulty in CTA interpretation, however, is often due to the presence of adjacent bone or calcified plaque which can influence stenosis measurements. MECT using calcium/bone subtraction has been proposed as a potential solution in these problem areas; however, the reconstructed images can result in overestimation of percent stenosis, even mistaking high-degree stenosis for occlusion when compared with contrast-enhanced MR angiography.[24] As such, corroboration with other modalities, including US, MRA, or confirmation with DSA is often still needed.

Active bleeding Spontaneous intracerebral hemorrhage is the second most common cause of stroke following ischemic stroke. Being able to identify those patients at highest risk for hematoma expansion is critical to guiding treatment goals, whether surgical or medical. Active contrast extravasation into a primary parenchymal hemorrhage on CT has long been associated with hematoma expansion and poor prognosis.[25] This CTA "spot sign" was shown to accurately predict hematoma expansion[26] though with the sensitivity of 51% and specificity of 85%.[27] By using MECT and iodine quantification in the hematoma, Tan and colleagues were able to more accurately quantify both focal and more diffuse contrast leakage within the hematoma, resulting in 71% sensitivity and 93% specificity.[28]

Computed Tomography Soft Tissue Neck

Technique and image quality

Optimal signal to noise ratio for CT soft tissue neck imaging is achieved at 65 keV, with 40 keV being optimal for tumor visualization.[29] Blended images of 80/150 Sn kVp demonstrated improved image quality at lower radiation dose in third-generation dual-source MECT scanners relative to 120 kVp SECT.[30] Significant metal and dental artifact reduction has been reported in multiple studies on VMI at 88 keV or higher energies.[31–33] Last, VNC images provide the accurate assessment of sialolithiasis.[34]

Pathology

Tumor visibility and characterization Poor contrast resolution is one of the most limiting factors of CT soft tissue neck imaging. This is often exacerbated in the sometimes cachectic patient with head and neck cancer with superimposed postsurgical scarring and posttreatment inflammation. By using the strong spectral properties of iodinated contrast, MECT with low-keV images can improve tumor visibility and allow distinction of tumor muscle interfaces in these patients, though at the cost of increased image noise[29] (**Fig. 10**).

Spine

Technique and image quality

Similar to MECT technique for other body parts, utilization of high-energy VMI has resulted in optimal image quality by reducing artifacts from spinal hardware. Two studies have advised dedicated energy level settings for evaluation of hardware–bone interface, spinal canal, and abdominal contents,[35,36] with noise-optimized

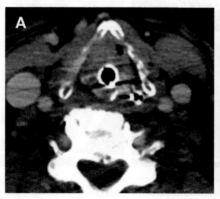
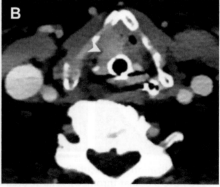

Fig. 10. Images of a 63-year-old intubated patient where low keV imaging at 50 keV (*B*) showed improved conspicuity of an incidental right vocal cord lesion (*yellow arrowhead* in *B*), which is not visible on conventional images (*A*).

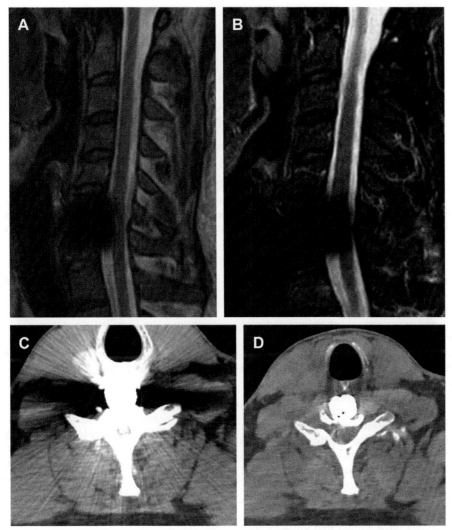

Fig. 11. Patient with susceptibility artifact from C6-7 ACDF hardware in MR imaging T2 (*A*) and STIR (*B*) sequences with persistent symptoms who subsequently underwent CT myelography. Beam-hardening artifact on CT limits assessment on conventional images (*C*), which is significantly reduced on 170 keV images with metal artifact reduction (MAR) (*D*).

VMI at 120 to 130 keV resulting in the least metallic artifacts and highest image quality. Combining high-energy VMI with metal artifact reduction software technique can further decrease artifacts (Fig. 11).

Pathology
For assessment of vertebral body compression fractures, CT has the benefit of depicting bony margins, whereas MR imaging is used to visualize marrow edema and assess acuity. Recent articles have indicated that MECT may be nearly as good as MR imaging at depicting bone marrow edema and lumbar disc herniation, potentially obviating the need for this additional examination.[37] Color-

coded VNCa imaging also yielded substantially higher diagnostic accuracy and confidence for assessing thoracic disk herniation compared with standard CT.[38]

APPLICATIONS IN EMERGENCY THORACIC AND ABDOMINAL IMAGING
Computed Tomography Angiography

Technique and image quality
CT angiograms of the chest and abdomen are among the most commonly performed cross-sectional imaging studies in the emergency department[39] to evaluate patients who present

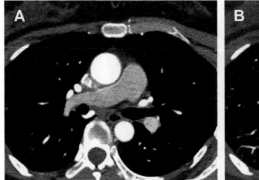
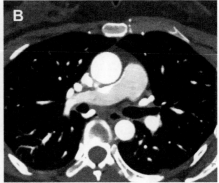

Fig. 12. A 45-year-old woman with chest pain. Conventional images from CT pulmonary angiogram (*A*) are suboptimal, with poor contrast enhancement, and attenuation at the pulmonary trunk of 180 HU. Reconstructed images at 40 keV (*B*) have significantly improved image quality, with attenuation at the pulmonary trunk of 612 HU.

with chest and abdominal pain as well as patients who sustain blunt and penetrating trauma.

Image quality is a frequent challenge in ER CTA studies, with many causes including motion, patient positioning, and poor contrast enhancement due to bolus timing or IV infiltration. This is especially common with CT pulmonary angiography (CTPA), where adequate enhancement of the pulmonary arterial tree is essential to make an accurate diagnosis, and repeat studies are not uncommonly performed.[40] Low-keV VMI, by accentuating iodine, will improve vascular enhancement in CTA studies and thereby improve image quality. The benefits of this technical advantage has been demonstrated in many CTA study types in thoracic and abdominal imaging, including CTPA,[41] aortic imaging,[42] evaluation of the abdominal vasculature,[43] and CT coronary angiography.[44]

Several studies have shown that low-keV VMI can be used to salvage nondiagnostic CTPA imaging, avoiding the need for a repeat study. Ghandour and colleagues[45] found that most of the CTPA studies with suboptimal enhancement could be salvaged with low-keV VMI, usually at 40 or 50 keV. Similarly, Bae and colleagues found that 78 of 79 suboptimally enhanced CTPA studies could reach diagnostic quality with low-keV VMI, with the highest CNR at 40 keV.[46] This same principle can be applied to other CTA studies, whereby reviewing low-keV images in an apparent suboptimal conventional CT angiogram renders a diagnostic quality study (Fig. 12).

Technique: contrast dose

Another potential technique advantage of using low-keV VMI is the ability to maintain image quality at a reduced dose of intravenous contrast in patients with renal insufficiency. For example, Dong and colleagues found that a low-contrast dose CTPA protocol using low-keV VMI allowed for superior intravascular enhancement, improved diagnostic confidence and comparable radiation dose when compared with a standard 120-kVp protocol.[47] These findings have been replicated in a variety of scan types in vascular imaging that are relevant to emergency radiologists: CTA imaging of the thoracic aorta,[48] coronary CT,[49,50] and imaging of the abdominal vasculature.[51–53] In

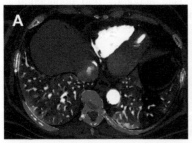
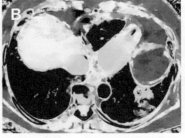
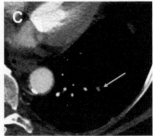

Fig. 13. CT pulmonary angiogram in 85-year-old woman with chest pain. No pulmonary embolism was detected by the radiologist on initial review; however, perfusion images (iodine overlay image, *A*; Z-effective image, *B*) show a perfusion defect in the left lower lobe. Subsequent review of conventional images revealed a subtle, subsegmental pulmonary embolism in the left lower lobe (*C*, orange *arrow*).

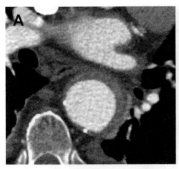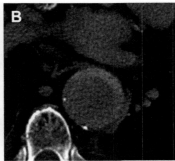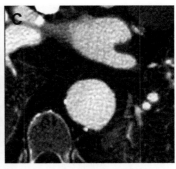

Fig. 14. 78-year-old man with chest pain. On contrast-enhanced CT, there is crescentic high density (measuring 69 HU) within the wall of the aorta (A). This appearance is suspicious for intramural hematoma (IMH); however, evaluation is incomplete without non-contrast images. VNC images (B) confirm the diagnosis of IMH, with high density in the wall of the aorta also measuring 69 HU. Iodine no water image (C) shows that there is no enhancement of the wall, with iodine content of 0 mg/mL.

addition, similar results have been shown with scan types that are not tailored to the vasculature, including contrast-enhanced body CT in children and young adults,[54] routine chest CT,[55] and routine abdominal CT.[56] If a patient with poor renal function requires an emergent contrast-enhanced study, a low-contrast dose protocol using VMI offers a potential tool for the radiologist to make the diagnosis while reducing risk to the patient.

Pathology

Pulmonary embolism and lung perfusion Beyond the technical advantages of low-VMI imaging in CTPA, MECT can also be used to aid diagnosis. In particular, iodine-selective imaging with MECT also allows for assessment of pulmonary parenchymal perfusion in patients with suspected pulmonary embolism or pulmonary angiopathy. Perfusion images with MECT have strong agreement with scintigraphy in a variety of clinical settings.[57,58] When perfusion is normal, this can increase diagnostic confidence that no pulmonary embolism is present; when abnormal, perfusion images can help radiologists localize pulmonary emboli. Perfusion of the lung parenchyma can be visualized with traditional color-coded iodine overlay images, or with "Z-effective" images: Z-effective images color code tissue based on atomic number, which accentuates the difference between normal and hypoperfused lung parenchyma (**Fig. 13**).

Intramural hematoma Intramural hematoma (IMH) can present a challenge in the ER setting, as it may be detected on a post-contrast scan in a patient without non-contrast imaging. In these cases, unless a follow-up non-contrast study or MR angiogram is performed, it can be difficult to determine if increased attenuation within the aortic wall is secondary to IMH or enhancement from

aortitis. In these cases, VNC and iodine overlay images can be used to avoid the need for a follow-up study. In a multicenter phantom and in vivo study, Si-Mohamed and colleagues demonstrated that for IMH, VNC images were comparable to TNC images in both CNR and diagnostic confidence.[59] In cases with suspected IMH, iodine-selective imaging can therefore be a helpful problem-solving tool to confirm the diagnosis (**Fig. 14**).

Endoleak Although most postoperative imaging in patients with repaired abdominal aortic aneurysms will occur in the outpatient setting, these patients will occasionally present to the ER with abdominal pain or other symptoms leading to CT imaging. It is not uncommon to see hyperdense material within an excluded aneurysm sac on a post-contrast study, which could represent endoleak or some other intrinsically dense material (eg, from prior embolization). Iodine-selective imaging with MECT allows for confident diagnosis of endoleak on a single phase acquisition.[60] In addition, VMI at low keV can accentuate endoleak, improving detection (**Fig. 15**).

Gastrointestinal bleeding CTA for suspected gastrointestinal bleeding is increasingly used in the ER setting, and MECT can be beneficial to optimize these studies and to problem solve in challenging cases. With low-keV VMI, iodine content will be accentuated, improving detection of sites of contrast extravasation.[61] With iodine selective images, iodine maps can be used to confirm iodine content within a site of extravasation; VNC images can also be used to potentially eliminate the need for a non-contrast acquisition.[62,63] Similarly, if a patient undergoing routine contrast-enhanced CT is found to have dense contents within the bowel lumen, iodine-selective

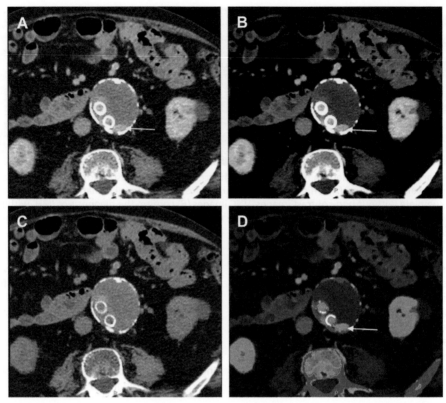

Fig. 15. A 87-year-old man with abdominal pain, and history of abdominal aortic aneurysm repair. On conventional images (*A*), there is high-density material within the aneurysm sac that is suspicious for endoleak (*yellow arrows*); this is more conspicuous on 50 keV images (*B*). On VNC (*C*) and iodine overlay (*D*) images, this is confirmed to contain iodine, consistent with type II endoleak.

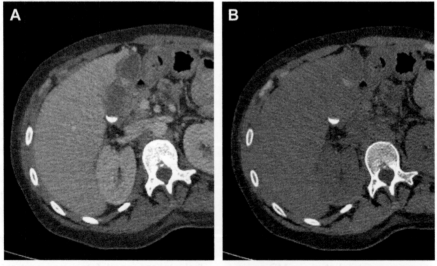

Fig. 16. Contrast-enhanced abdominal CT (*A*) in a 34-year-old woman on anticoagulation with anemia demonstrates dense material in the proximal duodenum. On VNC images (*B*), this material persists, confirming that it does not contain iodine and is therefore not a site of gastrointestinal (GI) bleeding. This likely represents ingested material such as bismuth.

images can be used to problem solve and determine if these contents contain iodine (**Fig. 16**).

Computed Tomography of the Chest, Abdomen, and Pelvis

Technique and image quality
One common misconception with MECT imaging is that imaging patients with two energy spectra will inherently lead to a higher radiation dose than single energy imaging. For routine ER imaging of the chest, abdomen, and pelvis, MECT has been shown to be similar or superior to SECT in image quality without an increase in radiation dose.[64,65]

As discussed in the CTA section, low-keV VMI can also be used in routine contrast-enhanced CT imaging to improve iodine enhancement CNR and improve overall image quality.[66,67] At our institution, low-keV imaging at 50 keV is sent to PACS for all contrast-enhanced CT.

Pathology
Solid organ lesions: detection Detection of benign and malignant lesions in the solid abdominal organs on abdominal CT requires maximizing contrast between the lesion and background organ parenchyma. This can be a particular challenge in the liver, pancreas, and spleen, where noise in normal parenchyma can make detection a challenge.

Low-keV VMI has been shown in a large body of research to improve detection of lesions in abdominal imaging, particularly in the liver and pancreas. In a study of 98 patients with colorectal cancer, Lenga and colleagues demonstrated significantly higher sensitivity and diagnostic

accuracy in detection of liver metastases with 40 keV images compared with conventional images.[68] De Cecco and colleagues found that noise-reduced 50 keV VMI have higher subjective image quality and diagnostic accuracy than conventional blended images in patients with hypervascular liver lesions.[69] In the pancreas, studies have shown the same benefit to using low-keV VMI.[70–72] Optimal CNR to evaluate pancreatic lesions is generally thought to be in the range of 40 to 55 keV.[73,74] Low-keV images therefore provide the radiologist with a powerful tool in abdominal imaging to improve lesion detection (**Fig. 17**).

Solid organ lesions: characterization
Incidental lesions in the abdominal organs are common on contrast-enhanced CT. Many of these will be indeterminate and incompletely characterized on single-phase CT studies, requiring follow-up with multiphase CT or MR imaging. This increases health care costs, patient anxiety, and potentially radiation exposure to the patient if a follow-up CT is performed.

MECT has the potential to characterize many incidental lesions at the time of detection and eliminate the need for advanced follow-up imaging. For example, it is common to find a renal lesion on contrast-enhanced CT with attenuation of over 20 HU, which could represent a Bosniak II cyst or a solid enhancing mass. According to follow-up guidelines published by the American College of Radiology (ACR), most of these lesions should be followed with renal mass protocol MR imaging or CT.[75] However, if the contrast-enhanced scan was performed with MECT, iodine-selective images can be used to triage the

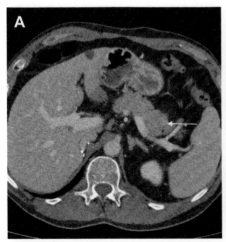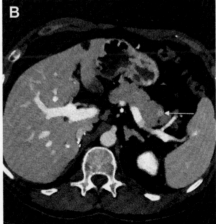

Fig. 17. A 54-year-old man with history of clear cell renal cell carcinoma. Subtle metastasis to the pancreatic tail (*yellow arrows*) is difficult to visualize on conventional images (*A*) and is easier to detect on 50 keV virtual monoenergetic images (*B*).

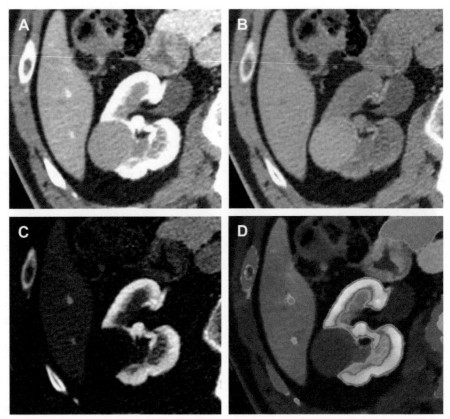

Fig. 18. A 75-year-old man with incidental hyperattenuating right renal lesion. The lesion measures 79 HU on conventional images (*A*). On virtual non-contrast images (*B*), the lesion measures 76 HU, compatible with a hemorrhagic cyst. The absence of iodine content is confirmed on gray scale and color-coded iodine-selective images, with iodine content of 0 mg/mL (*C, D*).

lesion. Studies have confirmed that iodine-selective imaging is accurate in determining whether a renal mass is enhancing or non-enhancing. In a 2019 systematic review and meta-analysis,[76] Salameh and colleagues showed pooled sensitivity and specificity of 97% and 95% of MECT in determining whether a mass was enhancing. An additional meta-analysis replicated

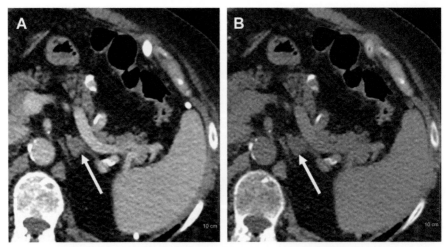

Fig. 19. A 80-year-old woman with indeterminate left adrenal lesion on contrast-enhanced CT, with attenuation of 70 HU (*A, white arrow*). On virtual non-contrast images, the attenuation is 8 HU, diagnostic of a benign lipid-rich adenoma (*B*). This diagnosis was confirmed on chemical shift MR imaging (not shown).

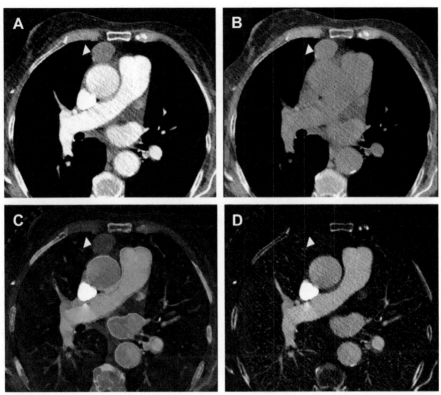

Fig. 20. A 93-year-old woman with incidental anterior mediastinal lesion on a CT performed for trauma (*yellow arrowheads*), which on conventional images (*A*) has an attenuation of 51 HU. On VNC images (*B*), the attenuation is also 51 HU, suggesting that this is a hemorrhagic/proteinaceous cyst rather than an enhancing mass. The lack of enhancement is confirmed on color-coded iodine overlay (*C*) and gray scale iodine no water (*D*) images; measured iodine content is 0 mg/mL.

these findings.[77] With iodine-selective images, a radiologist can quickly evaluate an indeterminate renal mass qualitatively for visible iodine content on an iodine-selective image. Indeterminate lesions can also be evaluated quantitatively by measuring iodine concentration on iodine-specific images or measuring attenuation on VNC images (**Fig. 18**).

Incidental, indeterminate adrenal lesions also present a common diagnostic dilemma. Although most of these are benign adenomas, the ACR recommends advanced imaging if they are above certain size thresholds or if detected in patients with a history of cancer.[78] For scans performed with MECT, these lesions can be triaged with evaluation of iodine-selective images. Research across vendor platforms has confirmed that if an adrenal lesion measures less than 10 HU on VNC images, it can be reliably characterized as a benign adenoma[79,80] (**Fig. 19**). However, VNC images will often slightly overestimate the attenuation of adrenal masses when compared with TNC images. In a meta-analysis including 170 patients

with 192 adrenal masses, Connolly and colleagues found that VNC images were 54% sensitive in diagnosing adrenal adenoma, but 100% specific with no false positives reported.[81] Therefore, there will be a subset of patients with adrenal masses that measure greater than 10 HU on VNC images which are subsequently shown to be lipid-rich adenomas on TNC or MR imaging.

Although renal and adrenal masses are the most extensively researched, the same principles apply to findings in other organ systems on thoracic and abdominal CT. If there is a lesion that is hyperattenuating and it is unclear to the radiologist whether iodine enhancement is present, the lesion can be evaluated with iodine-selective images (**Fig. 20**). Iodine-selective imaging has also been used to triage masses in the pancreas,[82] ovaries,[83] mediastinum,[84] thyroid,[85] and a variety of other clinical settings.

Organ perfusion in abdominal imaging
By improving iodine contrast, both low-keV VMI and iodine-selective images can assist the radiologist in the detection and characterization of organ

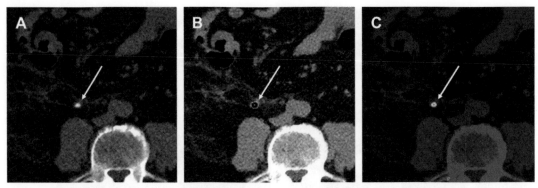

Fig. 21. A 70-year-old man with an obstructing calculus in the right mid ureter (*white arrows*) seen on conventional images (*A*). On a uric acid removed image (*B*), the stone is subtracted, compatible with a uric acid-based stone. This is confirmed on a color-coded uric acid overlay image (*C*), on which uric acid is color-coded in orange.

hypoperfusion and hyperperfusion in a variety of clinical settings. First and foremost among these is bowel ischemia; CT findings of ischemic bowel can be subtle, and yet detection is essential as ischemic bowel has high morbidity and mortality. Potretzke and colleagues compared MECT with conventional CT in a swine model of bowel ischemia and found improved conspicuity of bowel ischemia with 51-keV MECT images compared with traditional 120 kVp CT images.[86] In patients with small bowel obstruction, a study by Darras and colleagues showed that VMI (at 70 keV) maximized CNR of small bowel enhancement and improved diagnostic confidence in detection of bowel ischemia.[87] Similarly, in a different reader study of 60 consecutive patients with suspected acute bowel ischemia, iodine maps and 40 keV VMI increased conspicuity of ischemia and improved diagnostic accuracy.[88]

These principles can be applied to perfusion of other abdominal and pelvic organs. In patients with suspected pyelonephritis, low-keV VMI improved detection of inflamed renal parenchyma when compared with conventional images.[89] In patients with pancreatitis, low-keV VMI allows better assessment of tissue enhancement and demarcation of pancreatic inflammation and necrosis.[90] In suspected appendicitis, low-keV images improve SNR and CNR and are preferred by radiologists compared with conventional images.[91]

Stone assessment: urinary tract calculi
Determining the chemical composition of calculi can have an impact on management decisions, whereas uric acid-based stones may be managed medically with urine alkalization, calcium and struvite-based stones will often require more

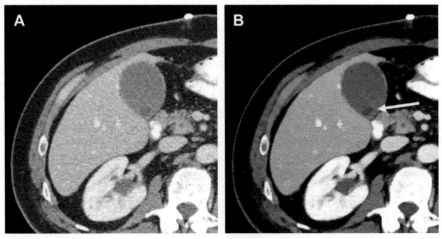

Fig. 22. A 53-year-old man with abdominal pain. On conventional images (*A*), there is a gallstone which is relatively isodense to surrounding bile and very difficult to visualize. The gallstone is much more conspicuous on 50 keV images (*B, yellow arrow*).

invasive management such as shock wave lithotripsy or percutaneous nephrolithotomy. On SECT, nearly all urinary tract calculi will appear hyperattenuating. Although attenuation measurements have been suggested as a method to distinguish uric acid-based stones from calcium-based stones,[92] this technique is not optimal for small stones due to challenges with ROI placement. In addition, the attenuation thresholds in the literature are variable and may differ depending on scan kVp and vendor.

Because of the different x-ray absorption behaviors of calcium and uric acid as a function of kVp, MECT has high accuracy in distinguishing calcium from uric acid-based stones; this has been confirmed in both in vivo and phantom studies across vendor platforms.[93–96] McGrath and colleagues reviewed many research papers with 662 patients and found that MECT was 88% sensitive and 98% specific in identifying stones that were uric acid-based.[97] A similar meta-analysis by Zheng and colleagues showed 96% sensitivity and 99% specificity for distinguishing uric acid and non-uric acid-based stones, and a sensitivity of 97% and specificity of 99% in distinguishing calcium-based from non-calcium-based stones.[98] MECT vendor platforms have different post-processed images that allow for stone visualization; some of these are in gray scale, whereas others are color-coded. These images allow radiologists to quickly determine whether a calculus is calcium or uric acid-based and include this information in the radiology report (Fig. 21).

Stone assessment: gallbladder and biliary tree
Many gallstones are noncalcified and isodense to surrounding bile on CT, rendering detection on conventional CT difficult or impossible. MECT can improve detection of noncalcified gallstones. Uyeda and colleagues showed that both low- and high-keV (40 and 190 keV) imaging improved conspicuity of noncalcified gallstones.[99] Therefore, in an ER patient with suspected gallstones or choledocholithiasis, low- or high-keV images can be quickly screened to improve detection of isodense stones[100] (Fig. 22).

SUMMARY

In conclusion, the authors have reviewed how MECT can be used for problem-solving in emergency radiology. The optimal use of MECT can improve detection of pathology, allow characterization of incidental lesions and other indeterminate findings, and change protocols to reduce contrast dose. With the increasing use of MECT scanners in emergency departments, radiologists should be aware of the fundamentals of this technology and how it can improve care in ER patients.

CLINICS CARE POINTS

- Virtual monogenergetic imaging at low keV can increase conspicuity of iodine content, therefore improving image quality of contrast enhanced CT studies and improving detection of pathology in ER imaging.
- Iodine selective imaging allows for iodine to be isolated within imaging, which can assess iodine content on a single phase acquisition.

DISCLOSURE

J.R. Wortman, United Imaging Intelligence, Consultant. M. Kunst: None.

REFERENCES

1. Paul J, Bauer RW, Maentele W, et al. Image fusion in dual energy computed tomography for detection of various anatomic structures–effect on contrast enhancement, contrast-to-noise ratio, signal-to-noise ratio and image quality. Eur J Radiol 2011; 80(2):612–9.
2. Neuhaus V, Abdullayev N, Große Hokamp N, et al. Improvement of Image Quality in Unenhanced Dual-Layer CT of the Head Using Virtual Monoenergetic Images Compared With Polyenergetic Single-Energy CT. Invest Radiol 2017;52(8):470–6.
3. Pomerantz SR, Kamalian S, Zhang D, et al. Virtual monochromatic reconstruction of dual-energy unenhanced head CT at 65-75 keV maximizes image quality compared with conventional polychromatic CT. Radiology 2013;266(1):318–25.
4. Park J, Choi YH, Cheon JE, et al. Advanced virtual monochromatic reconstruction of dual-energy unenhanced brain computed tomography in children: comparison of image quality against standard mono-energetic images and conventional polychromatic computed tomography. Pediatr Radiol 2017;47(12):1648–58.
5. Hixson HR, Leiva-Salinas C, Sumer S, et al. Utilizing dual energy CT to improve CT diagnosis of posterior fossa ischemia. J Neuroradiol J Neuroradiol 2016;43(5):346–52.
6. Lennartz S, Laukamp KR, Neuhaus V, et al. Dual-layer detector CT of the head: Initial experience in visualization of intracranial hemorrhage and hypodense brain lesions using virtual monoenergetic images. Eur J Radiol 2018;108:177–83.

7. Hu R, Daftari Besheli L, Young J, et al. Dual-Energy Head CT Enables Accurate Distinction of Intraparenchymal Hemorrhage from Calcification in Emergency Department Patients. Radiology 2016; 280(1):177–83.

8. Wiggins WF, Potter CA, Sodickson AD. Dual-Energy CT to Differentiate Small Foci of Intracranial Hemorrhage from Calcium. Radiology 2020; 294(1):129–38.

9. Naruto N, Tannai H, Nishikawa K, et al. Dual-energy bone removal computed tomography (BRCT): preliminary report of efficacy of acute intracranial hemorrhage detection. Emerg Radiol 2018;25(1): 29–33.

10. Ferda J, Novák M, Mírka H, et al. The assessment of intracranial bleeding with virtual unenhanced imaging by means of dual-energy CT angiography. Eur Radiol 2009;19(10):2518–22.

11. Khatri P, Wechsler LR, Broderick JP. Intracranial hemorrhage associated with revascularization therapies. Stroke 2007;38(2):431–40.

12. Gupta R, Phan CM, Leidecker C, et al. Evaluation of dual-energy CT for differentiating intracerebral hemorrhage from iodinated contrast material staining. Radiology 2010;257(1):205–11.

13. Bodanapally UK, Dreizin D, Issa G, et al. Dual-Energy CT in Enhancing Subdural Effusions that Masquerade as Subdural Hematomas: Diagnosis with Virtual High-Monochromatic (190-keV) Images. AJNR Am J Neuroradiol 2017;38(10): 1946–52.

14. von Kummer R, Allen KL, Holle R, et al. Acute stroke: usefulness of early CT findings before thrombolytic therapy. Radiology 1997;205(2): 327–33.

15. Barber PA, Demchuk AM, Zhang J, et al. Validity and reliability of a quantitative computed tomography score in predicting outcome of hyperacute stroke before thrombolytic therapy. ASPECTS Study Group. Alberta Stroke Programme Early CT Score. Lancet Lond Engl 2000;355(9216):1670–4.

16. Demeestere J, Wouters A, Christensen S, et al. Review of Perfusion Imaging in Acute Ischemic Stroke: From Time to Tissue. Stroke 2020;51(3): 1017–24.

17. Taguchi K, Itoh T, Fuld MK, et al. X-Map 2.0" for Edema Signal Enhancement for Acute Ischemic Stroke Using Non-Contrast-Enhanced Dual-Energy Computed Tomography. Invest Radiol 2018;53(7): 432–9.

18. Noguchi K, Itoh T, Naruto N, et al. A Novel Imaging Technique (X-Map) to Identify Acute Ischemic Lesions Using Noncontrast Dual-Energy Computed Tomography. J Stroke Cerebrovasc Dis Off J Natl Stroke Assoc 2017;26(1):34–41.

19. Mohammed MF, Marais O, Min A, et al. Unenhanced Dual-Energy Computed Tomography: Visualization of Brain Edema. Invest Radiol 2018; 53(2):63–9.

20. Leithner D, Mahmoudi S, Wichmann JL, et al. Evaluation of virtual monoenergetic imaging algorithms for dual-energy carotid and intracerebral CT angiography: Effects on image quality, artefacts and diagnostic performance for the detection of stenosis. Eur J Radiol 2018;99:111–7.

21. Cho ES, Chung TS, Oh DK, et al. Cerebral computed tomography angiography using a low tube voltage (80 kVp) and a moderate concentration of iodine contrast material: a quantitative and qualitative comparison with conventional computed tomography angiography. Invest Radiol 2012;47(2):142–7.

22. Zhang X, Pan T, Lu SS, et al. Application of Monochromatic Imaging and Metal Artifact Reduction Software in Computed Tomography Angiography after Treatment of Cerebral Aneurysms. J Comput Assist Tomogr 2019;43(6):948–52.

23. Josephson SA, Bryant SO, Mak HK, et al. Evaluation of carotid stenosis using CT angiography in the initial evaluation of stroke and TIA. Neurology 2004;63(3):457–60.

24. Korn A, Bender B, Brodoefel H, et al. Grading of carotid artery stenosis in the presence of extensive calcifications: dual-energy CT angiography in comparison with contrast-enhanced MR angiography. Clin Neuroradiol 2015;25(1):33–40.

25. Becker KJ, Baxter AB, Bybee HM, et al. Extravasation of radiographic contrast is an independent predictor of death in primary intracerebral hemorrhage. Stroke 1999;30(10):2025–32.

26. Delgado Almandoz JE, Yoo AJ, Stone MJ, et al. Systematic characterization of the computed tomography angiography spot sign in primary intracerebral hemorrhage identifies patients at highest risk for hematoma expansion: the spot sign score. Stroke 2009;40(9):2994–3000.

27. Demchuk AM, Dowlatshahi D, Rodriguez-Luna D, et al. Prediction of haematoma growth and outcome in patients with intracerebral haemorrhage using the CT-angiography spot sign (PREDICT): a prospective observational study. Lancet Neurol 2012;11(4):307–14.

28. Tan CO, Lam S, Kuppens D, et al. Spot and Diffuse Signs: Quantitative Markers of Intracranial Hematoma Expansion at Dual-Energy CT. Radiology 2019;290(1):179–86.

29. Lam S, Gupta R, Levental M, et al. Optimal Virtual Monochromatic Images for Evaluation of Normal Tissues and Head and Neck Cancer Using Dual-Energy CT. AJNR Am J Neuroradiol 2015;36(8):1518–24.

30. Suntharalingam S, Stenzel E, Wetter A, et al. Third generation dual-energy CT with 80/150 Sn kV for head and neck tumor imaging. Acta Radiol Stockh Swed 1987 2019;60(5):586–92.

31. De Crop A, Casselman J, Van Hoof T, et al. Analysis of metal artifact reduction tools for dental hardware in CT scans of the oral cavity: kVp, iterative reconstruction, dual-energy CT, metal artifact reduction software: does it make a difference? Neuroradiology 2015;57(8):841–9.

32. Bamberg F, Dierks A, Nikolaou K, et al. Metal artifact reduction by dual energy computed tomography using monoenergetic extrapolation. Eur Radiol 2011;21(7):1424–9.

33. Forghani R, Kelly HR, Curtin HD. Applications of Dual-Energy Computed Tomography for the Evaluation of Head and Neck Squamous Cell Carcinoma. Neuroimaging Clin N Am 2017;27(3): 445–59.

34. Pulickal GG, Singh D, Lohan R, et al. Dual-Source Dual-Energy CT in Submandibular Sialolithiasis: Reliability and Radiation Burden. AJR Am J Roentgenol 2019;213(6):1291–6.

35. Dangelmaier J, Schwaiger BJ, Gersing AS, et al. Dual layer computed tomography: Reduction of metal artefacts from posterior spinal fusion using virtual monoenergetic imaging. Eur J Radiol 2018; 105:195–203.

36. Martin SS, Wichmann JL, Scholtz JE, et al. Noise-Optimized Virtual Monoenergetic Dual-Energy CT Improves Diagnostic Accuracy for the Detection of Active Arterial Bleeding of the Abdomen. J Vasc Interv Radiol 2017;28(9):1257–66.

37. Booz C, Nöske J, Martin SS, et al. Virtual Noncalcium Dual-Energy CT: Detection of Lumbar Disk Herniation in Comparison with Standard Grayscale CT. Radiology 2019;290(2):446–55.

38. Koch V, Yel I, Grünewald LD, et al. Assessment of thoracic disk herniation by using virtual noncalcium dual-energy CT in comparison with standard grayscale CT. Eur Radiol 2021;31(12):9221–31.

39. Prologo JD, Gilkeson RC, Diaz M, et al. CT pulmonary angiography: a comparative analysis of the utilization patterns in emergency department and hospitalized patients between 1998 and 2003. AJR Am J Roentgenol 2004;183(4):1093–6.

40. Kline JA, Courtney DM, Beam DM, et al. Incidence and Predictors of Repeated Computed Tomographic Pulmonary Angiography in Emergency Department Patients. Ann Emerg Med 2009;54(1):41–8.

41. Apfaltrer P, Sudarski S, Schneider D, et al. Value of monoenergetic low-kV dual energy CT datasets for improved image quality of CT pulmonary angiography. Eur J Radiol 2014;83(2):322–8.

42. Beeres M, Trommer J, Frellesen C, et al. Evaluation of different keV-settings in dual-energy CT angiography of the aorta using advanced image-based virtual monoenergetic imaging. Int J Cardiovasc Imaging 2016;32(1):137–44.

43. Sudarski S, Apfaltrer P, Nance JW, et al. Optimization of keV-settings in abdominal and lower extremity dual-source dual-energy CT angiography determined with virtual monoenergetic imaging. Eur J Radiol 2013;82(10):e574–81.

44. Huang X, Gao S, Ma Y, et al. The optimal monoenergetic spectral image level of coronary computed tomography (CT) angiography on a dual-layer spectral detector CT with half-dose contrast media. Quant Imaging Med Surg 2020; 10(3):592–603.

45. Ghandour A, Sher A, Rassouli N, et al. Evaluation of Virtual Monoenergetic Images on Pulmonary Vasculature Using the Dual-Layer Detector-Based Spectral Computed Tomography. J Comput Assist Tomogr 2018;42(6):858–65.

46. Bae K, Jeon KN, Cho SB, et al. Improved Opacification of a Suboptimally Enhanced Pulmonary Artery in Chest CT: Experience Using a Dual-Layer Detector Spectral CT. AJR Am J Roentgenol 2018;210(4):734–41.

47. Dong J, Wang X, Jiang X, et al. Low-contrast agent dose dual-energy CT monochromatic imaging in pulmonary angiography versus routine CT. J Comput Assist Tomogr 2013;37(4):618–25.

48. Shuman WP, O'Malley RB, Busey JM, et al. Prospective comparison of dual-energy CT aortography using 70% reduced iodine dose versus single-energy CT aortography using standard iodine dose in the same patient. Abdom Radiol N Y 2017;42(3):759–65.

49. Raju R, Thompson AG, Lee K, et al. Reduced iodine load with CT coronary angiography using dual-energy imaging: a prospective randomized trial compared with standard coronary CT angiography. J Cardiovasc Comput Tomogr 2014;8(4): 282–8.

50. Carrascosa P, Leipsic JA, Capunay C, et al. Monochromatic image reconstruction by dual energy imaging allows half iodine load computed tomography coronary angiography. Eur J Radiol 2015;84(10):1915–20.

51. Agrawal MD, Oliveira GR, Kalva SP, et al. Prospective Comparison of Reduced-Iodine-Dose Virtual Monochromatic Imaging Dataset From Dual-Energy CT Angiography With Standard-Iodine-Dose Single-Energy CT Angiography for Abdominal Aortic Aneurysm. Am J Roentgenol 2016;207(6):W125–32.

52. He J, Wang Q, Ma X, et al. Dual-energy CT angiography of abdomen with routine concentration contrast agent in comparison with conventional single-energy CT with high concentration contrast agent. Eur J Radiol 2015;84(2):221–7.

53. Patino M, Parakh A, Lo GC, et al. Virtual Monochromatic Dual-Energy Aortoiliac CT Angiography With Reduced Iodine Dose: A Prospective Randomized Study. AJR Am J Roentgenol 2019;212(2):467–74.

54. Tabari A, Gee MS, Singh R, et al. Reducing Radiation Dose and Contrast Medium Volume With Application of Dual-Energy CT in Children and Young Adults. AJR Am J Roentgenol 2020;214(6): 1199–205.

55. Digumarthy SR, Singh R, Rastogi S, et al. Low contrast volume dual-energy CT of the chest: Quantitative and qualitative assessment. Clin Imaging 2021;69:305–10.

56. Lv P, Liu J, Chai Y, et al. Automatic spectral imaging protocol selection and iterative reconstruction in abdominal CT with reduced contrast agent dose: initial experience. Eur Radiol 2017;27(1): 374–83.

57. Dournes G, Verdier D, Montaudon M, et al. Dual-energy CT perfusion and angiography in chronic thromboembolic pulmonary hypertension: diagnostic accuracy and concordance with radionuclide scintigraphy. Eur Radiol 2014;24(1):42–51.

58. Meysman M, Everaert H, Buls N, et al. Comparison of ventilation-perfusion single-photon emission computed tomography (V/Q SPECT) versus dual-energy CT perfusion and angiography (DECT) after 6 months of pulmonary embolism (PE) treatment. Eur J Radiol 2015;84(9):1816–9.

59. Si-Mohamed S, Dupuis N, Tatard-Leitman V, et al. Virtual versus true non-contrast dual-energy CT imaging for the diagnosis of aortic intramural hematoma. Eur Radiol 2019;29(12):6762–71.

60. Javor D, Wressnegger A, Unterhumer S, et al. Endoleak detection using single-acquisition split-bolus dual-energy computer tomography (DECT). Eur Radiol 2017;27(4):1622–30.

61. Fulwadhva UP, Wortman JR, Sodickson AD. Use of Dual-Energy CT and Iodine Maps in Evaluation of Bowel Disease. RadioGraphics 2016;36(2): 393–406.

62. Wortman JR, Landman W, Fulwadhva UP, et al. CT angiography for acute gastrointestinal bleeding: what the radiologist needs to know. Br J Radiol 2017;90(1075):20170076.

63. Sun H, Hou XY, Xue HD, et al. Dual-source dual-energy CT angiography with virtual non-enhanced images and iodine map for active gastrointestinal bleeding: Image quality, radiation dose and diagnostic performance. Eur J Radiol 2015;84(5): 884–91.

64. Wortman JR, Shyu JY, Dileo J, et al. Dual-energy CT for routine imaging of the abdomen and pelvis: radiation dose and image quality. Emerg Radiol 2020;27(1):45–50.

65. Duan X, Ananthakrishnan L, Guild JB, et al. Radiation doses and image quality of abdominal CT scans at different patient sizes using spectral detector CT scanner: a phantom and clinical study. Abdom Radiol N Y 2020;45(10):3361–8.

66. Doerner J, Hauger M, Hickethier T, et al. Image quality evaluation of dual-layer spectral detector CT of the chest and comparison with conventional CT imaging. Eur J Radiol 2017;93:52–8.

67. Doerner J, Wybranski C, Byrtus J, et al. Intra-individual comparison between abdominal virtual mono-energetic spectral and conventional images using a novel spectral detector CT. PLoS One 2017;12(8):e0183759.

68. Lenga L, Lange M, Arendt CT, et al. Measurement Reliability and Diagnostic Accuracy of Virtual Monoenergetic Dual-Energy CT in Patients with Colorectal Liver Metastases. Acad Radiol 2020; 27(7):e168–75.

69. De Cecco CN, Caruso D, Schoepf UJ, et al. A noise-optimized virtual monoenergetic reconstruction algorithm improves the diagnostic accuracy of late hepatic arterial phase dual-energy CT for the detection of hypervascular liver lesions. Eur Radiol 2018;28(8):3393–404.

70. George E, Wortman JR, Fulwadhva UP, et al. Dual energy CT applications in pancreatic pathologies. Br J Radiol 2017;90(1080):20170411.

71. Clark ZE, Bolus DN, Little MD, et al. Abdominal rapid-kVp-switching dual-energy MDCT with reduced IV contrast compared to conventional MDCT with standard weight-based IV contrast: an intra-patient comparison. Abdom Imaging 2015; 40(4):852–8.

72. Frellesen C, Fessler F, Hardie AD, et al. Dual-energy CT of the pancreas: improved carcinoma-to-pancreas contrast with a noise-optimized monoenergetic reconstruction algorithm. Eur J Radiol 2015;84(11):2052–8.

73. Bellini D, Gupta S, Ramirez-Giraldo JC, et al. Use of a Noise Optimized Monoenergetic Algorithm for Patient-Size Independent Selection of an Optimal Energy Level During Dual-Energy CT of the Pancreas. J Comput Assist Tomogr 2017; 41(1):39–47.

74. Noda Y, Goshima S, Kaga T, et al. Virtual monochromatic image at lower energy level for assessing pancreatic ductal adenocarcinoma in fast kV-switching dual-energy CT. Clin Radiol 2020;75(4):320.e17–23.

75. Herts BR, Silverman SG, Hindman NM, et al. Management of the Incidental Renal Mass on CT: A White Paper of the ACR Incidental Findings Committee. J Am Coll Radiol JACR 2018;15(2):264–73.

76. Salameh JP, McInnes MDF, McGrath TA, et al. Diagnostic Accuracy of Dual-Energy CT for Evaluation of Renal Masses: Systematic Review and Meta-Analysis. AJR Am J Roentgenol 2019; 212(4):W100–5.

77. Bellini D, Panvini N, Laghi A, et al. Systematic review and meta-analysis investigating the diagnostic yield of dual-energy CT for renal mass

assessment. American Journal of Roentgenology 2019;212(5):1044-53.

78. Mayo-Smith WW, Song JH, Boland GL, et al. Management of Incidental Adrenal Masses: A White Paper of the ACR Incidental Findings Committee. J Am Coll Radiol JACR 2017;14(8):1038–44.

79. Helck A, Hummel N, Meinel FG, et al. Can single-phase dual-energy CT reliably identify adrenal adenomas? Eur Radiol 2014;24(7):1636–42.

80. Glazer DI, Maturen KE, Kaza RK, et al. Adrenal Incidentaloma Triage With Single-Source (Fast-Kilovoltage Switch) Dual-Energy CT. Am J Roentgenol 2014;203(2):329–35.

81. Connolly MJ, McInnes MDF, El-Khodary M, et al. Diagnostic accuracy of virtual non-contrast enhanced dual-energy CT for diagnosis of adrenal adenoma: A systematic review and meta-analysis. Eur Radiol 2017;27(10):4324–35.

82. Chu AJ, Lee JM, Lee YJ, et al. Dual-source, dual-energy multidetector CT for the evaluation of pancreatic tumours. Br J Radiol 2012;85(1018): e891–8.

83. Elsherif SB, Zheng S, Ganeshan D, et al. Does dual-energy CT differentiate benign and malignant ovarian tumours? Clin Radiol 2020;75(8):606–14.

84. Lee SH, Hur J, Kim YJ, et al. Additional value of dual-energy CT to differentiate between benign and malignant mediastinal tumors: an initial experience. Eur J Radiol 2013;82(11):2043–9.

85. Lee DH, Lee YH, Seo HS, et al. Dual-energy CT iodine quantification for characterizing focal thyroid lesions. Head Neck 2019;41(4):1024–31.

86. Potretzke TA, Brace CL, Lubner MG, et al. Early Small-Bowel Ischemia: Dual-Energy CT Improves Conspicuity Compared with Conventional CT in a Swine Model. Radiology 2014;275(1):119–26.

87. Darras KE, McLaughlin PD, Kang H, et al. Virtual monoenergetic reconstruction of contrast-enhanced dual energy CT at 70keV maximizes mural enhancement in acute small bowel obstruction. Eur J Radiol 2016;85(5):950–6.

88. Lourenco PDM, Rawski R, Mohammed MF, et al. Dual-Energy CT Iodine Mapping and 40-keV Monoenergetic Applications in the Diagnosis of Acute Bowel Ischemia. AJR Am J Roentgenol 2018; 211(3):564–70.

89. Marron D, Nahum GS, Gili D, et al. Low monoenergetic DECT detection of pyelonephritis extent. Eur J Radiol 2021;142:109837.

90. Dar G, Goldberg SN, Hiller N, et al. CT severity indices derived from low monoenergetic images at dual-energy CT may improve prediction of outcome in acute pancreatitis. Eur Radiol 2021; 31(7):4710–9.

91. Lev-Cohain N, Sosna J, Meir Y, et al. Dual energy CT in acute appendicitis: value of low mono-energy. Clin Imaging 2021;77:213–8.

92. Spettel S, Shah P, Sekhar K, et al. Using Hounsfield unit measurement and urine parameters to predict uric acid stones. Urology 2013;82(1):22–6.

93. Hidas G, Eliahou R, Duvdevani M, et al. Determination of renal stone composition with dual-energy CT: in vivo analysis and comparison with x-ray diffraction. Radiology 2010;257(2):394–401.

94. Primak AN, Fletcher JG, Vrtiska TJ, et al. Noninvasive differentiation of uric acid versus non-uric acid kidney stones using dual-energy CT. Acad Radiol 2007;14(12):1441–7.

95. Ananthakrishnan L, Duan X, Xi Y, et al. Dual-layer spectral detector CT: non-inferiority assessment compared to dual-source dual-energy CT in discriminating uric acid from non-uric acid renal stones ex vivo. Abdom Radiol N Y 2018;43(11): 3075–81.

96. Kordbacheh H, Baliyan V, Singh P, et al. Rapid kVp switching dual-energy CT in the assessment of urolithiasis in patients with large body habitus: preliminary observations on image quality and stone characterization. Abdom Radiol N Y 2019;44(3): 1019–26.

97. McGrath TA, Frank RA, Schieda N, et al. Diagnostic accuracy of dual-energy computed tomography (DECT) to differentiate uric acid from non-uric acid calculi: systematic review and meta-analysis. Eur Radiol 2020;30(5):2791–801.

98. Zheng X, Liu Y, Li M, et al. Dual-energy computed tomography for characterizing urinary calcified calculi and uric acid calculi: A meta-analysis. Eur J Radiol 2016;85(10):1843–8.

99. Uyeda JW, Richardson IJ, Sodickson AD. Making the invisible visible: improving conspicuity of non-calcified gallstones using dual-energy CT. Abdom Radiol 2017;42(12):2933–9.

100. Ratanaprasatporn L, Uyeda JW, Wortman JR, et al. Multimodality Imaging, including Dual-Energy CT, in the Evaluation of Gallbladder Disease. Radiogr Rev Publ Radiol Soc N Am Inc 2018;38(1):75–89.

Multienergy Computed Tomography Applications
Trauma

Hei Shun Yu, MD[a],*, Abhishek Keraliya, MD[a], Sachiv Chakravarti, BS[b], Jennifer W. Uyeda, MD[a]

KEYWORDS

- Multienergy CT • Trauma • Intracranial hemorrhage • Myocardial contusion • Solid organ injury
- Hollow viscus injury • Bone contusion

KEY POINTS

- Multienergy (ME) CT consists of simultaneous acquisition of images using low and high kilovolt peaks, which allows for differentiation of materials, given the different absorptive properties of materials.
- In the setting of neurotrauma, virtual monochromatic imaging has been used to reduce posterior fossa artifact, and bone subtraction has been used to increase conspicuity of extra-axial hemorrhage.
- Iodine-selective imaging is useful in the setting of chest trauma because iodine maps can increase conspicuity of myocardial contusion.
- Solid organ and hollow viscus injuries are made more conspicuous on ME CT using iodine maps and low kiloelectron volt virtual monochromatic imaging. Virtual noncontrast images have also been shown to be helpful in abdominopelvic trauma in cases where hyperattenuating material is present on postcontrast images and absent on virtual noncontrast images, suggesting active bleeding.
- Virtual noncalcium images and color overlay images help improve detection of subtle fractures and increase conspicuity of foci of active bleeding in the setting of musculoskeletal trauma.

INTRODUCTION

Trauma is the leading cause of death in the United States for patients younger than age 45.[1] Globally, trauma is responsible for 4.4 million deaths per year and accounts for billions of US dollars in health care costs.[2] The concept of the golden hour describes the first hour after a major trauma in which early treatment is most likely to improve clinical outcome.[3,4] In this narrow window of time, rapid and accurate diagnosis of injuries strongly influences management decisions. In hemodynamically stable patients, diagnostic imaging is often a major driver of these management decisions.

Trauma imaging typically includes multiple radiographs and computed tomography (CT) of the head, chest, abdomen, pelvis, and spine. Additional scan regions may be included based on the mechanism of injury. CT scan protocols are institution dependent and may include arterial phase imaging, single pass imaging versus anatomically segmented acquisition, split bolus techniques, and/or use of multienergy CT (ME CT).[5–9] The focus of this article is on the latter.

MULTIENERGY COMPUTED TOMOGRAPHY PRINCIPLES

Multienergy CT was first described in the late 1970s as a potentially useful tool given its ability to detect different tissue signatures.[10] Since its development, advances to ME CT technology

[a] Brigham and Women's Hospital, Emergency Radiology, 75 Francis Street, Boston, MA 02115, USA; [b] Johns Hopkins University, 3400 North Charles Street, Baltimore, MD 21218, USA
* Corresponding author.
E-mail address: hsyu@bwh.harvard.edu

Radiol Clin N Am 61 (2023) 23–35
https://doi.org/10.1016/j.rcl.2022.07.003
0033-8389/23/© 2022 Elsevier Inc. All rights reserved.

radiologic.theclinics.com

have allowed for its application from head to toe.[11–15] Different approaches for ME CT acquisition vary based on vendor and includes a dual-source ME CT, a single x-ray source that rapidly switches between low and high kilovolt peaks, and a detector-based system that uses a single x-ray tube and a layered detector that preferentially absorbs photons of different energy levels.[16–19] Regardless of the approach, ME CT uses information from two energy spectra, which differs from conventional CT images that use a single polychromatic x-ray beam. Multienergy data are used to optimize images, identify/differentiate materials, or quantify substances.[16,17,19]

Image optimization algorithms may be used to create virtual monoenergetic images and "blended" or "mixed" energy images. Virtual monoenergetic images are created with kiloelectron voltages ranging from 40 to 200 keV, depending on vendor. Lower kiloelectron volt images accentuate iodine content and improve image contrast, whereas higher kiloelectron volt image are used to reduce artifacts from metallic substances.[13,16] "Blended" or "mixed" images are weighted images that appear similar to standard image reconstructions. They combine data from the low-energy (high contrast, high noise) and high-energy (low contrast, low noise) acquisitions resulting in optimized contrast-to-noise ratio.[13,20]

Use of ME CT for identification/differentiation and quantification of substances are useful in the setting of trauma because material decomposition techniques can be used to evaluate iodine and calcium. Iodine is displayed as an iodine map, which only shows iodine content, or as an iodine overlay, which is a color-coded iodine image superimposed on a grayscale image and may increase conspicuity of an otherwise subtle finding on conventional CT (Fig. 1).[13,16,18] This technique allows quantification of content using direct measurements on the images.[16,21] Iodine content can also be removed from the images to create virtual unenhanced images. Calcium can be treated in a similar manner and can be subtracted from images to create virtual noncalcium images to detect bone edema.[13,16,18]

MULTIENERGY COMPUTED TOMOGRAPHY APPLICATION

The goal of imaging in trauma is to identify and determine the severity of injuries of the acutely injured patient.[5] Regardless of the type of injury, ME CT techniques have been shown to assist in this goal. Multienergy CT has helped in identification of hemorrhage on head CT and can also be used to troubleshoot when there is confusion about whether a finding is hemorrhage versus calcification (Figs. 2 and 3).[11,18,22,23] In the chest, ME CT has been useful for detection of cardiac contusion.[12,24,25] Multienergy CT has also been shown to be helpful in identifying solid organ, bowel, or mesenteric injuries. Application of ME CT techniques has also improved detection of fractures.[26–28] These clinical scenarios are further discussed in the following sections.

MULTIENERGY COMPUTED TOMOGRAPHY APPLICATION: NEUROTRAUMA

Multienergy CT is applied to neuroimaging for artifact reduction, material differentiation (specifically, calcium vs hemorrhage), bone subtraction, and iodine quantification and carotid plaque characterization.[11,21,29] The first three are most relevant in the setting of trauma.

On conventional head CT, the posterior fossa suffers from beam hardening, photon starvation, and scatter artifacts,[30] which may limit assessment for traumatic injury. Use of ME CT allows for reconstruction of virtual monochromatic images, which can limit these artifacts and improve soft tissue contrast. However, depending on the energy level selection, signal-to-noise ratio may suffer because there is a significant increase in noise at lower monochromatic energy levels.[11,31] In one study comparing reconstructions at multiple energy levels, images reconstructed at 75 keV demonstrated the peak level of reduction in posterior fossa artifact.[31] A subsequent study determined that interpretation of reconstructions performed at 80 and 100 keV had the highest sensitivity for detecting pathology when using MR imaging as a reference standard.[30] Of note, reconstruction algorithms for virtual monochromatic images differs among manufacturers and development of new algorithms may further reduce noise at lower energy levels. Therefore, determination of optimal monochromatic energy levels requires further investigation and comparison of equipment and software of different manufacturers.[11]

Material differentiation plays an important role in neurotrauma. On a noncontrast head CT, intracranial calcification and hemorrhage appear as hyperattenuating foci.[18,32] When intracranial high attenuation foci are identified in a trauma patient, it may be difficult to differentiate between hemorrhage and calcification without a comparison examination.[11,32] Using a three-material decomposition technique for calcium, reconstruction of calcium maps and virtual noncalcium images may be performed (see Figs. 2 and 3). Interpretation of these images may obviate interval follow-up imaging or clinical observation.[11,33] In

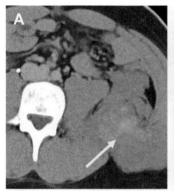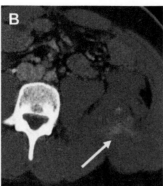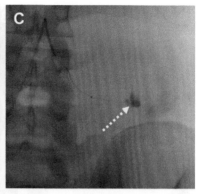

Fig. 1. An 18 year old presents status post stab injury with axial CT image (*A*) showing a faint hyperdensity in the left quadratus lumborum (*arrow*). Corresponding iodine overlay image (*B*) increases conspicuity of this finding (*arrow*) and is confirmed on subsequent angiogram (*C*) as active bleeding (*dashed arrow*) from a lumbar artery.

one study, blinded readers assessed single and ME CT to classify hyperattenuating foci. The authors found an increase in sensitivity, specificity, and accuracy to 96%, 100%, and 99%, respectively, compared with 74%, 95%, and 87%, respectively, on conventional CT for correct classification of hemorrhage.[32]

Bone subtraction is another useful ME CT technique for detection of extra-axial hemorrhage. Small acute extra-axial hemorrhages may be difficult to detect when they are located immediate subjacent to the inner table of the skull.[23] However, using bone subtraction, these hemorrhages are made more conspicuous (**Fig. 4**). Bone removal uses a binary system of classifying a voxel as behaving like calcium or iodine. Subsequently, signal from voxels identified as behaving like calcium are nulled.[11,22] In one study, blinded readers

assessed various types of intracranial hemorrhages without and with bone subtraction. Authors found that there was a significant improvement in detection of extra-axial hemorrhages and parenchymal contusions,[23] with 100% detection of extra-axial hemorrhages and contusions, compared with 61% and 65%, respectively, on conventional CT.

Traumatic head contusions are associated with iodine leak because of capillary fragmentation and disruption of the blood-brain barrier, which appears as hyperattenuation on contrast-enhanced examinations. Noncontrast head CT may identify contusions but often underestimates extent of injury.[34] Although it is not standard of care to perform CT angiography to evaluate traumatic brain injury, it is common for a follow-up head CT to be performed.[21] In these cases, there

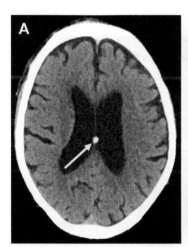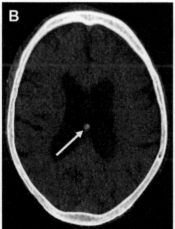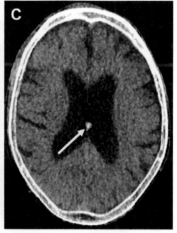

Fig. 2. A 90 year old status post fall with axial head CT (*A*) showing hyperdense focus along the septum pellucidum (*arrow*), which may represent calcium or hemorrhage. Calcium overlay image (*B*) and virtual noncalcium image (*C*) shows persistence of this finding on the noncalcium image and no corresponding calcium signal on the overlay image, which confirms that this is hemorrhage and not a calcified lesion (*arrow*).

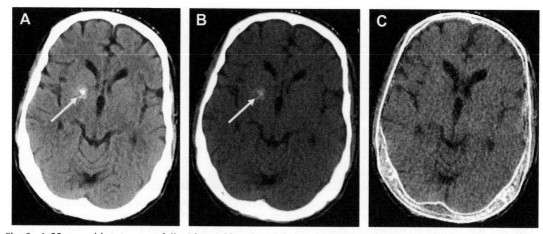

Fig. 3. A 66 year old status post fall with axial head CT (*A*) showing hyperdense focus in the right basal ganglia (*arrow*), which may represent calcium or hemorrhage. Calcium overlay image (*B*) shows persistence of this finding with corresponding calcium signal (*arrow*), which confirms that this is calcium and not hemorrhage. This is also confirmed by absence of the hyperdensity on virtual noncalcium image (*C*).

is typically residual contrast from the whole-body CT performed for the initial evaluation of the trauma patient. Acquisition of ME CT on this follow-up allows for iodine quantification, which has been applied to other parts of the body to accurately characterize lesions.[35–37] In one study, authors used this technique to quantify pseudohematoma volume and iodine quantity within the pseudohematoma and demonstrated correlation with mortality.[21]

MULTIENERGY COMPUTED TOMOGRAPHY APPLICATION: CHEST TRAUMA

Imaging of chest trauma is generally focused on identification of pulmonary parenchymal injuries, musculoskeletal injuries, pleural abnormalities, and aortic injuries, which are readily diagnosed

on conventional CT.[38] Cardiac injury, including myocardial contusion, pericardial rupture, myocardial rupture, papillary muscle injury, and coronary artery injury is more difficult to assess on conventional CT. This section focuses on myocardial contusion because the other injuries are rare or may be diagnosed based on clinical factors, such as hemodynamic instability.[12,25]

The diagnosis of myocardial contusion is difficult because some patients are symptomatic. Furthermore, troponins, electrocardiography, and transthoracic/transesophageal echocardiography may be normal unless injury is severe.[12] One case report describes a trauma patient found to have normal troponins, unrevealing electrocardiogram and echocardiography, and normal chest CT. Subsequent ME CT showed an area of myocardial contusion in the left ventricular wall.[24]

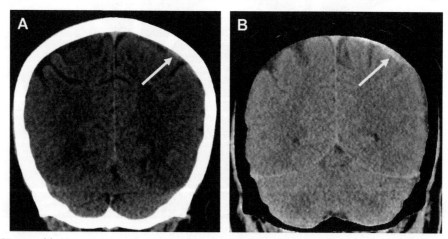

Fig. 4. A 35 year old status post assault with axial head CT (*A*) showing subtle hyperdense collection over the left cerebral convexity (*arrow*). Corresponding image with DE CT bone removal technique (*B*) increases conspicuity and shows the extent of the hemorrhage (*arrow*).

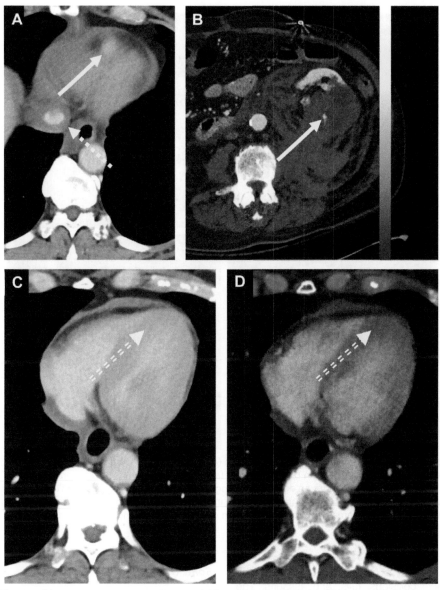

Fig. 5. A 61 year old presents status post motor vehicle collision with axial CT image (*A*) showing a faint outpouching from the anterior, inferior right ventricle and hemopericardium (*arrow*) and hematoma surrounding the inferior vena cava (*dashed arrow*). The outpouching is more conspicuous on corresponding image overlay image (*B*) confirming presence of pseudoaneurysm (*arrow*). In the operating room, a cardiac contusion was noted at the left ventricular apex, which is equivocally present on axial CT image (*C, arrow*) but is visible on iodine overlay image (*D, arrow*).

Conventional CT may be normal or may demonstrate an amorphous region of myocardial hypoenhancement, which may vary in size, shape, and density.[12,25] Although findings may be subtle, early identification of injuries helps with risk stratification and impacts management.[12] Multienergy CT is a potential tool for diagnosis of myocardial contusion because it is fast, available, and is able to identify extracardiac injury. Furthermore, application of ME CT techniques to create iodine maps increases conspicuity of subtle injuries (Fig. 5). In one study,

authors evaluated the utility of ME CT for diagnosis of mild blunt cardiac injury. Authors found high interobserver agreements among readers for presence of cardiac contusion, injury location, and size of injury.[12]

MULTIENERGY COMPUTED TOMOGRAPHY APPLICATION: ABDOMINOPELVIC TRAUMA

Abdominopelvic trauma is a significant cause of morbidity and mortality. Blunt trauma accounts for

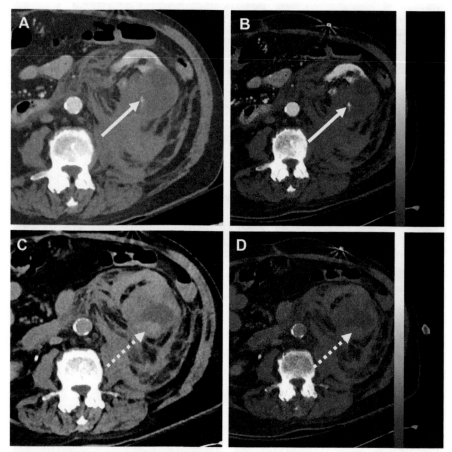

Fig. 6. A 62 year old status post fall with axial CT image (*A*) showing an AAST grade 4 renal injury with a hyperdense focus along the posterior margin of the midpole (*arrow*). The finding is present on corresponding iodine overlay image (*B, arrow*) and enlarges on delayed imaging as seen on axial CT image (*C, arrow*) confirming that it is active extravasation. Note that on axial iodine overlay image (*D*), only the anterior portion of the hyperdensity has iodine signal (*arrow*), whereas the posterior portion does not, suggesting the presence of blood clot.

70% of cases and is most commonly caused by motor vehicle collisions, falls, and assaults. The remaining 30% results from penetrating trauma, which includes gunshot and stab injuries.[5,9] CT is the modality of choice for the evaluation of abdominopelvic trauma with the goal of identifying injuries that impact patient management.

Various ME CT postprocessing techniques may assist in the evaluation of abdominopelvic trauma. As with imaging of the posterior fossa, abdominopelvic CT often suffers from streak artifact in the pelvis from orthopedic hardware. This may limit evaluation of pelvic structures or detection of free pelvic fluid in the trauma patient. In this scenario, ME CT may improve image quality by using images reconstructed from high kiloelectron volt levels to reduce beam hardening and photon starvation.[39,40] This technique may also be combined with vendor-specific metal artifact reduction algorithms.[41]

Solid Organ Injury

In the setting of blunt abdominopelvic, the most commonly injured solid organs are the spleen, liver, and kidneys. In these organs, parenchymal hematomas appear as geographic regions of relative hypoenhancement. Lacerations appear as hypoattenuating linear or branching lesions traversing the parenchyma. Subcapsular hematomas appear as hypoattenuating smooth collections outlining the contour of the injured organ.[9,13] The American Association for the Surgery of Trauma (AAST) has created injury grading scales for abdominopelvic organs, with injuries classified based on size, depth, and location of injury. The 2018 revision of the AAST solid organ injury grading scale now includes traumatic vascular injuries, including active contrast extravasation and contained vascular injuries, including

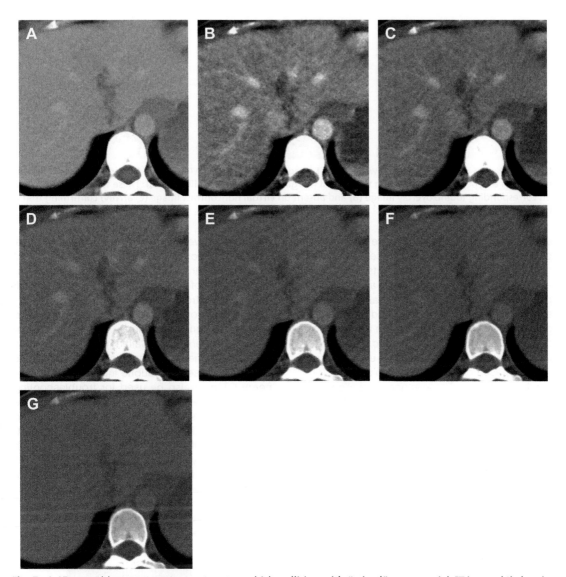

Fig. 7. A 15 year old presents status post motor vehicle collision with "mixed" energy axial CT image (*A*) showing an AAST grade 5 hepatic injury. On corresponding virtual monochromatic images at 40 keV (*B*), 50 keV (*C*), 60 keV (*D*), 70 keV (*E*), 80 keV (*F*), and 90 keV (*G*). The window and level are unchanged but there is decreasing conspicuity of the laceration as the energy levels increase.

pseudoaneurysm and arteriovenous fistula.[42] Active extravasation of contrast is defined as foci of extravascular contrast on arterial phase that enlarges on subsequent phases (**Fig. 6**). Contained vascular injuries are defined as circumscribed areas of extravascular contrast with similar attenuation to aorta on all phases.[43]

Identification of solid organ injury is not typically a diagnostic dilemma. However, in such settings as cardiogenic shock or poor contrast timing, the contrast bolus may not distribute properly, resulting in poor enhancement of the solid abdominal viscera.[44] These cases are difficult to evaluate

because injuries may not be apparent in a background of hypoenhancing parenchyma. Virtual monoenergetic imaging and iodine-selective images are useful in these cases to assess for parenchymal injury (**Fig. 7**). Studies have focused on the utility of ME CT in oncology for detection of hypovascular lesions and have shown improved visibility using lower kiloelectron volt images.[45–47] One study assessed the utility of virtual monoenergetic images for evaluation of hepatic and splenic lacerations. Authors found that 40-keV images had the highest contrast-to-noise ratio.[48] This principle may also be applied to pancreatic injury, which

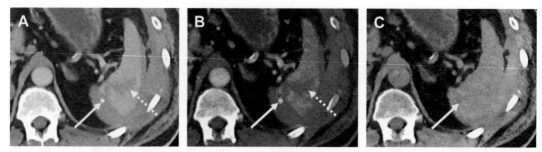

Fig. 8. A 68 year old status post fall with axial CT image (A) showing an AAST grade 4 splenic injury (dashed arrows) with a hyperdense focus along the medial margin of the spleen (solid arrows). These findings are present on corresponding iodine overlay image (B) and absent on virtual noncontrast image (C, arrow) confirming that it is active extravasation.

deserves special attention because the pancreatic phase occurs earlier. In these cases, assessment of pancreatic duct directly impacts patient management but may not be readily assessed if the pancreas is not imaged during peak parenchymal enhancement.[13] As with other solid abdominal organs, low kiloelectron volt images are used to increase conspicuity of pancreatic lacerations.[49] Iodine-selective images are also useful because they increase contrast between injured and uninjured parenchyma. These images also allow differentiation between active extravasation and hematoma, both of which appear hyperattenuating on virtual noncontrast images, but extravasation contains iodine.[13]

Identification of visceral vascular injury injuries is crucial because their presence is associated with failure of nonoperative management and may require angioembolization or laparotomy.[42,50,51] Multiple ME CT techniques may be useful to detect vascular injuries. For example,

iodine-selective and kiloelectron volt virtual monoenergetic images may improve visibility of subtle vascular injuries. Previous studies assessing the utility of ME CT for evaluation of endoleak have demonstrated that low kiloelectron volt virtual monochromatic reconstructions increased attenuation and conspicuity of extravascular contrast material.[52,53] Calcium subtraction may be used in patients with extensive atherosclerotic disease to assess for subtle injuries.[53,54] Multienergy CT may also be used for troubleshooting in cases where there is extravascular hyperdense material on a single phase (Fig. 8), which could represent calcification or extravascular contrast. Comparison of virtual noncontrast images with iodine overlay images helps determine the composition of the substance because contrast is only seen on the iodine overlay images and not the virtual noncontrast images. Bone or calcification is identified on virtual noncontrast images and iodine overlay images.[13]

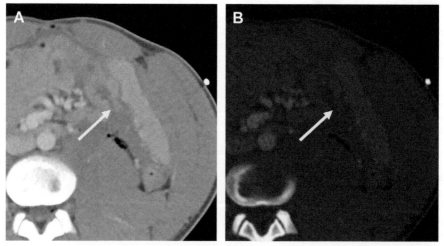

Fig. 9. A 22 year old presents status post gunshot wound with axial CT image (A) showing a subtle defect in a small bowel loop of the left abdomen (arrow). Corresponding iodine overlay image (B) improves visibility of the finding (arrow).

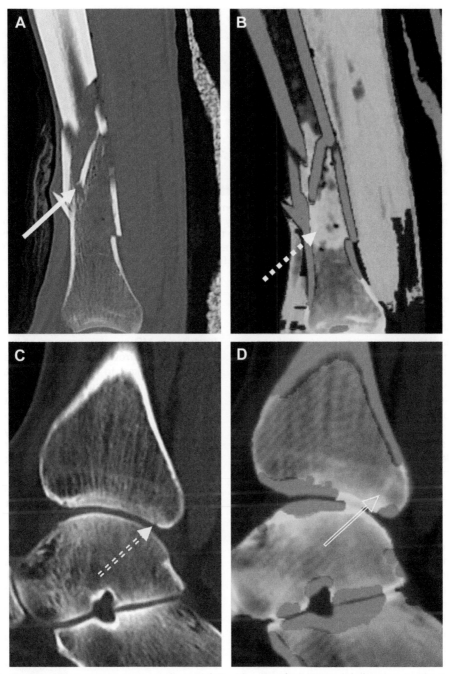

Fig. 10. A 45 year old presents status post slip and fall with sagittal CT image (*A*) showing a comminuted, displaced distal tibia fracture (*arrow*). Corresponding virtual noncalcium image with color overlay (*B*) shows bone marrow edema surrounding the fracture site (*arrow*). More inferiorly, there is a nondisplaced posterior malleolar fracture on sagittal CT image (*C, arrow*), which is subtle and more apparent on sagittal virtual noncalcium with color overlay image (*D, arrow*).

Bowel and Mesenteric Injury

The diagnosis of bowel and mesenteric injuries is critical for patient management and is difficult to diagnose clinically. Although there is a trend toward conservative management of solid organ injury, bowel and mesenteric injury is typically managed surgically because these injuries are associated with significant morbidity and mortality. Thus, contrast-enhanced CT of the abdomen and pelvis is the imaging modality of choice to determine which patients can be safely managed

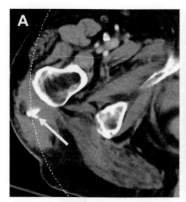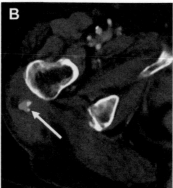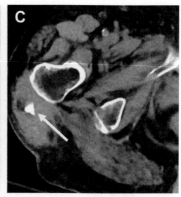

Fig. 11. A 96 year old status post fall with axial CT abdomen and pelvis image (*A*) showing a hematoma and hyperdense material over the right hip (*arrow*), which may represent active extravasation or bone fragment. Note that the hyperdense material is only partially included in the dual-energy field-of-view (*dashed line*). The portion of the finding within the dual-energy field-of-view is present on corresponding iodine overlay image (*B, arrow*) and absent on virtual noncontrast image (*C, arrow*) confirming that it is active extravasation.

without intervention.[55] However, diagnosis is difficult because specific findings, such as bowel wall discontinuity, extraluminal oral contrast, mesenteric hematoma, active extravasation, and mesenteric vessel injury, are uncommonly seen. Common findings, such as bowel wall thickening, mesenteric stranding, and free fluid, are sensitive but nonspecific.[55,56] The addition of ME CT has proven beneficial for assessment of bowel injury because bowel wall enhancement is more readily assessed and can assist in surgical planning (**Fig. 9**). Using virtual monoenergetic images and iodine-selective images, ME CT increases visibility of areas of diminished enhancement or bowel wall hyperemia. Virtual noncontrast images are used to increase conspicuity of intramural hematoma.[57] In one study, authors retrospectively assessed ME CT images of patients with surgically proven bowel injuries. Authors found that ME CT findings correlated with locations of injuries detected during surgery in all cases.[58] These techniques may also help with diffuse abnormalities, such as shock bowel, which is characterized by bowel wall thickening and mucosal hyperemia. In these patients, mucosal hyperemia and intramural hemorrhage may have a similar appearance. However, iodine-selective images show a lack of iodine uptake with the latter. Similarly, hyperattenuating ingested material is differentiated from mucosal hyperemia because it does not show iodine uptake on iodine-selective images.[13,59]

MULTIENERGY COMPUTED TOMOGRAPHY APPLICATION: MUSCULOSKELETAL TRAUMA

Diagnosis of displaced fractures poses no challenge on conventional radiography. However,

when a displaced fracture is not identified and high clinical suspicion for fracture persists, cross-sectional imaging may be obtained.[14] The reference standard for identification of nondisplaced fractures is MR imaging because of its ability to identify bone marrow lesions.[60,61] However, MR imaging is less likely to be performed in the emergency department because of limited availability and the longer duration of examination.[62] In contrast, CT is fast and readily accessible. In some cases, bone marrow lesions may also be identified as subtle regions of hyperattenuation.[14] Calcium subtraction can remove bony trabeculae, allow for direct assessment of underlying bone marrow, and increase visibility of bone marrow lesions (**Fig. 10**). Color overlay images may also be created to display bone marrow attenuation superimposed on anatomic CT images.[14,26,28]

Another common problem faced by radiologists occurs in the setting of fractures where there is adjacent hyperattenuating material, which may represent bone fragment or active extravasation of contrast. Using ME CT, these two materials are readily differentiated using iodine-selective and virtual noncontrast images (**Fig. 11**). Specifically, active extravasation of contrast would be present on iodine-selective images and absent on the virtual noncontrast images.[13]

SUMMARY

Imaging is critical in the setting of trauma because rapid and accurate assessment of the trauma patient impacts management and outcome. Advances in ME CT has added new tools to aid radiologists in these time-sensitive examinations by improving image quality and aiding in the differentiation of material composition. These techniques have been applied from head to toe, in the form of virtual noncontrast and noncalcium images, virtual monochromatic images, and iodine-selective images. Numerous studies have demonstrated the utility of ME CT images for aiding in detection and improving visibility of lesions.

CLINICS CARE POINTS

- Virtual monoenergetic imaging can be applied to reduce streak artifact in neuroimaging and can also be used to increase conspicuity of extravasated contrast in the setting of vascular injury.
- Iodine selective imaging increases conspicuity and radiologist confidence for detection of injuries in the chest, abdomen and pelvis.
- Material decomposition techniques can differentiate materials and characterize/confirm the presence of injury, as in the case of active bleeding or differentiation of calcium from hemorrhage. It can also be applied to improve detection of fracture and bone marrow lesions.

DISCLOSURE

The authors have nothing to disclose.

REFERENCES

1. Centers for Disease Control and Prevention, National Center for Injury Prevention and Control. Web-based injury statistics query and reporting system (WISQARS). 2020. Available at: https://www.cdc.gov/injury/wisqars. Accessed April 2022.
2. World Health Organization. Web-based injuries and violence fact sheet. 2021. https://www.who.int/newsroom/fact-sheets/detail/injuries-and-violence. [Accessed 21 April 2022].
3. Blow O, Magliore L, Claridge J, et al. The golden hour and the silver day: detection and correction of occult hypoperfusion within 24 hours improves outcome from major trauma. J Trauma Acute Care Surg 1999;47(5):964–9.
4. Howard JT, Kotwal RS, Santos-Lazada AR, et al. Reexamination of a battlefield trauma golden hour policy. J Trauma Acute Care Surg 2018;84:11–8.
5. Soto JA, Anderson SW. Multidetector CT of blunt abdominal trauma. Radiology 2012;265:678–93.
6. Hinzpeter R, Boehm T, Boll D, et al. Imaging algorithms and CT protocols in trauma patients: survey of Swiss emergency centers. Eur Radiol 2017;27:1922–8.
7. Nguyen D, Platon A, Shanmuganathan K, et al. Evaluation of a single-pass continuous whole-body 16-MDCT protocol for patients with polytrauma. Am J Roentgenol 2009;192:3–10.
8. Gomez E, Horton K, Fishman EK, et al. CT of acute abdominopelvic hemorrhage: protocols, pearls, and pitfalls. Abdom Radiol 2022;47:475–84.
9. Durso AM, Paes FM, Caban K, et al. Evaluation of penetrating abdominal and pelvic trauma. Eur J Radiol 2020;130:109187.
10. DiChiro G, Brooks R, Kessler R, et al. Tissue signatures with dual-energy computed tomography. Radiology 1979;131:521–3.
11. Potter CA, Sodickson AD. Dual-energy CT in emergency neuroimaging: added value and novel applications. Radiographics 2016;36:2186–98.
12. Sade R, Kantarci M, Ogul H, et al. The feasibility of dual-energy computed tomography in cardiac contusion imaging for mildest blunt cardiac injury. J Comput Assist Tomogr 2017;41:354–9.
13. Wortman JR, Uyeda JW, Fulwadhva UP, et al. Dual-energy CT for abdominal and pelvic trauma. Radiographics 2018;38:586–602.
14. Gosangi B, Mandell JC, Weaver MJ, et al. Bone marrow edema at dual-energy CT: a game changer in the emergency department. Radiographics 2020;40:859–74.
15. Aran S, Besheli LD, Karcaaltincaba M, et al. Applications of dual-energy CT in emergency radiology. Am J Roentgenol 2014;202:W314–24.
16. Johnson TRC. Dual-energy CT: general principles. Am J Roentgenol 2012;199:S3–8.
17. Parakh A, Lennartz S, An C, et al. Dual-energy CT images: pearls and pitfalls. RadioGraphics 2021;41:98–119.
18. D'Angelo T, Albrecht MH, Caudo D, et al. Virtual noncalcium dual-energy CT: clinical applications. Eur Radiol Exp 2021;5:1–13.
19. McCollough CH, Leng S, Yu L, et al. Dual- and multi-energy CT: principles, technical approaches, and clinical applications. Radiology 2015;276:637–53.
20. Mileto A, Ramirez-Giraldo JC, Marin D, et al. Nonlinear image blending for dual-energy MDCT of the abdomen: can image quality be preserved if the contrast medium dose is reduced? Am J Roentgenol 2014;203:838–45.
21. Bodanapally UK, Shanmuganathan K, Ramaswamy M, et al. Iodine-based dual-energy CT of traumatic hemorrhagic contusions: relationship to in-hospital mortality and short-term outcome. Radiology 2019;292:730–8.
22. Naruto N, Itoh T, Noguchi K. Dual energy computed tomography for the head. Jpn J Radiol 2018;36:69–80.
23. Naruto N, Tannai H, Nishikawa K, et al. Dual-energy bone removal computed tomography (BRCT): preliminary report of efficacy of acute intracranial hemorrhage detection. Emerg Radiol 2018;25:29–33.

24. Emet M, Saritemur M, Altuntas B, et al. Dual-source computed tomography may define cardiac contusion in patients with blunt chest trauma in. Am J Emerg Med 2015;33:865.e1–3.

25. Hammer MM, Raptis DA, Cummings KW, et al. Imaging in blunt cardiac injury: computed tomographic findings in cardiac contusion and associated injuries. Injury 2016;47:1025–30.

26. Bierry G, Venkatasamy A, Kremer S, et al. Dual-energy CT in vertebral compression fractures: performance of visual and quantitative analysis for bone marrow edema demonstration with comparison to MRI. Skeletal Radiol 2014;43:485–92.

27. Karaca L, Yuceler Z, Kantarci M, et al. The feasibility of dual-energy CT in differentiation of vertebral compression fractures. Br J Radiol 2016;89:20150300.

28. Kellock TT, Nicolaou S, Kim SSY, et al. Detection of bone marrow edema in nondisplaced hip fractures: utility of a virtual noncalcium dual-Energy CT application1. Radiology 2017;284:798–805.

29. Flores EJ, Abujudeh HH. Applications of dual-energy CT in emergency radiology. AJR Am J Roentgenol 2014;202:314–24.

30. Hixson HR, Leiva-Salinas C, Sumer S, et al. Utilizing dual energy CT to improve CT diagnosis of posterior fossa ischemia. J Neuroradiol 2016;43:346–52.

31. Pomerantz SR, Kamalian S, Zhang D, et al. Virtual monochromatic reconstruction of dual-energy unenhanced head CT at 65-75 keV maximizes image quality compared with conventional polychromatic CT. Radiology 2013;266:318–25.

32. Hu R, Besheli LD, Young J, et al. Dual-energy head CT enables accurate distinction of intraparenchymal hemorrhage from calcification in emergency department patients. Radiology 2016;280:177–83.

33. Wong WD, Mohammed MF, Nicolaou S, et al. Impact of dual-energy CT in the emergency department: increased radiologist confidence, reduced need for follow-up imaging, and projected cost benefit. Am J Roentgenol 2020;215:1528–38.

34. Baldon IV, Amorim AC, Marques Santana Larissa, et al. The extravasation of contrast as a predictor of cerebral hemorrhagic contusion expansion, poor neurological outcome and mortality after traumatic brain injury: a systematic review and meta-analysis. PLoS One 2020;15:1–12.

35. Yan WQ, Xin YK, Jing Y, et al. Iodine quantification using dual-energy computed tomography for differentiating thymic tumors. J Comput Assist Tomogr 2018;42:873–80.

36. Lee DH, Lee YH, Seo HS, et al. Dual-energy CT iodine quantification for characterizing focal thyroid lesions. Head Neck 2019;41:1024–31.

37. Kaltenbach B, Wichmann JL, Pfeifer S, et al. Iodine quantification to distinguish hepatic neuroendocrine tumor metastasis from hepatocellular carcinoma at dual-source dual-energy liver CT. Eur J Radiol 2018;105:20–4.

38. Costantino M, Gosselin MV, Primack SL. The ABC's of thoracic trauma imaging. Semin Roentgenol 2006;41:209–25.

39. Wellenberg RHH, Hakvoort ET, Slump CH, et al. Metal artifact reduction techniques in musculoskeletal CT-imaging. Eur J Radiol 2018;107:60–9.

40. Katsura M, Sato J, Akahane M, et al. Current and novel techniques for metal artifact reduction at CT: practical guide for radiologists. RadioGraphics 2017;38:450–61.

41. Long Z, DeLone DR, Kotsenas AL, et al. Clinical assessment of metal artifact reduction methods in dual-energy CT examinations of instrumented spines. Am J Roentgenol 2019;212:395–401.

42. Kozar RA, Crandall M, Shanmuganathan K, et al. Organ injury scaling 2018 update: spleen, liver, and kidney. J Trauma Acute Care Surg 2018;85:1119–22.

43. Uyeda JW, LeBedis CA, Penn DR, et al. Active hemorrhage and vascular injuries in splenic trauma: utility of the arterial phase in multidetector CT. Radiology 2014;270:99–106.

44. Sullivan IW, Hota P, Dako F, et al. Dependent layering of venous refluxed contrast: a sign of critically low cardiac output. Radiol Case Rep 2019;14:230–4.

45. Yamada Y, Jinzaki M, Tanami Y, et al. Virtual monochromatic spectral imaging for the evaluation of hypovascular hepatic metastases the optimal monochromatic level with fast kilovoltage switching dual-energy computed tomography. Invest Radiol 2012;47:292–8.

46. Sudarski S, Apfaltrer P, Nance JW, et al. Objective and subjective image quality of liver parenchyma and hepatic metastases with virtual monoenergetic dual-source dual-energy CT reconstructions. An analysis in patients with gastrointestinal stromal tumor. Acad Radiol 2014;21:514–22.

47. Nagayama Y, Iyama A, Oda S, et al. Dual-layer dual-energy computed tomography for the assessment of hypovascular hepatic metastases: impact of closing k-edge on image quality and lesion detectability. Eur Radiol 2019;29:2837–47.

48. Sun EX, Wortman JR, Uyeda JW, et al. Virtual monoenergetic dual-energy CT for evaluation of hepatic and splenic lacerations. Emerg Radiol 2019;26:419–25.

49. Ayoob AR, Lee JT, Herr K, et al. Pancreatic trauma: imaging review and management update. Radiographics 2021;41:58–74.

50. Federle M, Courcoulas A, Powell M, et al. Radiology blunt splenic injury in adults: clinical and CT criteria for management, with emphasis on active extravasation. Radiology 1998;206:137–42.

51. Anderson SW, Varghese JC, Lucey BC, et al. Blunt splenic trauma: delayed-phase CT for differentiation

of active hemorrhage from contained vascular injury in patients. Radiology 2007;243:88–95.

52. Maturen KE, Kaza RK, Liu PS, et al. 'Sweet spot'" for endoleak detection: optimizing contrast to noise using low keV reconstructions from fast-switch kVp dual-energy CT. J Comput Assist Tomogr 2012;36: 83–7.

53. Vlahos I, Godoy MCB, Naidich DP. Dual-energy computed tomography imaging of the aorta. J Thorac Imaging 2010;25:289–300.

54. Tran DN, Straka M, Roos JE, et al. Dual-energy CT discrimination of iodine and calcium: experimental results and implications for lower extremity CT angiography. Acad Radiol 2009;16:160–71.

55. Firetto MC, Sala F, Petrini M, et al. Blunt bowel and mesenteric trauma: role of clinical signs along with CT findings in patients' management. Emerg Radiol 2018;25:461–7.

56. Brody JM, Leighton DB, Murphy BL, et al. CT of blunt trauma bowel and mesenteric injury: typical findings and pitfalls in diagnosis. RadioGraphics 2000;20: 1525–36.

57. Wang TJ, Barrett S, Ali I, et al. Dual-energy CT in the acute setting: bowel trauma. Front Radiol 2022;2: 835834.

58. Baş S, Zarbaliyev E. The role of dual-energy computed tomography in locating gastrointestinal tract perforations. Cureus 2021;13:e15265.

59. Simonetti I, Verde F, Palumbo L, et al. Dual energy computed tomography evaluation of skeletal traumas. Eur J Radiol 2021;134:109456.

60. Wong AJN, Wong M, Kutschera P, et al. Dual-energy CT in musculoskeletal trauma. Clin Radiol 2021;76: 38–49.

61. Yang P, Wu G, Chang X. Diagnostic accuracy of dual-energy computed tomography in bone marrow edema with vertebral compression fractures: a meta-analysis. Eur J Radiol 2018;99:124–9.

62. Ai S, Qu M, Glazebrook KN, et al. Use of dual-energy CT and virtual non-calcium techniques to evaluate post-traumatic bone bruises in knees in the subacute setting. Skeletal Radiol 2014;43: 1289–95.

The Use of Enteric Contrast in the Emergency Setting

Mohamed Z. Rajput, MD[a,*], Suraj Kapoor, MD[a], Alec J. Wright, MD[a],
Daniel D. Friedman, MD[a], Michael N. Patlas, MD[b], Vincent M. Mellnick, MD[a]

KEYWORDS

- Emergency radiology • Enteric contrast • Oral contrast • Rectal contrast • Gastrointestinal leak
- Penetrating trauma • Appendicitis • Small-bowel obstruction

KEY POINTS

- Enteric contrast continues to play an important role in the imaging assessment of patients presenting to the emergency department, especially when combined with computed tomography in specific clinical situations to improve diagnostic accuracy.
- Enteric contrast is particularly helpful in assessing postoperative complications of abdominal surgeries such as anastomotic leaks and fistulas.
- Although not always administered routinely, enteric contrast can be useful to confirm bowel injuries in the setting of penetrating trauma. Enteric contrast can assist in the identification of the appendix in cases of suspected acute appendicitis. Enteric contrast is also effective at guiding operative versus nonoperative management of patients with small-bowel obstruction.
- Although enteric contrast is overall safe and well-tolerated, the benefits of using it should be weighed against potential risks to the patient, including the time required to administer enteric contrast potentially resulting in a delay in diagnosis.

INTRODUCTION

Diagnostic imaging plays an essential role in the management of patients presenting to the emergency department, as it facilitates rapid triage and diagnosis and can be used to guide the management of these often critically ill patients. For patients presenting to the emergency department with suspected acute abdominal pathology, multidetector computed tomography (CT) of the abdomen and pelvis remains the imaging examination of choice.[1] Historically, abdominopelvic CT had been performed routinely using enteric contrast to distend and opacify the gastrointestinal tract, aiding identification of intraluminal bowel masses as well as helping to differentiate bowel from intra-abdominal fluid collections and peritoneal or mesenteric lesions, among other entities.[2–5] Use of enteric contrast was particularly useful in the early generations of

CT scanners, where thicker slices and motion artifacts associated with longer scan times led to decreased spatial and contrast resolution, thus limiting diagnostic accuracy. However, as CT technology has improved over the years, becoming faster and better quality with the ability to generate thin reconstructions in multiple planes, the relative importance of enteric contrast has been called into question. In particular, the need for enteric contrast in the high-patient-volume setting of the emergency department, where issues related to cost, patient throughput, delays in patient care, and imaging turnaround times are assessed continuously, remains a source of ongoing debate. Although numerous studies have supported eliminating the routine use of enteric contrast in CT scanning,[5–10] there remains substantial concern that foregoing its use altogether will lead to interpretive errors and missed diagnoses.[2–4]

[a] Mallinckrodt Institute of Radiology, Washington University School of Medicine, 510 South Kingshighway Boulevard, St Louis, MO 63110, USA; [b] Department of Radiology, McMaster University, Hamilton General Hospital, Hamilton, ON L8L 2X2, Canada
* Corresponding author.
E-mail address: mrajput@wustl.edu

Radiol Clin N Am 61 (2023) 37–51
https://doi.org/10.1016/j.rcl.2022.09.002

This article reviews the role of enteric contrast in the emergency setting. An overview of different types of enteric contrast media is provided together with general protocol principles and issues to consider when administering enteric contrast. Specific applications and clinical situations to use enteric contrast in patients presenting to the emergency department are discussed.

Issues to Consider When Using Enteric Contrast Agents

Categories of enteric contrast media include positive, neutral, and negative agents. Positive contrast agents are higher attenuation than water and provide excellent contrast resolution between bowel and surrounding soft tissue structures.[11,12] Positive agents include barium sulfate and iodinated water-soluble contrast agents. High-osmolar, ionic iodinated water-soluble agents include diatrizoate meglumine/diatrizoate sodium (Gastrograffin or MD-Gastroview); low-osmolar, nonionic iodinated water-soluble agents include ioversol (Optiray) and iohexol (Omnipaque). Water-soluble agents are strongly preferred in emergency department patients and critically ill inpatients. Barium is contraindicated in known or suspected gastrointestinal perforation due to the risk of spillage into the peritoneum causing barium peritonitis, which water-soluble agents will not induce.

Neutral contrast media, which is similar to or slightly higher attenuation than water, can be used to distend the bowel lumen without obscuring the bowel mucosa and wall. Its primary function is in routine outpatient evaluation of inflammatory bowel disease via CT or MR enterography. Neutral contrast is typically not used in the emergency setting due to the large volumes required to achieve adequate bowel distention.[13] Likewise, negative contrast such as instilled air and carbon dioxide are also primarily reserved for outpatient indications such as colorectal cancer screening with CT colonography.

Contrast can be administered by mouth or by nonoral routes including gastric/enteric catheters or introduced via the rectum or ostomy stoma. The route chosen will depend on the clinical question to be addressed. Abdominal radiography following administration of a small volume of water-soluble contrast through a preexisting enteral nutrition catheter, including gastrostomy and gastro-jejunostomy tubes, is often performed to assess a suspected malpositioned catheter or to confirm appropriate placement before usage.

Specific protocols that provide information on the precise timing and amounts of enteric contrast to be administered are largely practice-specific. At our institution, we typically administer a dilute water-soluble contrast agent and perform CT imaging approximately 30 min to 1 h afterward to assess potential pathology in the upper gastrointestinal tract. However, we generally wait at least 2 h after administration before performing scans intended to assess distal small-bowel pathology. Although this time interval typically ensures sufficient intraluminal opacification, thereby increasing the likelihood of a diagnostic study, it can be extended in patients with delayed intestinal transit from ileus or bowel obstruction. In other cases, contrast agents can be administered per rectum or through an ostomy. They are administered by a radiologist with the patient on the CT table using an appropriately sized Foley or other flexible rubber catheter. Adequate retrograde opacification of the area of clinical concern is confirmed via either topogram or a single slice transaxial ("scout") image that is reviewed before full scanning. In pediatric patients, enteric contrast is typically diluted based on the patient's age and/or weight to minimize the risk of streak artifact on CT that may obscure important findings. Of note, inappropriately diluted high-osmolar agents can promote dangerous fluid shifts and electrolyte disturbances in neonates and small children. In these patients, the use of dilute low-osmolar agents with lower risk profiles may be the preferred alternative.[14]

There are several issues to keep in mind when considering the use of enteric contrast. First, one needs to be certain that the patient is willing and able to cooperate with oral or rectal administration of the contrast agents. It may be difficult to obtain the necessary level of cooperation when performing studies on pediatric patients or adults with combative behavior. Some patients refuse to drink oral contrast, particularly barium and high-osmolar iodinated agents, because of their unpleasant taste; flavoring agents can be added to help mitigate this problem. Likewise, orally administered contrast or contrast delivered via gastric tube should be used with caution in patients at high risk for aspiration (eg, elderly patients, patients with suspected bowel obstruction, and trauma patients with altered mentation) (Fig. 1).[15–18] Large volumes of aspirated barium can elicit pneumonitis or pneumonia.[19] Aspiration of high-osmolar iodinated agents can also result in pneumonitis, as well as life-threatening flash pulmonary edema when aspirated in high quantities. In this patient population, low-osmolar agents should be preferentially considered. Other adverse effects associated with the use of enteric contrast agents include nausea, vomiting, abdominal pain, and, rarely, anaphylactic shock.[20]

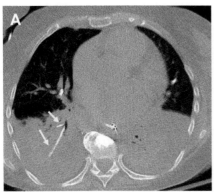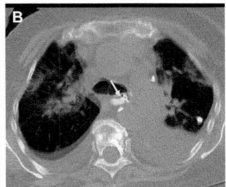

Fig. 1. Aspirated enteric contrast. A 68-year-old woman with Roux-en-Y gastric bypass complicated by perforation after attempted nasogastric tube placement, status post jejunal perforation repair, presenting with persistent leukocytosis and fevers. Transaxial CT images of the abdomen and pelvis obtained following administration of 30 mL of water-soluble enteric contrast through her preexisting nasogastric tube (*A, B*) show linear high attenuating material in the right lower lobe bronchial tree (*A: solid arrows*), compatible with aspirated contrast. Retained enteric contrast in the distended esophagus (*B: solid arrow*) likely refluxed from the stomach into the airway.

In some situations, the presence of enteric contrast may actually compromise the quality of a CT examination. For example, extravasation of intravenous contrast agents into the bowel lumen may be obscured by positive enteric contrast in patients with acute gastrointestinal tract bleeding (**Fig. 2**). The use of positive enteric contrast might also obscure the bowel wall in cases of suspected bowel ischemia and/or intramural hemorrhage, thus limiting the quality of the assessment.

Clinical Applications

Evaluation of anastomotic leaks, fistula, abscesses, and perforations in the gastrointestinal tract

Many patients seek evaluation and care in the emergency department following abdominal surgery for a myriad of reasons, ranging from causes that are self-limiting to potentially life-threatening. Postoperative complications of abdominal surgeries are frequently associated with significant morbidity, including peritonitis, sepsis, and death.[21,22] Although many complications are common to all types of abdominal surgeries, some are unique to the surgical procedure performed.[23] Anastomotic leaks, which are typically diagnosed during the first few days or weeks following surgery, are among the most significant and serious postoperative complications of abdominal surgery, with mortality as high at 50% if left undiagnosed.[24] A clinician may be alerted to the possibility of an anastomotic leak based on the development of signs and symptoms that include fever, unexplained leukocytosis, and the presence of gas, purulent, enteric, and/or fecal discharge

from the patient's surgical drains. Signs of anastomotic leakage on CT can be nonspecific and overlap with anticipated postsurgical findings, including the presence of intraperitoneal and peri-anastomotic air and/or fluid.

Extravasation of enteric contrast has been identified as the most specific sign of an anastomotic leak.[25,26] CT combined with enteric contrast provides the best diagnostic assessment for identifying the presence and location of a leak with excellent anatomic detail as well as showing additional important findings that may be otherwise clinically unsuspected (**Fig. 3**).[25,26] Knowledge of the type of surgery and anastomoses performed is critical before determining the appropriate method for administering enteric contrast. To evaluate suspected leaks from esophageal, gastric, or small-bowel anastomoses, including patients following bariatric surgery, enteric contrast is administered orally or via an enteric tube, followed by an appropriate delay before scanning to ensure contrast has reached the anastomotic site. Rectal administration of contrast should be performed to assess suspected left colonic or rectal anastomotic leaks (**Fig. 4**). Either oral or rectal contrast can be used when evaluating potential anastomotic leaks involving the right colon. Of note, the use of balloon catheters should be avoided in patients with recently-created low anal or rectal anastomoses to minimize the risk of iatrogenic disruption.[26]

Another common postoperative complication of abdominal surgery is the formation of intra-abdominal fluid collections or abscesses, which can also be associated with anastomotic leaks.[27] These collections can often interdigitate between

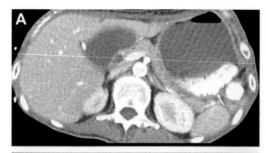

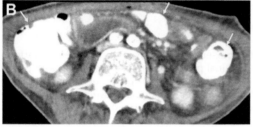

Fig. 2. Active gastrointestinal bleeding assessment obscured by enteric contrast. A 77-year-old man with abdominal pain and melena, who had a CT with oral contrast at an outside hospital the day prior. Multiphasic CT of the abdomen and pelvis without and with intravenous contrast was performed. Venous phase transaxial CT images (*A*, *B*) show a large volume of enteric contrast in the stomach and throughout the remainder of the gastrointestinal tract (*solid arrows*), limiting detection of active gastrointestinal bleeding. Subsequent upper endoscopy showed multiple actively bleeding gastric ulcers.

small-bowel loops, and, by mimicking the appearance of fluid-filled bowel, may go undetected by the radiologist. Opacifying adjacent bowel loops with enteric contrast can thereby help increase the conspicuity of these extraluminal collections and help guide percutaneous drainage.

Fistulas from the gastrointestinal tract to the abdominal wall can also develop from chronic inflammation related to abdominal surgery but are also seen in penetrating Crohn's disease and malignancies.[28] Fistulas can also be associated with fluid collections or abscesses. CT performed with enteric contrast, either orally administered or injected through a visible sinus tract penetrating the skin surface, may help delineate the size, extent, and patency of a fistula (**Fig. 5**). Similar to assessing for an anastomotic leak, if oral contrast is given, an appropriate delay before scanning should be ensured to allow for passage of contrast to the site of suspected fistula.

In the absence of recent abdominal surgery or intervention, nontraumatic perforation of the gastrointestinal tract can also be readily diagnosed by CT. Direct imaging findings include extraluminal gas (which may be concentrated at the site of perforation) and focal discontinuity of the bowel wall.[29,30] Although extravasation of enteric contrast is highly specific for a diagnosis, gastrointestinal perforation is often not clinically suspected a priori. Although most cases of gastrointestinal perforation are identified on CT without using enteric contrast, administering it can be useful in a follow-up study to confirm the site of perforation (**Fig. 6**). Moreover, in recent years, several institutions have adopted CT with oral contrast to evaluate for suspected esophageal perforation in patients presenting to the emergency department. Fluoroscopic esophagram, which is generally considered the imaging test of choice for detecting esophageal perforation, may be challenging to perform in the time and resource-limited setting of the emergency department, particularly after-hours and overnight when the necessary radiology staff may be scarce (**Fig. 7**).[31] CT with oral contrast has been shown to have a high negative predictive value similar to that of fluoroscopy, and shows even greater sensitivity than fluoroscopy, for diagnosing esophageal perforation.[31] In contrast to fluoroscopy, CT can also be used to evaluate for

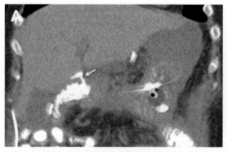
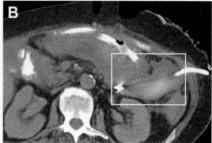

Fig. 3. Duodenal leak. A 74-year-old woman with duodenal perforation status post repair, presenting with increasing surgical drain output. Coronal CT image of the upper abdomen obtained without intravenous contrast (*A*) shows extraluminal enteric contrast extending through a defect in the superior aspect of the duodenal first segment, confirming a persistent duodenal leak (*solid arrow*). Dilute enteric contrast material is also present within a drained collection in the left upper quadrant (box), explaining the increased drain output.

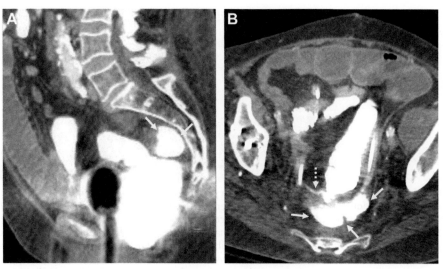

Fig. 4. Anastomotic dehiscence/leak following colorectal surgery. A 72-year-old woman with a sigmoid stricture status post-low anterior resection and primary anastomosis 6 days ago, presenting with postoperative leukocytosis. Sagittal (A) and transaxial (B) CT images of the pelvis performed with intravenous and rectal contrast show a large amount of extraluminal enteric contrast in the presacral space (*solid arrows*) near the location of the surgical drains. Enteric contrast appears to extend directly from the colorectal anastomosis (*B: dashed arrow*), confirming postoperative anastomotic dehiscence/leak.

extra-esophageal abnormalities that may be contributing to the patient's symptoms. Protocols vary by institution but typically include pre-contrast imaging, supine post-contrast imaging performed immediately after administration of enteric contrast orally or via gastric tube placed into the esophagus, and, if needed, prone post-contrast imaging.[32]

Penetrating Abdominal Trauma

Trauma is a leading cause of death worldwide and accounts for one in every 10 deaths.[33,34] CT remains the primary cross-sectional imaging modality used to evaluate traumatic injuries in hemodynamically stable patients as it provides highly accurate assessments of a wide spectrum

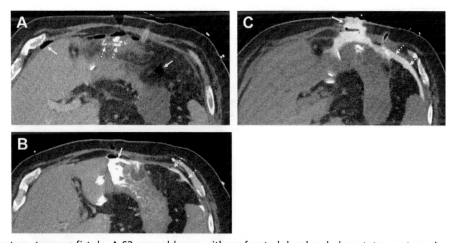

Fig. 5. Gastrocutaneous fistula. A 63-year-old man with perforated duodenal ulcer status post repair and gastrojejunostomy, presenting after leakage from his midline abdominal incision. Initial transaxial CT images of the abdomen and pelvis with intravenous contrast and without enteric contrast (A) show a small amount of pneumoperitoneum in the upper abdomen (*solid arrows*). High-density suture material at the gastrojejunal anastomosis (*dashed arrows*). The examination was repeated after the administration of enteric contrast with transaxial CT images of the abdomen and pelvis (B, C) showing leakage of contrast from the site of the gastrojejunal anastomosis (*B: solid arrow*) into the peritoneal space (*B, C: dashed arrows*) and through the midline wound (*C: solid arrow*), indicative of a gastrocutaneous fistula.

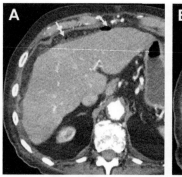 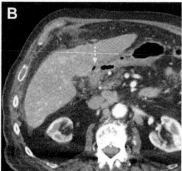 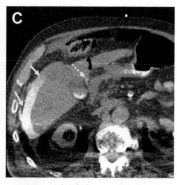

Fig. 6. Perforated gastric ulcer. An 87-year-old man with prostate cancer presenting with abdominal pain. Transaxial CT images of the abdomen and pelvis with intravenous contrast (*A, B*) show small-volume pneumoperitoneum (*solid arrows*) with locules of extraluminal gas concentrated along the pylorus, suggesting perforated peptic ulcer disease (*B: dashed arrow*). Transaxial CT image of the abdomen and pelvis obtained the next day with oral contrast only (*C*) shows interval increase in perihepatic free fluid tracking along the right paracolic gutter containing extravasated enteric contrast (*solid arrows*). A small tract of contrast in the right upper quadrant (*dashed arrow*) is seen communicating between the pyloric perforation and the perihepatic fluid collection.

of injuries sustained by this patient cohort.[35,36] Injuries to the abdomen are the third most common type of trauma following injuries to the head and extremities. Most abdominal injuries are caused by blunt trauma as opposed to penetrating mechanisms.[37] Injuries to the bowel, in particular, can be a source of misdiagnosis and lead to complicated outcomes including peritonitis, sepsis, and death.[38–41]

Routine administration of enteric contrast in the CT evaluation of patients with blunt abdominal trauma is no longer recommended, with previous studies showing no added benefit to its usage in identifying bowel injury.[42,43] Enteric contrast has been shown to be useful in assessing penetrating abdominal injuries, but not without controversy. Developed in the early 2000s, the "triple contrast"

protocol that combines intravenous, oral, and rectal contrast has been shown to be highly accurate and specific for identifying surgically important bowel injuries from penetrating trauma. Triple contrast can be particularly valuable when the clinical team requires diagnostic certainty of a bowel injury to forgo nonoperative management and proceed with laparotomy.[44] Extravasated enteric contrast is a direct sign of bowel injury, with specificity near 100% and near complete agreement and inter-observer reliability.[45] However, as with other indications for abdominopelvic imaging in the emergency setting, routine use of enteric contrast in penetrating abdominal trauma has been called into question. Although highly specific, leakage of enteric contrast alone has poor sensitivity and is seen in only 15% to 29%

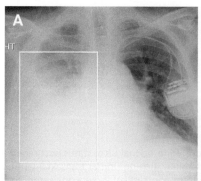 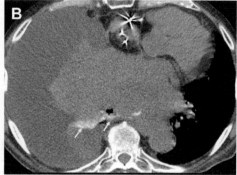

Fig. 7. Esophageal rupture. An 81-year-old man with chest pain after undergoing esophagogastroduodenoscopy and esophageal dilation of an esophageal stricture. Chest radiograph (*A*) reveals a large right-sided pleural effusion (box) that was new from a prior examination. Transaxial CT image of the chest with oral contrast (*B*) shows leakage of contrast from the distal esophagus into the right pleural space (*arrow*), confirming iatrogenic esophageal rupture.

of patients with penetrating bowel injury, and in an even fewer 2% to 6% of all patients scanned.[41,45,46] Furthermore, many bowel injuries can be accurately identified through a combination of direct and indirect signs other than extravasated enteric contrast, including evidence of a wound tract extending to the bowel wall, focal wall thickening, and free intraperitoneal fluid and/or hemorrhage.[45] Relying on enteric contrast leak to confirm bowel injury can also underestimate partial thickness serosal injures that may also require repair.[47]

Using enteric contrast in this patient cohort is also not without disadvantages and risks, foremost being the time delay required administering enteric contrast, and, in the case of orally administered contrast, time needed for transit and opacification of the small bowel. This poses an issue in trauma patients who can become rapidly unstable, potentially requiring immediate surgical intervention before CT can be obtained. Although the impact of these delays on patient outcomes is not completely understood, it has been shown that even short delays in identifying penetrating injuries to the colon and rectum are associated with increased morbidity and mortality.[48–50] Unsurprisingly, the use of enteric contrast varies greatly by institution, underscored by a recent survey of members from the American Society of Emergency Radiology in which most of the respondents reported that they do not routinely administer enteric contrast when evaluating penetrating abdominal injury.[51] At this time, The American College of Radiology does not offer specific recommendations on the use of enteric contrast in patients with penetrating trauma.[52]

At our institution, we use a single (intravenous) contrast protocol when evaluating blunt and penetrating trauma, reserving oral and/or rectal contrast in the setting of penetrating trauma as a problem-solving tool for equivocal cases in which a follow-up scan is either requested or deemed necessary to maximize diagnostic accuracy.[20] Enteric contrast may be helpful when evaluating penetrating stab wounds, as these injuries can be subtle, and their full extent may not be clear (**Fig. 8**). Enteric contrast is also helpful in patients with multiple penetrating abdominal injuries where retracing wound tracts can be particularly challenging. We find rectal contrast valuable in identifying penetrating colorectal injuries, which result not only from direct trauma but also from foreign bodies and iatrogenic causes (**Fig. 9**). In particular, rectal contrast can help distinguish extraperitoneal versus intraperitoneal rectal injuries for purposes of pre-surgical planning; extraperitoneal injuries are managed with fecal diversion only, whereas

intraperitoneal injuries require both fecal diversion and primary surgical repair.[53] Enteric contrast is also helpful for confirming traumatic esophageal injuries, which are extremely rare, but when do occur, are much more often from penetrating rather than blunt mechanisms (**Fig. 10**).[54]

Appendicitis

Appendicitis is a common surgical emergency in patients presenting to the emergency department, particularly among children and young adults.[55–58] Historically, clinical symptoms and signs were used alone to diagnose appendicitis. Today, though, imaging plays an essential role in the diagnosis of appendicitis and associated complications including perforation, obstruction, and abscess formation. Imaging is also used to identify alternative causes of abdominal pain once appendicitis has been excluded. Although ultrasound is used initially to assess for appendicitis in some patient populations, namely pediatric and pregnant patients, sonographic visualization of the appendix may be difficult for numerous reasons, including operator technique, obscuring bowel gas, or limited acoustic window due to body habitus. In contrast, CT is both highly sensitive and specific in diagnosing appendicitis and is thus the preferred imaging modality used to evaluate for appendicitis in most patients presenting to the emergency department.

Traditionally, oral and/or rectally-administered enteric contrast was used in the CT assessment of appendicitis; nonfilling of a dilated appendix (>6 mm) is a highly sensitive sign of appendiceal obstruction and appendicitis (**Fig. 11**).[59,60] Furthermore, luminal obstruction may precede inflammatory changes, including periappendiceal fat stranding and fluid, identified on CT.[61] Nonfilling of the most distal aspect of the appendix can suggest the frequently-challenging diagnosis of tip appendicitis (**Fig. 12**). Luminal filling throughout the length of the appendix with enteric contrast also confidently excludes appendicitis with high specificity (**Fig. 13**).[61] Positive enteric contrast can help differentiate the appendix from surrounding small-bowel loops and prominent coursing vessels that may mimic the appendix, as well as help identify periappendiceal fluid collections separate from bowel. This can be particularly helpful when assessing pediatric patients with comparatively low levels of intra-abdominal visceral fat compared with older patients, which typically serves as a natural contrast agent and facilitates visualization of the appendix.[62]

However, there are several potential disadvantages to administering enteric contrast to assess

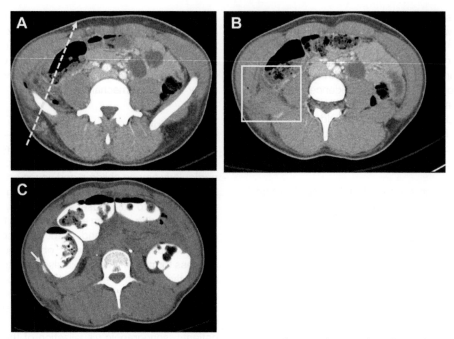

Fig. 8. Penetrating colonic injury. An 18-year-old man presenting after a stab wound to the back. Transaxial CT images of the abdomen and pelvis with intravenous contrast (*A*, *B*) show a penetrating wound tract in the right flank (*dashed arrow*) with retroperitoneal gas and hemorrhage abutting the ascending colon and cecum (box), suspicious for colonic injury. Follow up study with rectally administered enteric contrast confirmed a full thickness injury to the ascending colon evidenced by a small amount of extraluminal contrast (*solid arrow*).

for appendicitis. First, pediatric patients, who represent a large proportion of those ultimately diagnosed with appendicitis, may not tolerate oral contrast because of its unpleasant taste or because of concomitant abdominal pain, nausea, and vomiting. Rectal contrast may also not be well-tolerated in this patient cohort because of the discomfort associated with a rectal catheter and colonic distention with contrast. The time interval required for the transit of oral contrast to the cecum before CT scanning can delay diagnosis and potentially increase the risk of appendiceal perforation.[63,64] The use of oral contrast may also delay the induction of general anesthesia required for surgical management of appendicitis.[65] Moreover, once oral contrast reaches the cecum, it does not opacify a normal appendix in 8% to 31% of cases.[66]

Numerous recent studies with both adults and pediatric patients have shown the similar performance of enteric and nonenteric contrast protocol CT in diagnosing appendicitis.[10,62,65–69] This is likely due at least in part to the improved resolution and image quality provided by new CT

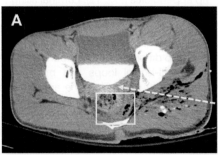
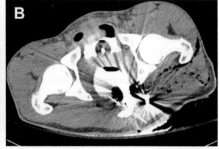

Fig. 9. Penetrating rectal injury. A 21-year-old-man presenting after gunshot wound to the pelvis. Initial CT image of the abdomen and pelvis with intravenous contrast (*A*) shows a wound tract in the left hemipelvis (*dashed arrow*) with multiple bullet fragments in the left gluteal muscles. Perirectal hemorrhage and gas is also seen (box), highly suspicious for rectal injury. Subsequent CT of the pelvis after instilling rectal contrast (*B*) shows a large transmural defect in the posterior rectum (*solid arrows*).

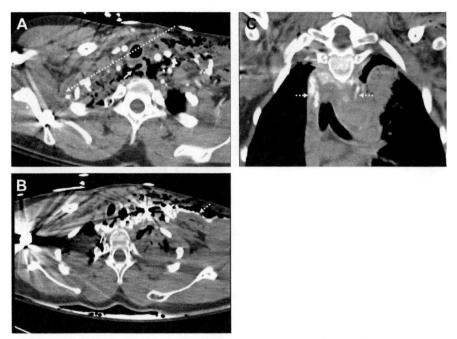

Fig. 10. Penetrating esophageal injury. A 23-year-old woman presenting after gunshot wound to the left chest. Transaxial CT image of the chest with intravenous contrast (*A*) shows a large bullet tract across the lower neck/upper chest, crossing the thoracic inlet (*dashed arrow*), with a focal discontinuity in the upper esophagus (*solid arrow*), highly suspicious for esophageal injury. Repeat chest CT images following administration of water-soluble oral contrast (*B, C*) confirm a full-thickness esophageal injury with extraluminal contrast extending from the site of injury (B: solid *arrow*) into the mediastinum (*C: dashed arrows*) and neck soft tissues (*B: dashed arrow*).

technologies that facilitate identification of the appendix without the need for enteric contrast.[62] Nonetheless, enteric contrast is still used routinely in cases of suspected appendicitis at some institutions, and on a case-by-case basis at others.

Small-Bowel Obstruction

Small-bowel obstruction is a common cause of acute abdominal pain in patients presenting to the emergency department, with the potential for high morbidity and mortality. Although most

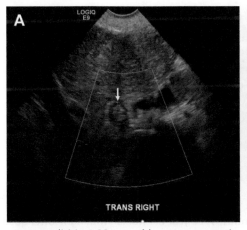
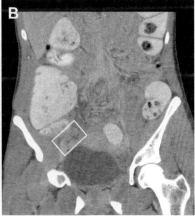

Fig. 11. Acute appendicitis. A 28-year-old woman presenting with pelvic pain. Transvaginal sonogram initially obtained (*A*) showed normal ovaries and uterus (not included) but did reveal a tubular echogenic structure in the right lower quadrant with bowel signature (*solid arrow*). CT following the administration of rectal contrast was subsequently performed (*B*). There is adequate instillation of contrast retrograde through the colon to the cecum. The appendix was identified arising off the base of the cecum, which did not fill with enteric contrast (box). The diagnosis of appendicitis was confirmed at surgery.

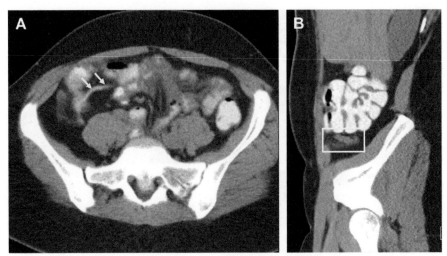

Fig. 12. Tip appendicitis. A 45-year-old woman with right lower quadrant pain. Transaxial CT image of the abdomen and pelvis with oral contrast (*A*) shows a normal-appearing, nondilated proximal appendix filled entirely with enteric contrast (*solid arrow*). Careful review of the sagittal reformat image (*B*), however, shows nonfilling of a thickened, minimally dilated appendiceal tip with periappendiceal fat stranding (box), indicating tip appendicitis.

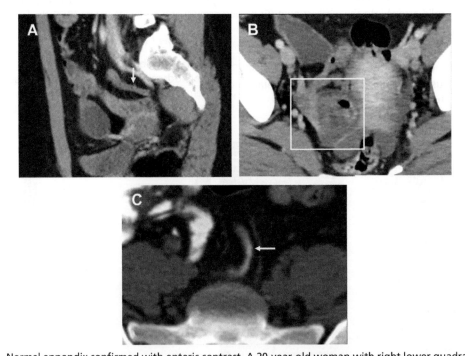

Fig. 13. Normal appendix confirmed with enteric contrast. A 20-year-old woman with right lower quadrant pain. Sagittal CT image of the pelvis (*A*) shows a normal, nondilated proximal appendix (*solid arrow*). Transaxial CT image of the pelvis (*B*) shows free fluid, small-bowel loops, and the right adnexa, which were difficult to separate from the tip of the appendix (box). Owing to ongoing clinical concern for appendicitis, a repeat examination was performed after administration of oral contrast (*C*). The appendix is clearly depicted anterior to the sacrum and contains oral contrast throughout its length, confirming a normal appendix and no acute appendicitis (*solid arrow*).

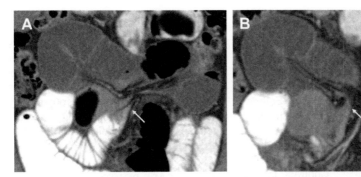

Fig. 14. Closed-loop small-bowel obstruction. A 68-year-old man with abdominal pain and inability to pass stool or gas. Coronal CT image of the abdomen and pelvis with enteric contrast (*A*) shows a tapered small-bowel contour with abrupt end of the oral contrast column (*solid arrow*). Additional coronal CT image more posterior (*B*) shows clustered loops of dilated small bowel not opacified with enteric contrast, with two transition points originating from the same point (*solid arrows*), indicating a closed loop obstruction. A closed loop small-bowel obstruction secondary to adhesions was identified at surgery.

small-bowel obstructions develop secondary to intra-abdominal adhesions, other causes include hernias, neoplasms, inflammatory bowel disease, and foreign bodies.[70] CT is the primary imaging modality used to diagnose small-bowel obstruction and has largely replaced abdominal radiography for this indication. CT can identify the precise location of a bowel obstruction, its severity (low- or high-grade), and often its underlying cause. Intravenous contrast is used whenever possible to help identify signs of bowel ischemia, including bowel wall thickening and hypoenhancement.[70]

Enteric contrast can play an important role in the diagnosis and management of patients with small-bowel obstruction. Typically, enteric contrast is not initially administered to patients with suspected small-bowel obstruction before obtaining CT, as many of these patients are experiencing nausea and/or vomiting limiting any oral intake. In addition, positive intraluminal contrast may potentially obscure the bowel wall and imaging signs of ischemia on CT. Though if enteric contrast had been administered because small-bowel obstruction was not suspected, it may help delineate the transition point of an obstruction where intraluminal contrast abruptly stops.

Patients with small-bowel obstruction who do not require emergent surgery can be managed with gastric decompression and intravenous fluids. Many surgeons, including those at our institution, also use a water-soluble contrast (WSC)

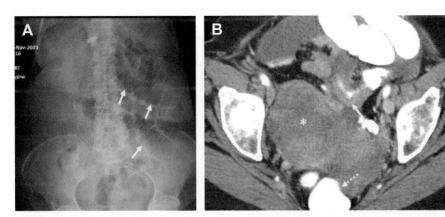

Fig. 15. Malignant partial small-bowel obstruction. An 82-year-old woman with nausea and vomiting. Abdominal radiograph (*A*) shows multiple dilated, gas-filled small-bowel loops in the left hemiabdomen (*solid arrows*), suggestive of a small-bowel obstruction. Enteric contrast was administered through a gastric tube, and transaxial CT image of the abdomen and pelvis subsequently obtained (*B*) shows a transition point in the left lower quadrant (*solid arrow*) adjacent to a large solid right adnexal mass (*asterisk*), later biopsied as ovarian adenocarcinoma. Contrast is seen beyond the transition point in the rectum (*dashed arrow*), indicative of a partial, rather than complete, obstruction.

challenge to predict the likelihood of successful conservative therapy.[71] Water-soluble enteric contrast, typically 40 to 150 mL of a high-osmolar iodinated agent, is administered orally or via gastric tube, and follow-up abdominal radiographs are obtained 8 and 24 h later to assess its transit through the gastrointestinal tract. Enteric contrast reaching the colon at least 24 h after administration has been shown to be >95% sensitive and specific in predicting resolution of adhesive small-bowel obstruction and successful nonoperative management.[72,73] Contrast failing to reach the colon at 24 h indicates a higher grade of obstruction likely requiring surgical intervention.

Although CT imaging is not typically performed as part of the WSC challenge, it may be useful as an ancillary tool, particularly in cases where visualization of contrast in the colon on abdominal radiographs becomes difficult due to dilutional effects or large patient body habitus. As a problem-solving tool in patients who are deemed poor surgical candidates, enteric contrast can also help confirm the presence of a closed-loop small-bowel obstruction, where a loop of bowel is obstructed both distally and proximally. Enteric contrast will be unable to transit within this localized region of small-bowel dilation (Fig. 14). Identifying a closed-loop small-bowel obstruction is critical, as the affected segment of bowel is at high risk of ischemia. The WSC challenge may also have a therapeutic effect in alleviating small-bowel obstruction, although the data attesting to this point is less conclusive.[72–77] The WSC challenge is also highly sensitive for differentiating between small-bowel obstruction and ileus in postoperative patients.[78] Although most studies have focused on patients with small-bowel obstruction secondary to adhesions, the WSC challenge may also help guide the management of nonadhesive obstructions, including malignant small-bowel obstruction and obstruction due to abdominal wall hernias (Fig. 15).[79–81]

SUMMARY

In conclusion, enteric contrast continues to play an important role in the imaging assessment of patients presenting to the emergency department. Although it may no longer be required to ensure diagnostic accuracy on a routine basis, enteric contrast remains valuable, particularly when used in a targeted fashion to address specific clinical questions on a case-by-case basis. Enteric contrast is safe and well-tolerated by most patients with a low risk of serious side effects. A recent survey revealed that most patients (89%) would prefer to drink oral contrast, even with

only the slightest likelihood that this will improve diagnostic accuracy, rather than accepting a risk of a missed finding.[82] Radiologists report increased diagnostic confidence and reader reliability in cases in which any type of enteric contrast is used for CT imaging.[83] This can be particularly important in the emergency setting, where one encounters critical, life-threatening pathologies requiring confident and accurate diagnoses on a routine basis.

CLINICS CARE POINTS

- Targeted use of enteric contrast for CT imaging in patients presenting to the emergency department is helpful in specific clinical scenarios, especially when assessing for gastrointestinal tract perforation or complications following abdominal surgery.

DISCLOSURE

None of the authors have any disclosures.

REFERENCES

1. Alabousi A, Patlas MN, Sne N, et al. Is oral contrast necessary for multidetector computed tomography imaging of patients with acute abdominal pain? Can Assoc Radiol J 2015;66(4):318–22.
2. Megibow AJ. Oral contrast utilization for abdominal/pelvic CT scanning in today's emergency room setting. Abdom Radiol 2017;42(3):781–3.
3. Winter T. A plea for oral contrast administration in CT for emergency department patients. Am J Roentgenol 2010;195(1). https://doi.org/10.2214/AJR.10.4223.
4. Sokhandon F. Oral contrast administration for abdominal and pelvic CT scan in emergency setting: is there a happy medium? Abdom Radiol 2017;42(3):784–5.
5. Lee SY, Coughlin B, Wolfe JM, et al. Prospective comparison of helical CT of the abdomen and pelvis without and with oral contrast in assessing acute abdominal pain in adult Emergency Department patients. Emerg Radiol 2006;12(4):150–7.
6. Huynh LN, Coughlin BF, Wolfe J, et al. Patient encounter time intervals in the evaluation of emergency department patients requiring abdominopelvic CT: Oral contrast versus no contrast. Emerg Radiol 2004;10(6):310–3.
7. Razavi SA, Johnson JO, Kassin MT, et al. The impact of introducing a no oral contrast abdominopelvic CT

examination (NOCAPE) pathway on radiology turn around times, emergency department length of stay, and patient safety. Emerg Radiol 2014;21(6): 605–13.

8. Levenson RB, Camacho MA, Horn E, et al. Eliminating routine oral contrast use for CT in the emergency department: Impact on patient throughput and diagnosis. Emerg Radiol 2012;19(6):513–7.

9. Wang ZJ, Chen KS, Gould R, et al. Positive enteric contrast material for abdominal and pelvic CT with automatic exposure control: What is the effect on patient radiation exposure? Eur J Radiol 2011;79(2). https://doi.org/10.1016/j.ejrad.2011.03.059.

10. Anderson SW, Soto JA, Lucey BC, et al. Abdominal 64-MDCT for suspected appendicitis: The use of oral and IV contrast material versus IV contrast material only. Am J Roentgenol 2009;193(5):1282–8.

11. Marks WM, Goldberg HI, Moss AA, et al. Intestinal pseudotumors: A problem in abdominal computed tomography solved by directed techniques. Gastrointest Radiol 1980;5(1):155–60.

12. Shirkhoda A. Diagnostic pitfalls in abdominal CT. Radiographics 1991;11(6):969–1002.

13. Griffey RT, Fowler KJ, Theilen A, et al. Considerations in Imaging Among Emergency Department Patients With Inflammatory Bowel Disease. Ann Emerg Med 2017;69(5):587–99. https://doi.org/10.1016/j.annemergmed.2016.04.010.

14. Callahan MJ, Talmadge JM, MacDougall R, et al. The use of enteric contrast media for diagnostic CT, MRI, and ultrasound in infants and children: A practical approach. Am J Roentgenol 2016;206(5): 973–9.

15. Lim-Dunham JE, Narra J, Benya EC, et al. Aspiration after administration of oral contrast material in children undergoing abdominal CT for trauma. Am J Roentgenol 1997;169(4):1015–8.

16. Federle MP, Peitzman A, Krugh J. Use of oral contrast material in abdominal trauma CT scans: Is it dangerous? J Trauma 1995;38(1):51–3.

17. Donnelly LF, Frush DP, Frush KS. Aspirated contrast material contributing to respiratory arrest in a pediatric trauma patient. Am J Roentgenol 1998;171(2):471–3.

18. Trulzsch DV, Penmetsa A, Karim A, et al. Gastrografin-induced aspiration pneumonia: A lethal complication of computed tomography. South Med J 1992;85(12):1255–6.

19. ACR Committee on Drugs and Contrast Media, ACR Manual on Contrast Media, 105, 2021. Available at: http://www.acr.org/~/media/ACR/Documents/PDF/QualitySafety/Resources/ContrastManual/2013_Contrast_Media.pdf. Accessed February 01, 2022.

20. Jawad H, Raptis C, Mintz A, et al. Single-contrast CT for detecting bowel injuries in penetrating abdominopelvic trauma. Am J Roentgenol 2018;210(4):761–5.

21. Gorgun E, Remzi FH. Complications of Ileoanal Pouches. Clin Colon Rectal Surg 2004;17(1):43–55.

22. Bertelsen CA, Andreasen AH, Jørgensen T, et al. Anastomotic leakage after anterior resection for rectal cancer: Risk factors. Color Dis 2010;12(1): 37–43.

23. O'Malley RB, Revels JW. Imaging of Abdominal Postoperative Complications. Radiol Clin North Am 2020;58(1):73–91.

24. Guillem JG, Cohen AM. Current issues in colorectal cancer surgery. Semin Oncol 1999;26(5):505–13.

25. Kauv P, Benadjaoud S, Curis E, et al. Anastomotic leakage after colorectal surgery: diagnostic accuracy of CT. Eur Radiol 2015;25(12):3543–51.

26. Samji KB, Kielar AZ, Connolly M, et al. Anastomotic Leaks After Small- and Large-Bowel Surgery: Diagnostic Performance of CT and the Importance of Intraluminal Contrast Administration. Am J Roentgenol 2018;210(6):1259–65.

27. Weinstein S, Osei-Bonsu S, Aslam R, et al. Multidetector CT of the postoperative colon: Review of normal appearances and common complications. Radiographics 2013;33(2):515–32.

28. Tonolini M, Magistrelli P. Enterocutaneous fistulas: a primer for radiologists with emphasis on CT and MRI. Insights Imaging 2017;8(6):537–48.

29. Kothari K, Friedman B, Grimaldi GM, et al. Nontraumatic large bowel perforation: spectrum of etiologies and CT findings. Abdom Radiol 2017;42(11): 2597–608.

30. Hainaux B, Agneessens E, Bertinotti R, et al. Accuracy of MDCT in predicting site of gastrointestinal tract perforation. Am J Roentgenol 2006;187(5): 1179–83.

31. Wei CJ, Levenson RB, Lee KS. Diagnostic utility of CT and fluoroscopic esophagography for suspected esophageal perforation in the emergency department. Am J Roentgenol 2020;215(3): 631–8.

32. Norton-Gregory AA, Kulkarni NM, O'connor SD, et al. CT esophagography for evaluation of esophageal perforation. Radiographics 2021;41(2): 447–61.

33. Oyeniyi BT, Fox EE, Scerbo M, et al. Trends in 1029 Trauma Deaths at a Level 1 Trauma Center. Injury 2017;48(1):5.

34. Mock C, Joshipura M, Arreola-Risa C, et al. An estimate of the Number of Lives that Could be Saved through Improvements in Trauma Care Globally. World J Surg 2012;36(5):959–63.

35. Wolfman NT, Bechtold RE, Scharling ES, et al. Blunt upper abdominal trauma: evaluation by CT. Am J Roentgenol 1992;158(3):493–501.

36. Wing VW, Federle MP, Morris JA, et al. The clinical impact of CT for blunt abdominal trauma. Am J Roentgenol 1985;145(6):1191–4.

37. Kumar A, Panda A, Gamanagatti S. Blunt pancreatic trauma: A persistent diagnostic conundrum? World J Radiol 2016;8(2):159.

38. Inaba K, Branco BC, Moe D, et al. Prospective evaluation of selective nonoperative management of torso gunshot wounds: When is it safe to discharge? J Trauma Acute Care Surg 2012;72(4):884–91.

39. Múnera F, Morales C, Soto JA, et al. Gunshot Wounds of Abdomen: Evaluation of Stable Patients with Triple-Contrast Helical CT. Radiology 2004; 231(2):399–405.

40. Chiu WC, Shanmuganathan K, Mirvis SE, et al. Determining the need for laparotomy in penetrating torso trauma: a prospective study using triple-contrast enhanced abdominopelvic computed tomography. J Trauma 2001;51(5):860–9.

41. Shanmuganathan K, Mirvis SE, Chiu WC, et al. Triple-contrast helical CT in penetrating torso trauma: A prospective study to determine peritoneal violation and the need for laparotomy. Am J Roentgenol 2001; 177(6):1247–56.

42. Stafford RE, McGonigal MD, Weigelt JA, et al. Oral contrast solution and computed tomography for blunt abdominal trauma: A randomized study. Arch Surg 1999;134:622–7.

43. Lee CH, Haaland B, Earnest A, et al. Use of positive oral contrast agents in abdominopelvic computed tomography for blunt abdominal injury: Meta-analysis and systematic review. Eur Radiol 2013; 23(9):2513–21.

44. Paes FM, Durso AM, Pinto DS, et al. Diagnostic performance of triple-contrast versus single-contrast multi-detector computed tomography for the evaluation of penetrating bowel injury. Emerg Radiol 2022; 0123456789. https://doi.org/10.1007/s10140-022-02038-0.

45. Saksobhavivat N, Shanmuganathan K, Boscak AR, et al. Diagnostic accuracy of triple-contrast multi-detector computed tomography for detection of penetrating gastrointestinal injury: a prospective study. Eur Radiol 2016;26(11):4107–20.

46. Shanmuganathan K, Mirvis SE, Chiu WC, et al. Penetrating torso trauma: Triple-contrast helical CT in peritoneal violation and organ injury - A prospective study in 200 patients. Radiology 2004;231(3): 775–84.

47. Sharpe JP, Magnotti LJ, Weinberg JA, et al. Applicability of an established management algorithm for colon injuries following blunt trauma. J Trauma Acute Care Surg 2013;74(2):419–25.

48. Shatnawi NJ, Bani-Hani KE. Management of civilian extraperitoneal rectal injuries. Asian J Surg 2006; 29(1):11–6.

49. Gumus M, Kapan M, Onder A, et al. Factors affecting morbidity in penetrating rectal injuries: a civilian experience. Turkish J Trauma Emerg Surg 2011;17(5):401–6.

50. Girgin S, Gedik E, Uysal E, et al. Independent risk factors of morbidity in penetrating colon injuries. Ulus Travma ve Acil Cerrahi Derg 2009;15(3):232–8.

51. Ozimok CJ, Mellnick VM, Patlas MN. An international survey to assess use of oral and rectal contrast in CT protocols for penetrating torso trauma. Emerg Radiol 2019;26(2):117–21.

52. Broder JS, Hamedani AG, Liu SW, et al. Emergency Department contrast practices for abdominal/pelvic computed tomography - A national survey and comparison with the American College of Radiology Appropriateness Ariteria. J Emerg Med 2013;44(2): 423–33.

53. Naeem M, Hoegger MJ, Petraglia FW, et al. CT of penetrating abdominopelvic trauma. Radiographics 2021;41(4):1064–81.

54. Xu AA, Breeze JL, Paulus JK, et al. Epidemiology of traumatic esophageal injury: An analysis of the national Trauma Data Bank. Am Surg 2019;85(4): 342–9.

55. Chien M, Habis A, Glynn L, et al. Staged imaging pathway for the evaluation of pediatric appendicitis. Pediatr Surg Int 2016;32(7):671–8.

56. Saito JM, Yan Y, Evashwick TW, et al. Use and accuracy of diagnostic imaging by hospital type in pediatric appendicitis. Pediatrics 2013;131(1). https://doi.org/10.1542/peds.2012-1665.

57. Garcia EM, Camacho MA, Karolyi DR, et al. ACR Appropriateness Criteria® Right Lower Quadrant Pain-Suspected Appendicitis. J Am Coll Radiol 2018;15(11):S373–87.

58. Kharbanda AB, Taylor GA, Bachur RG. Suspected appendicitis in children: Rectal and intravenous contrast-enhanced versus intravenous contrast-enhanced CT. Radiology 2007;243(2):520–6.

59. Rao PM, Rhea JT, Novelline RA, et al. Helical CT combined with contrast material administered only through the colon for imaging of suspected appendicitis. AJR Am J Roentgenol 1997;169(5): 1275–80.

60. Mullins ME, Kircher MF, Ryan DP, et al. Evaluation of suspected appendicitis in children using limited helical CT and colonic contrast material. Am J Roentgenol 2001;176(1):37–41.

61. Tang SJ, Pickhardt PJ, Kim DU, et al. Positive Oral Contrast Solution at MDCT for Suspected Acute Appendicitis in Adults: Rate of Appendiceal Luminal Filling of Normal and Inflamed Appendixes. Am J Roentgenol 2019;213(5):W211–7.

62. Farrell CR, Bezinque AD, Tucker JM, et al. Acute appendicitis in childhood: oral contrast does not improve CT diagnosis. Emerg Radiol 2018;25(3): 257–63.

63. Papandria D, Goldstein SD, Rhee D, et al. Risk of perforation increases with delay in recognition and surgery for acute appendicitis. J Surg Res 2013; 184(2):723–9.

64. Bickell NA, Aufses AH, Rojas M, et al. How time affects the risk of rupture in appendicitis. J Am Coll Surg 2006;202(3):401–6.

65. Ramalingam V, Bates DDB, Buch K, et al. Diagnosing acute appendicitis using a nonoral contrast CT protocol in patients with a BMI of less than 25. Emerg Radiol 2016;23(5):455–62.

66. Rao PM, Rhea JT, Novelline RA, et al. Helical CT technique for the diagnosis of appendicitis: Prospective evaluation of a focused appendix CT examination. Radiology 1997;202(1):130–44.

67. Anderson SW, Rhea JT, Milch HN, et al. Influence of body habitus and use of oral contrast on reader confidence in patients with suspected acute appendicitis using 64 MDCT. Emerg Radiol 2010;17(6):445–53.

68. Kepner AM, Bacasnot JV, Stahlman BA. Intravenous contrast alone vs intravenous and oral contrast computed tomography for the diagnosis of appendicitis in adult ED patients. Am J Emerg Med 2012;30(9):1765–73.

69. Wadhwani A, Guo L, Saude E, et al. Intravenous and Oral Contrast vs Intravenous Contrast Alone Computed Tomography for the Visualization of Appendix and Diagnosis of Appendicitis in Adult Emergency Department Patients. Can Assoc Radiol J 2016;67(3):234–41.

70. Patel K, Zha N, Neumann S, et al. Computed Tomography of Common Bowel Emergencies. Semin Roentgenol 2020;55(2):150–69.

71. Chang KJ, Marin D, Kim DH, et al. ACR Appropriateness Criteria® Suspected Small-Bowel Obstruction. J Am Coll Radiol 2020;17(5):S305–14.

72. Branco BC, Barmparas G, Schnüriger B, et al. Systematic review and meta-analysis of the diagnostic and therapeutic role of water-soluble contrast agent in adhesive small bowel obstruction. Br J Surg 2010;97(4):470–8.

73. Ceresoli M, Coccolini F, Catena F, et al. Water-soluble contrast agent in adhesive small bowel obstruction: A systematic review and meta-analysis of diagnostic and therapeutic value. Am J Surg 2016;211:1114–25.

74. Zielinski MD, Haddad NN, Cullinane DC, et al. Multi-institutional, prospective, observational study comparing the Gastrografin challenge versus standard treatment in adhesive small bowel obstruction. J Trauma Acute Care Surg 2017;83(1):47–54.

75. Scotté M, Mauvais F, Bubenheim M, et al. Use of water-soluble contrast medium (gastrografin) does not decrease the need for operative intervention nor the duration of hospital stay in uncomplicated acute adhesive small bowel obstruction? A multi-center, randomized, clinical trial (Adhesive Small. Surgery (United States) 2017;161:1315–25.

76. Vather R, Josephson R, Jaung R, et al. Gastrografin in prolonged postoperative ileus: A double-blinded randomized controlled trial. Ann Surg 2015;262(1):23–30.

77. Biondo S, Miquel J, Espin-Basany E, et al. A Double-Blinded Randomized Clinical Study on the Therapeutic Effect of Gastrografin® in Prolonged Postoperative Ileus after Elective Colorectal Surgery. World J Surg 2016;40(1):206–14.

78. Khasawneh MA, Ugarte MLM, Srvantstian B, et al. Role of Gastrografin Challenge in Early Postoperative Small Bowel Obstruction. J Gastrointest Surg 2014;18(2):363–8.

79. Khasawneh MA, Eiken PW, Srvantstyan B, et al. Use of the Gastrografin challenge in patients with a history of abdominal or pelvic malignancy. Surg (United States) 2013;154(4):769–76.

80. D'Agostino R, Ali NS, Leshchinskiy S, et al. Small bowel obstruction and the gastrografin challenge. Abdom Radiol 2018;43(11):2945–54.

81. Hunter Lanier M, Ludwig DR, Ilahi O, et al. Prognostic Value of Water-Soluble Contrast Challenge for Nonadhesive Small Bowel Obstruction. J Am Coll Surg 2022;234(2):121–8.

82. Woolen SA, Maturen KE, Nettles A, et al. Patient-Centered Assessment of the Value of Oral Contrast Material. J Am Coll Radiol 2017;14(12):1626–31.

83. Kammerer S, Höink AJ, Wessling J, et al. Abdominal and pelvic CT: is positive enteric contrast still necessary? Results of a retrospective observational study. Eur Radiol 2015;25(3):669–78.

Update on the Role of Imaging in Detection of Intimate Partner Violence

Anji Tang, MD[a,b], Andrew Wong, MD, PhD[a,b], Bharti Khurana, MD[a,b],*

KEYWORDS

- Intimate partner violence • Nonaccidental trauma • Domestic violence
- Longitudinal imaging history

KEY POINTS

- Intimate partner violence (IPV) is defined as physical, sexual, or psychological aggression inflicted by a current or former partner.
- Radiologists have the unique opportunity to overcome many patient- and clinician-related barriers to IPV diagnosis because of their ability to generate unbiased objective reports.
- Longitudinal imaging review may increase sensitivity for the detection of IPV. Machine learning and natural language processing are powerful tools to facilitate longitudinal imaging review.
- Radiologists should discuss the suspicion of IPV with ordering physicians and add it to the report once the patient safety plan is established. Interdisciplinary collaboration is critical.
- Although less common, IPV occurs in men and older adults, with unique injury patterns and greater severity at presentation.

INTRODUCTION
Definition

Intimate partner violence (IPV) is defined by the Centers for Disease Control and Prevention as a current or former partner stalking or inflicting physical, sexual, or psychological aggression on the victim.[1]

Prevalence, Incidence, and Epidemiology

IPV is a highly prevalent issue in the United States. In a 2011 report by the National Intimate Partner and Sexual Violence Survey, which sampled English and Spanish speaking adults 18 years or older, one in five women and one in seven men disclosed severe physical violence by an intimate partner in their lifetimes,[2] resulting in injury, post-traumatic stress, and required medical care.[1]

Globally, 20% of homicides are perpetrated by intimate partners or family members, with women comprising most victims.[3] The National Violent Death Reporting System from 2003 to 2014 revealed more than half of all female homicides in the United States were IPV-related.[4]

Although IPV occurs in all age groups regardless of sex, ethnicity, and social status, it most often affects patients aged 18 to 24 years.[1] Women outnumber men,[5] and most victims suffer an IPV episode by age 25.[5] Gender and racial/ethnic minorities are disproportionately affected. Studies have shown higher rates of IPV in Alaska Native/Native American women and immigrants.[5] Members of same-sex relationships, transgender women, and human trafficking survivors also frequently experience IPV.[5]

Funding: Brigham Research Institute.
Nonrelevant disclosures: GE HealthCare Research, Book Royalties Cambridge University Press, Section Editor, Emergency Radiology, UptoDate Walters Kluwer, and ROKIT Health Care Consulting.
[a] Department of Radiology, Brigham and Women's Hospital, 75 Francis Street, Boston, MA 02115, USA;
[b] Trauma Imaging Research and Innovation Center, Brigham and Women's Hospital, Harvard Medical School, 75 Francis Street, Boston, MA 02115, USA
* Corresponding author.
E-mail address: bkhurana@bwh.harvard.edu
Twitter: @anjitweet (A.T.); @andrewwongmdphd (A.W.); @KhuranaBharti (B.K.)

Radiol Clin N Am 61 (2023) 53–63
https://doi.org/10.1016/j.rcl.2022.07.004

Nature of the Problem

There are many barriers to accurate and timely detection of IPV in the clinical setting. Patients may underreport IPV or not seek help because they fear retaliation from the partner or breach of confidentiality,[6] or are limited by economic dependency, learned helplessness, or attachment to the abusive relationship.[7] Patients may internalize stigma, feeling self-blame and embarrassment.[8] Societal stigmas include fear of judgment from family members and cultural prejudices, depicting the victim as unassertive and dependent. Elderly patients and patients in same-sex relationships can experience intersectional stigma, being devalued for their age or sexuality.[8] Clinician-related barriers include lack of time, inappropriate assessment of patients' population risk of IPV exposure, apprehension about offending the patient or partner, and discomfort with discussing IPV.[6] Clinicians may feel insufficiently trained, unsure how to document in the medical record, or frustrated when patients do not follow their advice.[9] Finally, patients and clinicians may feel powerless to enact change,[6] especially if social work services are not immediately at their disposal.[9] IPV creates economic burdens for society as a whole, averaging $103,767 per female victim and $23,414 per male victim, with collective lifetime costs of up to $1.3 trillion.[10]

Screening in the health care setting is problem-ridden. Prior studies show that even when women were asked to complete screening questionnaires before clinical visits, a large proportion were lost to follow-up,[11] and follow-through was poor.[12] Improper screening techniques can negatively affect the patient. Issuing advice without training in IPV advocacy and an appropriate safety plan may make the patient vulnerable to immediate harm. For instance, the perpetrator may harm the victim for disclosing the information and attempting to leave. Documentation of IPV can have legal ramifications, affecting child custody. Finally, breaching confidentiality can expose the patient to social stigma and discrimination from insurers and employers.[13] IPV victims can experience loss of status and economic discrimination. They may be perceived as risky tenants, leading to decreased access to housing, or face discrimination by the judicial system in the form of negative police response or inadequate prosecution.[8]

COVID-19 and Exacerbation of Intimate Partner Violence

IPV has become more prevalent with worldwide stresses caused by the COVID-19 pandemic,[14] which has changed the course of IPV for the worse by exacerbating well-known risk factors for IPV, including financial stress, substance abuse, isolation, and psychiatric disorders. COVID-19-related economic difficulty has disproportionately affected women, with increased unemployment and increased caregiving needs related to school closures.[15] Rates of alcohol and drug use have increased during the pandemic,[16] whereas lockdowns and social distancing have heightened social isolation and psychiatric illness.[17] In particular, social restrictions have reduced victims' ability to report IPV (eg, lack of online police reporting options) and access shelters[18,19] and made physical separation from the abuser more difficult.[20]

Nonradiologic screening methods are handicapped by telemedicine visits, which limit the sensitivity of the physical examination to evaluate injuries (eg, bruises) and preclude open communication between the clinician and potential victim.[20] With virtual visits, lack of privacy may preclude IPV screening during telehealth calls, nonverbal cues may be limited, and physicians overwhelmed by pandemic-driven patient volume may overlook or misinterpret IPV-related injuries.[14] IPV-centric programs have become restricted because many health care facilities prioritize COVID-related cases, whereas strained victim shelters struggle to accommodate more residents.[20]

Imaging shows the pandemic has increased IPV frequency and severity, with increased severity likely related to delay in seeking assistance.[14] Gosangi and colleagues[14] compared IPV victims reporting during the first 7 weeks of the pandemic with the same period for the last 3 years and found an increase in incidence of deep injuries, injuries with high-risk mechanisms, and injuries with increased severity. These trends necessitate increased vigilance from health care personnel to take appropriate action.[21]

Radiologic imaging has been crucial in bypassing barriers to IPV screening and identification. Radiologists are well-equipped in the face of new challenges, such as COVID-19, having the unique advantage of avoiding bias by only assessing the patient's current and past imaging, mitigating underreporting by discerning mismatches between image findings and provided clinical history,[22] and operating under a setting of physical isolation of the victim from accompanying partner and third parties.[23]

DISCUSSION

Radiologists have expanded their role in the identification of IPV by stepping beyond the confines of simply reporting traumatic findings, rather interpreting them in the context of four major considerations.[22]

Location and Imaging Patterns Specific to Intimate Partner Violence

IPV impacts soft tissues and the axial and appendicular skeleton. An analysis of 1.65 million emergency department (ED) visits documented by the National Electronic Injury Surveillance System All Injury Program (NEISS-AIP) from 2005 through 2013 revealed multiorgan involvement (**Fig. 1**).[24] Injury breakdown based on radiology reports also reveals a multisystem spectrum of injuries (**Fig. 2**).

Upper extremity

Upper extremity injury is an important category of IPV because it could be reflective of defensive injuries.[25] A review of upper extremity fractures in the NEISS-AIP sustained by women aged 15 to 64 over a decade, showed that the most frequently fractured parts were the fingers (34%), hand (22%), and wrist (14%), followed by the forearm (13%), and shoulder (9%). The elbow and humerus (each 4%) were least frequently fractured.[26] Similar patterns were seen among upper extremity injuries in patients reporting physical IPV to a tertiary trauma center in the Northeast over 5 years, among whom fractures accounted for 52% and soft tissue injuries 39% of all injuries. The hand was most frequently

injured, and phalanges most frequently fractured, followed by the forearm (radius and ulna); displaced and comminuted fractures were rare,[27] similar to prior studies.[25,28] Notably, dislocation/subluxations were the least frequent category of all injury types,[27] indicating most injuries were arguably less apparent on clinical examinations. The greater frequency of nondisplaced, noncomminuted fractures among IPV victims may be secondary to the lower energy injury mechanisms involved, compared with higher energy mechanisms in accidental trauma, such as motor vehicle collisions.[27]

Face

The face is one of the most easily accessible targets of IPV,[29,30] accounting for 83% of assault cases.[30] Out of all facial injuries recorded in patients reporting IPV at a tertiary trauma center in the Northeast over a 5-year period,[31] left-sided injuries were more common, and the midface was most frequently targeted, similar to prior studies and reflecting the right-handed dominance of the general population.[29,30] The most commonly observed fractures were of the nasal bone (30% of all fractures), mandible (11%), and orbit (10%) (**Fig. 3**).[31] Unsurprisingly, nasal fractures predominated, the nose being the most prominent projection of the face.[29,30] Prior studies have similarly reflected mandibular and nasal fractures as the most frequent sites, and zygomatic fractures as the second or third most common site.[29,30] Few fractures were displaced or comminuted, with 95% having none or minimal displacement.[31]

Other locations

Lower extremity injuries comprised the third most common location after upper extremities and the face in patients reporting IPV to a tertiary trauma center in the Northeast over 5 years. Injuries of the foot followed by the ankle were most common, especially fractures of the metatarsals. Results had a slight gender dichotomy, with more displaced fractures in men, slightly higher fraction of femoral and ankle fractures, and upper leg soft tissue injuries in men, and slightly higher proportion of metatarsal fractures in women.[32] Thoracic (including cardiovascular) and abdominal injuries comprised smaller albeit nonnegligible fractions of injuries in victims of physical abuse (24% and 10%, respectively).[33] Finally, spine injuries accounted for a smaller proportion of total IPV-related injuries. All injuries were classified as AO type A, and most frequently localized to the upper lumbar spine (L1 and L2).[34] Although rare, spine and thoracoabdominal injuries are still important to identify, because they are strategic sites targeted by assailants purposefully avoiding the face.

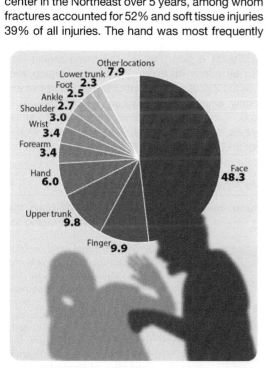

Other locations
Lower trunk **7.9**
Foot **2.3**
Ankle **2.5**
Shoulder **2.7**
Wrist **3.0**
3.4
Forearm **3.4**
Hand **6.0**
Upper trunk **9.8**
Finger **9.9**
Face **48.3**

Fig. 1. Distribution of IPV injuries as seen by orthopedic surgeons in the ED. (*From* Matoori S, Khurana B, Balcom MC, et al. Addressing intimate partner violence during the COVID-19 pandemic and beyond: how radiologists can make a difference. Eur Radiol. 2021;31(4):2126-2131.)

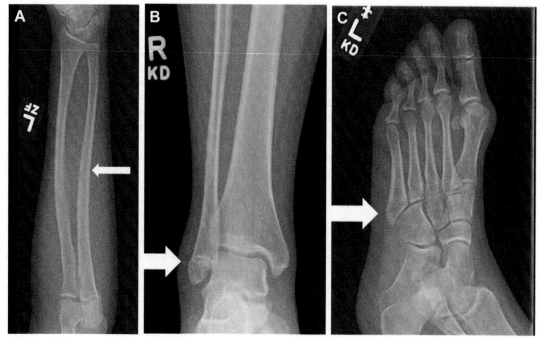

Fig. 2. A 25-year-old woman reporting assault by boyfriend (initially reported falling down stairs). (A) Nondisplaced fracture (arrow) of the left ulna mid-diaphysis. (B) Minimally displaced right fibula fracture (arrow) 6 months before ulnar fracture. (C) Nondisplaced base of fifth metatarsal fracture (arrow) of the left foot 3 months before fibular fracture. (From Khurana B, Sing D, Gujrathi R, et al. Recognizing Isolated Ulnar Fractures as Potential Markers for Intimate Partner Violence. J Am Coll Radiol. 2021;18(8):1108-1117.)

Synchronous and recurrent injuries

Synchronous injuries (concurrent but affecting different body parts) are predominantly seen in the face and extremities,[33] with craniofacial injuries especially common. For example, 41% of patients with synchronous injuries among IPV patients with upper extremity injuries suffered concomitant head and face injuries,[27] and 24% of patients with vertebral injuries sustained concurrent craniofacial injuries.[34] This percentage was reduced in IPV victims with lower extremity injuries, accounting for only 4.5% of patients.[32] Recurrent IPV episodes are also common.

Although a greater percentage feature injuries of a different region (Fig. 4), the same region can also be reinjured. Injury of the same region was seen in 22% of patients with IPV-related upper extremity injuries, half of whom injured the same hand,[27] and 30% of patients with lower extremity injuries, again with most (72%) occurring in the foot and ankle.[32]

Old Injuries of Different Body Parts

Crucial to early detection of IPV has been the comprehensive review of longitudinal imaging for

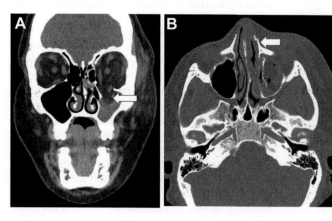

Fig. 3. Example of nasal and orbital maxillofacial fracture. A 35-year-old woman strangulated and hit on the face by her boyfriend. (A) Acute comminuted inferiorly displaced left inferomedial orbital wall fracture (arrow) requiring surgical repair. (B) Minimally displaced left nasal bone fracture (arrow). (From Gosangi B, Park H, Thomas R, et al. Exacerbation of Physical Intimate Partner Violence during COVID-19 Pandemic. Radiology. 2021;298(1):E38-E45.)

each patient, which not only includes current and prior imaging that provides data across different time points, but also accounts for all imaging listed in a patient's record, rather than only anatomically related studies.[33] For instance, if a patient is being evaluated for facial fracture, longitudinal imaging analysis incorporates data from not only all current and prior face computed tomography (CT), but every relevant radiologic examination the patient has undergone, such as radiographs of the extremities, or CT of the trunk. Among patients identified as IPV victims via longitudinal imaging review, radiologists predicted IPV earlier than the patients' self-reported date in 62% of victims of any type of abuse, and 53% of victims of physical abuse, by a median of 64 months in the former group, and 69.3 months in the latter. Longitudinal imaging review identified a greater proportion of moderate and high suspicion cases of IPV for both groups compared with review of only anatomically related studies.[33]

Injuries Inconsistent with the History

Patients frequently seek treatment of IPV-related injuries without attributing to IPV.[25] Conversely, not all suspicious injuries are IPV-related. Differentiating IPV-related from non-IPV-related causes is essential for the specificity of detection and pinpointing radiologic findings inconsistent with provided clinical history.

Intimate partner violence versus trauma

A case control study comparing injuries between 185 known IPV victims and 555 age- and sex-matched control subjects from the general population presenting to the ED (excluding the IPV cohort) found the proportion of patients with soft tissue injuries, fracture of any chronicity, obstetric-gynecologic findings (ie, intrauterine growth restriction, subchorionic hematoma, failed pregnancy, retained products of conception), and orbital hematoma was significantly greater in the IPV cohort.[35] Specifically, acute nasal bone and orbital fracture, and fracture of an extremity (whether subacute, chronic, or age-indeterminate) were significantly more frequent in the IPV group. Extremity fractures accounted for most fractures in the control group, whereas craniofacial fractures accounted for most in the IPV group,[35] suggesting a difference in injury mechanism.

Isolated ulnar fractures are potentially indicative of IPV. A query of patients aged 18 to 50 at three level I trauma centers from 2005 to 2019 using key phases "ulnar fracture" or equivalents, or procedural billing codes yielded a cohort with isolated ulnar fractures, among whom one-third were confirmed or suspected IPV victims.[36] This is consistent with prior studies' findings of isolated ulnar fractures being associated with direct blows.[25] Comparing the group of confirmed and suspected IPV with the non-IPV group demonstrated a significant association of IPV with nondisplaced fractures and a greater number of ED visits.[36]

In another review of upper extremity fractures sustained by women in the NEISS-AIP, the most common site for IPV and being accidently struck

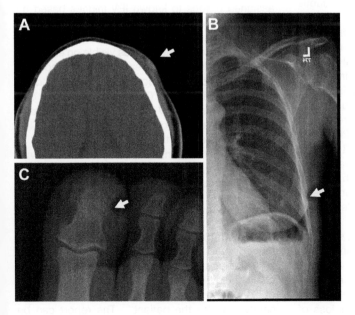

Fig. 4. Recurrent injuries to different organs. A 51-year-old woman with metachronous IPV injuries over 9 years. (*A*) Frontoparietal subgaleal hematoma (*arrow*). (*B*) Left seventh rib fracture (*arrow*). (*C*) Nondisplaced great toe distal tuft fracture (*arrow*).

(ie, striking or being struck by an object, as opposed to accidental fall) was the phalanges. Finger fractures accounted for a smaller percentage of accidental fall-related upper extremity fractures. The odds of phalangeal fracture were much higher in accidental striking and IPV than accidental fall, the odds of shoulder fracture were higher in IPV than accidental striking, and the odds of forearm fracture were higher in fall and IPV than accidental striking. The authors encouraged radiologists to discuss the possibility of IPV with the ordering physician in any woman presenting with a finger fracture because of fall and a shoulder/forearm fracture with a vague history of accidental striking.[26]

Overall, although progress has been made, it remains difficult to differentiate accidental and non-accidental trauma in adults, and more studies are needed in this direction.

High Imaging Utilization

Tracking the number and types of imaging studies obtained may shed light on IPV status. IPV victims undergo four times more imaging studies than age- and sex-matched control subjects.[35] Associations have been reported between IPV and decreased numbers of screening studies (eg, mammography, dual energy x-ray absorptiometry). Another study of isolated ulnar fractures found that cancellations of screening studies were more frequent in the IPV group.[36]

ROLE FOR MR IMAGING

In addition to radiography and CT, advanced modalities, such as MR imaging, can illuminate subtle and chronic findings, especially head and neck injuries. Common mechanisms include concussive traumatic brain injuries and strangulation, which can lead to hypoxic brain injury,[37] cervical vascular injury, neck soft tissue injury, and intramuscular hemorrhage.[25] Diffusion tensor imaging may shed light on long-term neurologic sequelae of traumatic brain injuries similar to recurrent concussions in football players. A study of 20 female IPV victims who underwent diffusion MR imaging found a negative correlation between brain injury score and fractional anisotropy, which is high within white matter and low in gray matter or cerebrospinal fluid.[38] This suggests a possible correlation between traumatic brain injuries and the victim's white matter brain structure. A separate study of six women from domestic violence shelters who underwent 7-T brain MR imaging, including three women with prior concussive head trauma and three control subjects who never experienced blunt force head trauma or loss of consciousness, revealed significant differences in resting state connectivity in victims of head trauma.[39] Specifically there was a difference in the default mode connectivity/network, a marker of brain activity during non-goal-oriented tasks that is suppressed during goal orientation.[39] Head trauma survivors showed higher outflow to default mode connectivity/network regions and cortical arousal and resting state default mode connectivity/network activation.[39]

INTIMATE PARTNER VIOLENCE SCREENING DURING IMAGING VISITS

Imaging visits are often underused as a screening opportunity. The increased frequency of imaging encounters in IPV victims may be seen as greater willingness to reach out in protected health care environments.[40] Narayan and colleagues[41] explored this possibility by adding a question about safety in the home to the intake questionnaire at outpatient breast imaging sites from June 2016 to December 2017. Out of 68,158 patients surveyed, 71 indicated feeling unsafe (0.1%), and these individuals were referred to the Helping Abuse and Violence End Now program, a free and confidential supplier of services for abuse victims ranging from counseling to advocacy.[41] Other imaging facilities may consider similar approaches.

QUANTIFYING FINDINGS

In addition to descriptive findings, efforts are increasing to add quantifiable metrics and standardize diagnosis. Gosangi and colleagues[14] assigned grades to known IPV injuries based on anatomic location and injury depth. Mild injuries (grade I) ranged from no visible external injuries to superficial extremity injuries visible on examination, whereas very severe injuries (grade IV) encompassed deep visceral injuries inflicted by sharp or blunt trauma (Table 1).[14] Park and colleagues[33] graded IPV likelihood by categorizing suspicion levels as low, moderate, and high (Table 2) based on the presence of injuries in anatomic distributions commonly seen in IPV victims, injuries across time points, and obstetric complications on imaging.

MULTIDISCIPLINARY COLLABORATION

Once the radiologist diagnoses IPV, findings must be conveyed to the ordering clinician, and appropriate steps taken to address them. The radiologist should refrain from incorporating suspicion of IPV in the report unless there is an established safety plan for the patient.[41] The report can be

Table 1 Criteria for grading IPV severity	
Grades of IPV	Injuries
Grade I/mild	No visible external injuries Superficial injuries involving extremities on physical examination, such as contusion, abrasion, bruise, swelling, and so forth Superficial soft tissue swelling involving extremities
Grade II/ moderate	Superficial injuries in the central torso (chest and abdomen) Multiple superficial injuries involving the torso and extremities Subgaleal hematoma and facial hematoma
Grade III/severe	Extremity fractures Single rib fracture Intramuscular hematomas Soft tissue stab wounds
Grade IV/very severe	Organ or visceral injury secondary to stab or blunt trauma Pneumothorax/ hemothorax Pneumoperitoneum/ hemoperitoneum Facial fractures Skull fractures Spine fractures Two or more rib fractures Strangulation marks over the neck Burns Gunshot wound

Adapted from Gosangi B, Park H, Thomas R, et al. Exacerbation of Physical Intimate Partner Violence during COVID-19 Pandemic. Radiology. 2021;298(1):E38-E45.

Table 2 Objective criteria to aid the radiologist in systemic assignment of IPV likelihood	
Likelihood	Criteria
Low	Absence of any findings
Moderate	1. Single injury known to be highly associated with IPV (eg, facial swelling, isolated ulnar fracture as defensive injury, nasal bone fracture, periorbital fracture). 2. Two extremity and/or axial injuries on different occasions. 3. A disproportionate number of radiologic studies of known target and defensive body areas in IPV, such as extremity radiographs, head and face CT, despite their negative impression for injury. 4. Recurrent obstetric complications (different pregnancies): failed pregnancy, intrauterine growth retardation, subchorionic hematoma.
High	1. Two or more injuries known to be highly associated with IPV (eg, facial swelling, isolated ulnar fracture as defensive injury, nasal bone fracture, periorbital fracture). 2. More than 2 injuries in the same or different anatomic region at other times (acute and chronic). 3. More than 2 obstetric complications (different pregnancies): failed pregnancy, intrauterine growth retardation, subchorionic hematoma. 4. Combination of 2 or more criteria for the moderate likelihood.

accessed by the abusive partner leading to escalation of violence and inability for the victim to receive appropriate health care support. A network of clinicians and social workers is necessary to manage the downstream ramifications. For example, plastic surgeons may be the primary subspecialty consulted in the ED for hand and head/face trauma. Abbate Ford and colleagues[42] detail several cases of IPV-related trauma in the ED at a tertiary trauma center in the Northeast, including an orbital floor fracture resulting from blunt trauma to the face requiring open reduction and internal fixation, and a dorsal hand laceration requiring suturing and splinting of the thumb.

Whether or not an IPV victim requires medical or surgical intervention, referral to specialized resources is key.

USING MACHINE LEARNING FOR INTIMATE PARTNER VIOLENCE DETECTION

Manual review of radiologic studies is time consuming, subjective, and error-prone because of subspecializations and silos. Radiologists may fail to take into account all necessary findings in a report or available reports because of sheer volume, or subjectively apply criteria to determine whether one injury supports a low versus high likelihood of IPV. Artificial intelligence and machine learning are increasingly popular tools in radiology that aid human interpretation with computer engineering algorithms. Two neural network models were recently trained using natural language processing techniques (which extracted relevant information from unstructured texts) and a publicly available clinical contextual word embedding model (ClinicalBERT) to predict the date of IPV occurrence based on 34,642 radiology reports from 1479 IPV and control patients.[43] The best model in the study predicted IPV a median of 3.08 years before the patient's self-reported date, with high specificity (95%) and moderate sensitivity (64%).

INTIMATE PARTNER VIOLENCE IN OLDER ADULTS AND MEN

Although the most vulnerable age groups for IPV lean toward younger cohorts, older victims make up a small yet nonnegligible fraction of the at-risk population (Fig. 5). A study of all injuries coded as IPV in the NEISS-AIP from 2005 to 2015 defining older adults as greater than 60 years old and adult patients as less than 60 years old found that older adults accounted for 1.8% of IPV visits. Older adults were more frequently male, experienced more trunk injuries, and were more likely to be hospitalized (15.7% vs 4.2%) than younger patients, suggesting greater injury severity at presentation. Compared with younger patients, a greater percentage of older adults suffered lacerations (40.6% vs 14.2%). Alarmingly, older women were more likely to suffer internal organ injury, especially of the head.[44]

Data from the NEISS-AIP from the same time period showed that men accounted for 17.2% for all injury visits related to IPV. Compared with women, men were more likely to be older, and a greater percentage were Black (40.5% vs 28.8%). A significantly higher percentage of cutting, fire/burn injuries, and gunshot wounds were noted in men, and a significantly higher number of male patients required hospitalization, reflecting greater injury severity at presentation. These findings reflect significant underreporting in men because of social stigma and societal norms. Men are less likely to seek help because they might not recognize IPV as criminal and may see IPV as unmasculine or fear being ridiculed. It is imperative for radiologists to recognize unique injury patterns related to IPV in older adult and

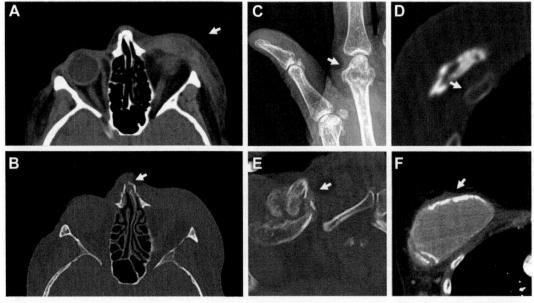

Fig. 5. IPV in older adults. A 67-year-old woman found down by emergency medical services who had been struck by her partner. (*A*) Left periorbital hematoma (*arrow*). (*B*) Acute nasal bone fractures (*arrow*). (*C*) Second metacarpal head fracture (*arrow*). (*D*) Acute displaced right fifth rib fracture (*arrow*). (*E*) Chronic healing right clavicle fracture (*arrow*). (*F*) Acute intracapsular and extracapsular implant rupture (*arrow*).

male victims to facilitate identification and timely intervention.[45]

SUMMARY

IPV is a prevalent national crisis with challenges to timely detection and management. Radiologists can circumvent patient- and clinician-related barriers to IPV screening and identification. COVID-19 spurred an increase in IPV incidence and posed new challenges to health care providers. Efforts are being made to systematically differentiate imaging stigmata of IPV-related injuries from accidental trauma, and quantify degree of severity and suspicion. Longitudinal imaging review of all current and prior imaging rather than review of only anatomically related studies has been shown to be advantageous in early detection of IPV, and machine learning is emerging as a powerful means to efficiently and accurately review large imaging volumes. Advanced modalities, such as MR imaging, have proven insightful as an addition to traditional modalities. It is important not to overlook IPV even in populations that are less frequently afflicted, such as older adult and male victims, because of a greater risk of injury severity.

CLINICS CARE POINTS

- Imaging studies confirm IPV is a multisystem process, affecting the face, extremities, and spine, among others. Maxillofacial injuries tend to localize to the left side and midface. Injuries of the hand, foot, and ankle are most common in the extremities. Although less common, spine injuries are important to detect because they may be strategic locations targeted by assailants wishing to avoid the face.

- Differentiating IPV from accidental trauma remains a challenge and requires more case control studies. Isolated ulnar fractures in women are potentially indicative of IPV. A significantly greater odds of finger fractures are seen in IPV compared with falls. Similarly, odds of shoulder and forearm fractures are greater in IPV compared with accidental striking/being struck by an object.

- Longitudinal imaging review consisting of all radiologic studies is more sensitive at detecting IPV compared with review of current and prior imaging of only anatomically related studies.

- Machine learning natural language processing algorithms have great potential for analyzing large volumes of radiology reports to further aid longitudinal imaging review and allow radiologists to detect IPV earlier than patients' self-reported date.

- MR imaging may be useful in illuminating the subtle neuroanatomic changes of IPV traumatic brain injury victims.

DISCLOSURE

No disclosure for A. Tang and A. Wong.

REFERENCES

1. Miller E, McCaw B. Intimate partner violence. N Engl J Med 2019;380(9):850–7.
2. Breiding MJ, Smith SG, Basile KC, et al. Prevalence and characteristics of sexual violence, stalking, and intimate partner violence victimization–national intimate partner and sexual violence survey, United States, 2011. MMWR Surveill Summ 2014;63(8):1–18.
3. Available at: https://www.unodc.org/documents/data-and-analysis/gsh/Booklet_4.pdf [No title]. Accessed January 17, 2022.
4. Petrosky E, Blair JM, Betz CJ, et al. in Homicides of adult women and the role of intimate partner violence - United States, 2003-2014. MMWR Morb Mortal Wkly Rep 2017;66(28):741–6.
5. Dicola D, Spaar E. Intimate partner violence. Am Fam Physician 2016;94(8):646–51.
6. Intimate Partner Violence Screening. Available at: https://www.ahrq.gov/ncepcr/tools/healthier-pregnancy/fact-sheets/partner-violence.html. Accessed January 17, 2022.
7. Hien D, Ruglass L. Interpersonal partner violence and women in the United States: an overview of prevalence rates, psychiatric correlates and consequences and barriers to help seeking. Int J Law Psychiatry 2009;32(1):48–55.
8. Overstreet NM, Quinn DM. The intimate partner violence stigmatization model and barriers to help-seeking. Basic Appl Soc Psych 2013;35(1):109–22.
9. Colarossi L, Breitbart V, Betancourt G. Barriers to screening for intimate partner violence: a mixed-methods study of providers in family planning clinics. Perspect Sex Reprod Health 2010;42(4):236–43.
10. Peterson C, Kearns MC, McIntosh WL, et al. Lifetime economic burden of intimate partner violence among U.S. adults. Am J Prev Med 2018;55(4):433–44.
11. MacMillan HL, Wathen CN, Jamieson E, et al. Screening for intimate partner violence in health

care settings: a randomized trial. JAMA 2009; 302(5):493–501.

12. Nelson HD, Bougatsos C, Blazina I. Screening women for intimate partner violence: a systematic review to update the U.S. Preventive Services Task Force recommendation. Ann Intern Med 2012; 156(11):796–808. W - 279, W - 280, W - 281, W - 282.

13. Liebschutz JM, Rothman EF. Intimate-partner violence: what physicians can do. N Engl J Med 2012;367(22):2071–3.

14. Gosangi B, Park H, Thomas R, et al. Exacerbation of physical intimate partner violence during COVID-19 pandemic. Radiology 2021;298(1):E38–45.

15. Parolin Z. Unemployment and child health during COVID-19 in the USA. Lancet Public Health 2020; 5(10):e521–2.

16. Taylor S, Paluszek MM, Rachor GS, et al. Substance use and abuse, COVID-19-related distress, and disregard for social distancing: a network analysis. Addict Behav 2021;114:106754.

17. Hossain MM, Sultana A, Purohit N. Mental health outcomes of quarantine and isolation for infection prevention: a systematic umbrella review of the global evidence. Epidemiol Health 2020;42: e2020038.

18. Evans ML, Lindauer M, Farrell ME. A pandemic within a pandemic: intimate partner violence during Covid-19. N Engl J Med 2020;383(24):2302–4.

19. Cannon CEB, Ferreira R, Buttell F, et al. COVID-19, intimate partner violence, and communication ecologies. Am Behav Scientist 2021;65(7):992–1013. https://doi.org/10.1177/0002764221992826.

20. Matoori S, Khurana B, Balcom MC, et al. Intimate partner violence crisis in the COVID-19 pandemic: how can radiologists make a difference? Eur Radiol 2020;30(12):6933–6.

21. Boserup B, McKenney M, Elkbuli A. Alarming trends in US domestic violence during the COVID-19 pandemic. Am J Emerg Med 2020; 38(12):2753–5.

22. Khurana B, Seltzer SE, Kohane IS, et al. Making the "invisible" visible: transforming the detection of intimate partner violence. BMJ Qual Saf 2020;29(3): 241–4.

23. Matoori S, Khurana B, Balcom MC, et al. Addressing intimate partner violence during the COVID-19 pandemic and beyond: how radiologists can make a difference. Eur Radiol 2021; 31(4):2126–31.

24. Loder RT, Momper L. Demographics and fracture patterns of patients presenting to US emergency departments for intimate partner violence. J Am Acad Orthop Surg Glob Res Rev 2020;4(2). https://doi.org/10.5435/JAAOSGlobal-D-20-00009.

25. Alessandrino F, Keraliya A, Lebovic J, et al. Intimate partner violence: a primer for radiologists to make

the "invisible" visible. Radiographics 2020;40(7): 2080–97.

26. Khurana B, Raja A, Dyer GSM, et al. Upper extremity fractures due to intimate partner violence versus accidental causes. Emerg Radiol 2022;29(1):89–97.

27. Thomas R, Dyer GSM, Iii Tornetta P, et al. Upper extremity injuries in the victims of intimate partner violence. Eur Radiol 2021;31(8):5713–20.

28. Bhandari M, Dosanjh S, Tornetta P 3rd, et al, Violence Against Women Health Research Collaborative. Musculoskeletal manifestations of physical abuse after intimate partner violence. J Trauma 2006;61(6):1473–9.

29. Bhole S, Bhole A, Harmath C. The black and white truth about domestic violence. Emerg Radiol 2014; 21(4):407–12.

30. Arosarena OA, Fritsch TA, Hsueh Y, et al. Maxillofacial injuries and violence against women. Arch Facial Plast Surg 2009;11(1):48–52.

31. DPS 2021. Available at: https://dps2021.rsna.org/exhibit/?exhibit=SDP-HN-13. Accessed January 17, 2022.

32. Gosangi B, Lebovic J, Park H, et al. Imaging patterns of lower extremity injuries in victims of intimate partner violence (IPV). Emerg Radiol 2021;28(4): 751–9.

33. Park H, Gujrathi R, Gosangi B, et al. Longitudinal imaging history in early identification of intimate partner violence. Eur Radiol 2021. https://doi.org/10.1007/s00330-021-08362-2.

34. Watane GV, Gosangi B, Thomas R, et al. Incidence and characteristics of spinal injuries in the victims of intimate partner violence (IPV). Emerg Radiol 2021;28(2):283–9.

35. George E, Phillips CH, Shah N, et al. Radiologic findings in intimate partner violence. Radiology 2019; 291(1):62–9.

36. Khurana B, Sing D, Gujrathi R, et al. Recognizing isolated ulnar fractures as potential markers for intimate partner violence. J Am Coll Radiol 2021;18(8): 1108–17.

37. Meyer JE, Jammula V, Arnett PA. Head trauma in a community-based sample of victims of intimate partner violence: prevalence, mechanisms of injury and symptom presentation. J Interpers Violence 2021. 8862605211016362.

38. Valera EM, Cao A, Pasternak O, et al. White matter correlates of mild traumatic brain injuries in women subjected to intimate-partner violence: a preliminary study. J Neurotrauma 2019;36(5):661–8.

39. Karakurt G, Whiting K, Jones SE, et al. Alth among the victims of intimate partner violence: a case-series exploratory study. Front Psychol 2021;12:710602.

40. Flores EJ, Narayan AK. The role of radiology in intimate partner violence. Radiology 2019;291(1):70–1.

41. Narayan AK, Lopez DB, Miles RC, et al. Implementation of an intimate partner violence screening

assessment and referral system in an academic women's imaging department. J Am Coll Radiol 2019;16(4 Pt B):631–4.

42. Abbate Ford O, Khurana B, Sinha I, et al. The plastic surgeon's role in the COVID-19 crisis: regarding domestic violence. Cureus 2021; 13(1):e12650.

43. Chen IY, Alsentzer E, Park H, et al. Intimate partner violence and injury prediction from radiology reports. Pac Symp Biocomput 2021;26:55–66.

44. Khurana B, Loder RT. Injury patterns and associated demographics of intimate partner violence in older adults presenting to U.S. emergency departments. J Interpers Violence 2021. 88626052 11022060.

45. Khurana B, Hines DA, Johnson BA, et al. Injury patterns and associated demographics of intimate partner violence in men presenting to U.S. emergency departments. Aggress Behav 2021. https://doi.org/ 10.1002/ab.22007.

Elder Abuse

Mihan Lee, MD, PhD[a],*, Aisara Chansakul, MPH[a], Jessica A. Rotman, MD[b],
Anthony Rosen, MD[a]

KEYWORDS

• Elder abuse • Assault • Geriatrics

KEY POINTS

• Imaging correlates of elder abuse are poorly characterized, limiting radiologists' contributions to elder abuse assessments, especially in emergent medical settings.
• Elder abuse victims are most likely to sustain radiographically visible injuries to the face, upper extremities, and head.
• Most common injury patterns characterized to date include nasal bone fractures, upper extremity fractures, rib fractures, and subdural hematomas.
• As with child abuse, it is critical to interpret injuries within a clinical context to assess whether the extent of injury is concordant with the reported mechanism.
• Particular challenges to the radiologic assessment of elder abuse include broad overlap in the appearance of abusive injuries with accidental injuries and limited communications with frontline clinical providers.

INTRODUCTION

Elder abuse is a form of domestic abuse, defined as "physical, sexual, or psychological abuse, as well as neglect, abandonment, and financial exploitation of an older person... either in a relationship where there is an expectation of trust, and/or when an older person is targeted based on age." [1] The prevalence of elder abuse has been estimated to be approximately 10% in community-dwelling adults and approximately 20% among residents of nursing homes.[2–5] Moreover, many victims suffer from multiple types of abuse concurrently.[6,7] This article focuses on imaging findings of physical elder abuse.

Elder abuse has severe medical consequences and has been linked to dementia, depression, and overall mortality.[8] It also carries a heavy financial burden, estimated in the billions of dollars annually in increased direct medical costs.[9,10] This is only expected to increase in future years due to the anticipated growth of the geriatric population.[1] Despite the urgency of this problem, elder abuse continues to be deeply underdiagnosed,

with as few as 1 in 24 cases of elder abuse identified and reported to the authorities.[11,12]

The health care system, particularly the emergency department (ED), may offer an important opportunity to identify elder abuse and initiate intervention.[13,14] Many abused older adults are isolated, and an ED visit for acute injury or illness may be the only time they leave their homes.[4]

In child abuse, diagnostic radiologists have played a major role in developing strategies to improve identification in the ED. Imaging correlates of child abuse have been extensively characterized,[15–17] and it is not uncommon for the pediatric radiologist, rather than the pediatrician or emergency physician, to raise the first alarm for abuse.[17] In stark contrast, emergency radiologists currently play a very limited role in the detection of elder abuse.[2,18,19] Significant knowledge gaps remain on how to use imaging to assess for potential abuse, and most radiologists in the United States do not receive training in elder abuse identification.[13] This article seeks to describe imaging findings in physical elder abuse that have been characterized and offer commentary on particular challenges to the radiologic

[a] Weill Cornell Medical Center, 525 East 68th Street, New York, NY 10282, USA; [b] Unity Health Toronto, 36 Queen St East, Toronto, ON M5B 1W8, Canada
* Corresponding author.
E-mail address: mrl9006@nyp.org

Radiol Clin N Am 61 (2023) 65–70
https://doi.org/10.1016/j.rcl.2022.08.001

assessment of elder abuse as well as potential future research directions that may aid radiologists in integrating this assessment into their practice.

IMAGING FINDINGS

Similar to the radiographic assessment of child abuse in pediatric radiology, current knowledge regarding the role of radiologists in elder abuse detection centers on the incorporation of clinical history and context. For example, the radiographic finding of a "mechanism mismatch," that is, an injury or fracture pattern inconsistent with the mechanism being described by the patient or their caregivers, is a critical finding that should trigger concern for potential elder abuse.[20,21] Clinical providers informing radiologists about how the patient purportedly sustained injuries is critical for radiologists to comment on whether their injuries are concordant.

Another critical piece of history in evaluating a mechanism mismatch is the functional status of the patient. In assessments for child abuse, patients' developmental stage is always compared with the reported mechanism of injury. Developmentally impossible scenarios, such as a 2-month-old rolling off the bed, raise red flags. In older adults, functional or ambulatory status is more difficult to infer from the patient's age alone, and often is not documented in clinical notes or available to radiologists at the time of study interpretation. However, open and two-way communications with frontline providers can help radiologists make this assessment and raise concerns when warranted.

Preliminary studies of geriatric assault, used as a proxy for physical elder abuse, have shown that elder victims of assault sustain distinct patterns of injury, with positive imaging findings primarily localized to the face, head, and upper extremities, in that order—in fact, up to three-quarters of acute traumatic findings were reported to occur within these regions.[13,22–25] This finding appeared to be in keeping with the limited information about mechanisms of injury available from the clinical notes, which suggests that elders were most commonly punched/hit (apparently about the face), followed closely by being pushed to the ground (where they would plausibly catch or brace themselves on the upper extremities).[23] Of note, facial fractures appear to be significantly more common than intracranial injury,[22] probably reflecting a propensity for abusers to strike at victims' faces. The most commonly fractured facial bones are the nasal bones, followed by maxillary and orbital fractures[23,24] (see illustrative case in Fig. 1). Another important observation was that facial and head injuries in elder were significantly

lateralized to the left side, likely a consequence of facing predominantly right-handed assailants; this imaging finding has also been described in studies of intimate partner violence.[26]

Patterns of elder abuse-related injury in the extremities are more variable, though there is a marked predominance of injuries to the upper extremities over the lower extremities. This likely reflects a variety of mechanisms, including falling or being pushed to the floor and breaking impact with an outstretched hand, as well as possibly attempting to block direct blows. Wrist and forearm fractures are particularly common, such as the classic Colles fracture (Fig. 2). "Nightstick" fractures may also occur, when a victim pronates and flexes at the elbow to block an overhead blow, exposing the ulna to direct impact (Fig. 3). A distal ulnar diaphyseal fracture has also been described as a relatively specific finding in elder abuse.[20]

Rib fractures are another common injury found in victims of elder abuse; however, they are extremely common in the elder population in general, making it particularly difficult to assess whether or not these reflect abuse or benign trauma (see later discussion). Similarly, subdural hematomas were the most common intracranial injury (Fig. 4). These are also very prevalent in older patients and can be seen in relatively minor impact injuries due to brain parenchymal atrophy and the increased propensity to tear bridging cortical veins.

Soft tissue injuries are undoubtedly a critical component of elder abuse and likely comprise the majority of injuries sustained. Although few studies have focused on this issue, one reported that up to 72% of elder abuse victims sustain soft tissue injuries, such as hematomas, particularly on the head, neck, lateral right arm, or posterior torso.[27] Radiographic literature on these injuries is limited. First, they may not be radiographically apparent or well characterized on imaging and, secondly, they are best assessed at bedside and imaging may not be ordered.

Of note, injuries are often detected as secondary or incidental findings on studies of non-dedicated body parts, especially in elderly patients who may be poor historians secondary to dementia or other illness, or provide incomplete histories regarding their injuries in an attempt not to disclose abuse. In these situations, it is critical that the radiologist scrutinize all aspects of the study—the "edges of the film" of a radiograph and the scout and the first and last slices on a CT—and to recommend further dedicated imaging if an additional injury is suspected. This fact also highlights how important it can be for primary teams to convey, along with their

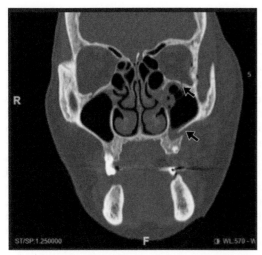

Fig. 1. Coronal CT of the face demonstrates acute fractures of the left maxillary bone and the left orbital floor (*black arrows*).

imaging requisition, information about the patient's presentation and clinical state, including the reliability of their reported history, so that the radiologist can be on the alert.

Elder Neglect

A subset of elder abuse with physical manifestations is elder neglect, which is substantially more prevalent than direct assaultive injuries. Previous work has characterized several "red flags" for elder neglect, including weight loss,[7] decubitus ulcers,[28,29] poor hygiene, malnutrition, and dehydration.[30] However, these entities may also occur as a result of common geriatric illnesses, and, thus no specific radiographic findings have been described. This can result not only from willful neglect but also from caregivers who are unaware or uneducated about elders' care needs. For example, elderly patients may not be taken regularly to see doctors, may be left to wander unsupervised resulting in frequent falls, or bedbound patients may not be turned appropriately, resulting in decubitus ulcers or gangrene.

Although these injuries would usually be apparent at bedside, frontline clinicians have noted that radiologists could help to assess the extent and the age of soft tissue injuries, particularly in cases where a thorough physical examination is difficult. Radiologists may also be well-positioned to note a repeated pattern of similar injuries, as imaging studies are reviewed in comparison with multiple prior examinations that may not have yet been brought to the attention of the frontline clinicians; this can highlight both repetitive issues (such as multiple presentations with

fractures) or slowly progressive ones (such as worsening cachexia or decubitus ulcers). Rigorous review of imaging, in conjunction with further efforts to improve and streamline communication, is a critical direction for future work.

CHALLENGES

Several challenges have been described in characterizing more sensitive and specific imaging correlates of elder abuse, in comparison to the pediatric population, who often sustain specific and identifiable injuries in the setting of non-accidental trauma because of their small size and the unique features of skeletally immature bones.[17,31,32] By contrast, in the geriatric population, entities like deconditioning, gait instability, and osteoporosis can all make elderly patients significantly more likely to fracture from relatively minor mechanisms of injury.[7,21] Healed or healing fractures, particularly of the ribs, are very common in older patients, and seen so commonly that radiologists may not even consistently choose to describe them in reports. Moreover, in older adult patients, there is broad overlap between patterns of injury that result from abusive trauma (such as a direct blow) and those that result from an accident or mild impact (such as a fall from standing in an osteoporotic patient). Therefore, radiologists assessing cases of elder trauma may not know whether to include, or even how to go about stating, their concern for abuse.

This lack of knowledge about evidence-based imaging correlates for abuse has also posed an obstacle to designing training curricula on elder abuse for students, residents, and continuing medical education. Radiologists currently receive neither formal nor informal training in elder abuse identification,[13] which stands in stark contrast to the rigorous training almost all describe in recognizing child abuse. In the absence of specific lesions that radiologists can be taught to recognize as "flags" for elder abuse, nearly all radiology programs have chosen to omit the topic until better evidence is available. As a result, radiologists can feel even less prepared and qualified to provide meaningful insights on cases with concern for abuse when asked for their assessment by frontline clinicians. In interview-based qualitative studies, both radiologists and emergency medicine physicians reported believing that a lack of adequate training led them to miss cases of elder abuse and expressed a desire for more training on the subject.[2,13]

A final obstacle to radiologic characterization is an established clinical workflow in which radiologists occupy a much more peripheral place than

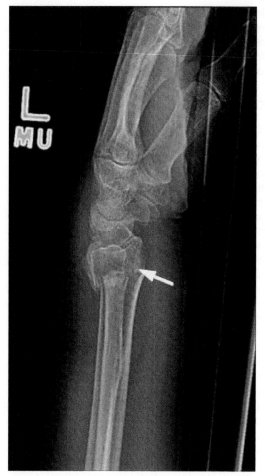

Fig. 2. Lateral radiograph of the left wrist demonstrates an acute transverse fracture of the distal radius with mild impaction and dorsal displacement (*white arrow*).

mechanism mismatch in older patients is done predominantly by bedside assessment, with radiologists often given minimal history. In one interview-based study, frontline providers from various fields, including emergency medicine physicians and geriatricians, stated that they did not regard radiology as a source of additional or new information in cases of trauma, but rather thought of imaging only as a confirmatory measure or to assess extent of injury.[21] Moreover, these providers stated that they did not routinely make it a practice to provide detailed history or clinical context. Although these barriers have been characterized in studies from large academic centers, they would only be heightened and accentuated in many other practice settings, such as private practice or smaller community hospitals, where radiologists are not physically embedded into clinical care teams.

FUTURE DIRECTIONS

Future research, which is already ongoing, must continue to seek definitive imaging correlates of elder abuse to aid radiologists in confidently contributing to detection. Also, researchers and clinical leaders should explore the workflow and context within which radiologists work and develop changes to help them partner more effectively with frontline clinicians in an elder abuse assessment. Although radiographic injury patterns in victims of geriatric assault have begun to be described, these patterns are still emerging and as yet nonspecific. Better characterizing these patterns can help diagnostic radiologists improve their ability to identify cases of potential intentional injury among cases of purportedly accidental trauma, and ultimately serve as a first step in improving their sensitivity for physical elder abuse. In this way, radiologists may become better incorporated into the multidisciplinary effort to detect and manage elder abuse, alongside emergency medicine physicians, geriatricians, and social workers.

To address gaps in training, modules on elder abuse detection should be incorporated into radiology educational curricula, as well as continuing medical education. The literature supports face-to-face training on abuse for health professionals as more effective in increasing knowledge than distributing written information.[5] Therefore, an important future direction may be designing and piloting hands-on training modules for radiologists to gain exposure to elder abuse and its detection and management strategies. For these trainings to be evidence-based and relevant, these efforts must evolve alongside ongoing research

their counterparts in pediatrics. Although suspicious features such as identifying "mismatches" between the reported mechanism of trauma and the radiographic injury can be key to abuse assessments, this potential is severely limited by gaps in communication between frontline providers and radiologists. Communication between radiologists and front-line clinicians is often very limited due to a multitude of factors, including time constraints, delayed medical charting, and difficult-to-navigate electronic medical record (EMRs). As a result, information conveyed on imaging requisitions remains minimal and shallow, continually limiting the contribution that radiologists can make to an abuse assessment. Unlike in pediatrics, where radiologists are always hyper-aware of the reported mechanism of injury and are able to make an assessment of whether the injury findings fit, the evaluation of a

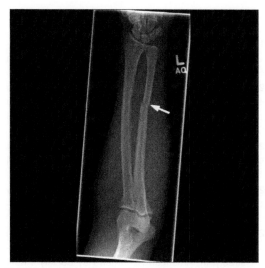

Fig. 3. AP radiograph of the left forearm demonstrates an acute minimally displaced fracture of the ulnar diaphysis (*white arrow*), compatible with a "nightstick fracture."

investigating imaging findings related elder abuse, and incorporate these findings into practice as it is published.

Meanwhile, both cultural and practical modifications to current workflow are necessary to improve communication between radiology and other clinical teams, and to ensure that radiologists have access to the clinical information necessary for them to perform meaningful abuse assessments. Emphasizing to frontline clinicians the potential of radiologists to contribute to elder abuse detection,

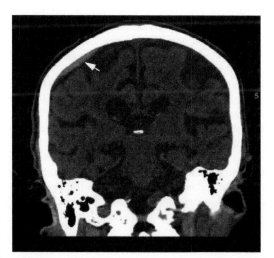

Fig. 4. Coronal CT of the head demonstrates a small hyperdense crescentic fluid collection overlying the right frontoparietal lobe (*white arrow*), compatible with acute subdural hemorrhage.

and particularly the value while ordering imaging of providing information about injury mechanism and functional status, is critical. This can serve to better define the role of radiologists, and disrupt the conception that evaluation for elder abuse involves exclusively bedside assessment. In addition, clinicians and radiologists should be encouraged to discuss any concerns or suspicion of elder abuse in real time, and to collaborate on assessment. Electronic medical records may be modified to facilitate and support this cultural shift. Finally, care must be taken to adopt channels of communication that neither unduly slow workflow, nor cause premature alarm and distress to families. Pilot programs are needed to test, modify, and develop them into working protocols. Implementing these strategies can serve as vital first steps to integrating radiologists into the effort to detect and initiate treatment for elder abuse.

CLINICS CARE POINTS

- Radiologists should be aware that, while knowledge about the most common patterns of injury in elder abuse is still emerging, the most likely injured body parts are the head, face, and upper extremities, and that facial injuries may have the propensity to be left-sided.

DISCLOSURE

The authors report no financial conflicts of interest.

REFERENCES

1. Connolly M, Brandl B, Breckman R. The elder justice roadmap: a stakeholder initiative to respond to an emerging health, justice, financial and social crisis. [Internet]. Department of Justice. 2014. https://www.justice.gov/file/852856/download. [Accessed 22 September 2022].
2. Rosen T, Hargarten S, Flomenbaum NE, et al. Identifying Elder Abuse in the Emergency Department: Toward a Multidisciplinary Team-Based Approach. Ann Emerg Med 2016;68(3):378–82.
3. Burnes D, Pillemer K, Caccamise PL, et al. Prevalence of and Risk Factors for Elder Abuse and Neglect in the Community: A Population-Based Study. J Am Geriatr Soc 2015;63(9):1906–12.
4. Touza Garma C. Influence of health personnel's attitudes and knowledge in the detection and reporting of elder abuse: An exploratory systematic review. Psychosoc Interv 2017;26(2):73–91.

5. Cooper C, Selwood A, Blanchard M, et al. Abuse of people with dementia by family carers: representative cross sectional survey. BMJ 2009;338(2):b155.

6. Acierno R, Hernandez MA, Amstadter AB, et al. Prevalence and Correlates of Emotional, Physical, Sexual, and Financial Abuse and Potential Neglect in the United States: The National Elder Mistreatment Study. Am J Public Health 2010;100(2):292–7.

7. Lachs MS, Pillemer K. Elder abuse. Lancet Lond Engl 2004;364(9441):1263–72.

8. Lachs MS. The Mortality of Elder Mistreatment. JAMA 1998;280(5):428.

9. MetLife Mature Market Institute, The National Committee for the Prevention of Elder Abuse, The Center for Gerontology at Virginia Polytechnic Institute and State University. Broken Trust: Elders, Family & Finances. [Internet]. 2009. Available from: https://www.giaging.org/documents/mmi-study-broken-trust-elders-family-finances.pdf Accessed 22 September 2022, 2009.

10. National Center on Elder Abuse. Research: Statistics/Data. [Internet]. https://ncea.acl.gov/whatwedo/research/statistics.html#42. Accessed 22 September 2022.

11. Yaffe MJ, Wolfson C, Lithwick M. Professions show different enquiry strategies for elder abuse detection: Implications for training and interprofessional care. J Interprof Care 2009;23(6):646–54.

12. Heyborne RD. Elder Abuse: Keeping the Unthinkable in the Differential. Acad Emerg Med 2007; 14(6):566–7.

13. Rosen T, Bloemen EM, Harpe J, et al. Radiologists' Training, Experience, and Attitudes About Elder Abuse Detection. AJR Am J Roentgenol 2016; 207(6):1210–4.

14. Kahan FS, Paris BEBE. Why elder abuse continues to elude the health care system. Mt Sinai J Med N Y 2003;70(1):62–8.

15. Kleinman PK, editor. Diagnostic imaging of child abuse. 3rd edn. Cambridge, United Kingdom; New York: Cambridge University Press; 2015. p. 730.

16. Offiah A, van Rijn RR, Perez-Rossello JM, et al. Skeletal imaging of child abuse (non-accidental injury). Pediatr Radiol 2009;39(5):461–70.

17. Section on Radiology. Diagnostic imaging of child abuse. Pediatrics 2009;123(5):1430–5.

18. Cooper C, Selwood A, Livingston G. Knowledge, Detection, and Reporting of Abuse by Health and Social Care Professionals: A Systematic Review. Am J Geriatr Psychiatry 2009;17(10):826–38.

19. Samaras N, Chevalley T, Samaras D, et al. Older Patients in the Emergency Department: A Review. Ann Emerg Med 2010;56(3):261–9.

20. Wong NZ, Rosen T, Sanchez AM, et al. Imaging Findings in Elder Abuse: A Role for Radiologists in Detection. Can Assoc Radiol J J Assoc Can Radiol 2017;68(1):16–20.

21. Lee M, Rosen T, Murphy K, et al. A role for imaging in the detection of physical elder abuse. J Am Coll Radiol 2018;15(11):1648–50.

22. Murphy K, Waa S, Jaffer H, et al. A Literature Review of Findings in Physical Elder Abuse. Can Assoc Radiol J 2013;64(1):10–4.

23. Lee, Lee, MR; Gogia, K; Rotman, JA, et al. Clinical and Radiographic Findings in Geriatric Assault [abstract]. In: American Roentgen Ray Society Virtual annual Meeting, April 18–22, 2021; virtual.

24. Rosen T, LoFaso VM, Bloemen EM, et al. Identifying injury patterns associated with physical elder abuse: analysis of legally adjudicated cases. Ann Emerg Med 2020;76(3):266–76.

25. Ziminski CE, Wiglesworth A, Austin R, et al. Injury patterns and causal mechanisms of bruising in physical elder abuse. J Forensic Nurs 2013;9(2):84–91.

26. Gujrathi R, Tang A, Thomas R, et al. Facial injury patterns in victims of intimate partner violence. Emerg Radiol 2022;1–11.

27. Wiglesworth A, Austin R, Corona M, et al. Bruising as a marker of physical elder abuse. J Am Geriatr Soc 2009;57(7):1191–6.

28. Fulmer T. Elder Abuse and Neglect Assessment. J Gerontol Nurs 2003;29(6):4–5.

29. Dyer CB, Connolly M-T, McFeeley P. The Clinical and Medical Forensics of Elder Abuse and Neglect [Internet]. National Academies Press (US); 2003 https://ncea.ahttps://ncea.acl.gov/What-We-Do/Research/Statistics-and-Data.aspx. Accessed 22 September 2022.

30. Harrell R, Toronjo CH, McLaughlin J, et al. How geriatricians identify elder abuse and neglect. Am J Med Sci 2002;323(1):34–8.

31. Raissaki M, Veyrac C, Blondiaux E, et al. Abdominal imaging in child abuse. Pediatr Radiol 2011;41(1):4–16.

32. Nimkin K, Spevak MR, Kleinman PK. Fractures of the hands and feet in child abuse: imaging and pathologic features. Radiology 1997;203(1):233–6.

Oncologic Emergencies in the Head and Neck

Carlos Zamora, MD, PhD[a],*, Mauricio Castillo, MD[b], Paulo Puac-Polanco, MD, MSc[c,d],
Carlos Torres, MD, FRCPC[e]

KEYWORDS

• Head • Neck • Cancer • Emergencies • MRI • CT

KEY POINTS

• Patients with head and neck cancers are susceptible to emergencies related to tumor infiltration, systemic disorders, or treatment complications.
• Hematologic disorders are common in patients with cancer and result in hypercoagulable states or hemorrhage.
• Infections in patients with cancer are secondary to immunocompromise, complications from surgery, or use of indwelling devices.

INTRODUCTION

Head and neck cancers are an important cause of morbidity and mortality, with an estimated 562,328 new cases and 277,597 deaths worldwide in 2020.[1] Patients are susceptible to a wide range of emergencies caused by tumor infiltration of critical structures, impaired immune status, bleeding or thrombosis, or treatment complications. They can also be affected by metabolic derangements secondary to systemic effects from cancer, paraneoplastic syndromes, or chemotherapy. Because the neck houses life-sustaining structures, emergencies in this region have dire consequences. Maxillofacial complications are important because of their potential to propagate to the orbits and intracranially. Here, we present an overview of imaging findings of various emergencies that occur in patients with head and neck cancer. We discuss their pathophysiological mechanisms and review clinical features that aid in diagnosis.

IMAGING TECHNIQUE

Computed tomography (CT) is the mainstay for the evaluation of acute complications in the head and neck. It is fast and appropriate for patients who are sick and unstable and can identify conditions necessitating urgent surgery or airway management. Compared with CT, MRI has superior tissue contrast but is reserved for conditions that require further characterization in patients who are stable. Administration of contrast material is important when infection is suspected, and it may help discriminate it from enhancing tumor.

For further evaluation of intra- and extracranial conditions, contrast-enhanced MRI is superior to CT. In the neck and maxillofacial structures, both contrast-enhanced CT and MRI have appropriate roles but CT is preferred in the acute setting. MRI evaluation of inflammatory or infectious complications in the neck, maxillofacial structures, and orbits, requires the use of fat suppression

[a] Division Head of Neuroradiology, Department of Radiology, University of North Carolina School of Medicine, CB 7510, Old Infirmary Building, 101 Manning Drive, Chapel Hill, NC 27599-7510, USA; [b] Division of Neuroradiology, Department of Radiology, University of North Carolina School of Medicine, CB 7510, Old Infirmary Building, 101 Manning Drive, Chapel Hill, NC 27599-7510, USA; [c] Department of Radiology, McMaster University, St. Joseph's Healthcare, Hamilton, Ontario, Canada; [d] Department of Radiology, Juravinski Innovation Tower, Level 0, Room T0113, 50 Charlton Avenue East, Hamilton, Ontario L8N 4A6, Canada; [e] Department of Radiology, Radiation Oncology and Medical Physics, University of Ottawa, Box 232, General Campus Room 1466e, 501 Smyth Road, Ottawa, Ontario K1H 8L6, Canada
* Corresponding author.
E-mail address: carlos_zamora@med.unc.edu

Radiol Clin N Am 61 (2023) 71–90
https://doi.org/10.1016/j.rcl.2022.08.002

techniques for T2 and postcontrast T1 sequences to better show edema and enhancement, respectively, but artifacts from hemorrhage, metallic clips, and radiation seeds may hinder interpretation.

CT arteriography (CTA) and/or venography (CTV) are the initial studies when there is concern for vascular complications such as active bleeding, occlusion, pseudoaneurysm, or thrombosis. Catheter angiography is the gold standard to show active extravasation and arteriovenous shunting that can be difficult to visualize on CTA when it involves small vessels. Catheter angiography can also provide a route for endovascular treatment when indicated.

INTRACRANIAL COMPLICATIONS

Neurologic complications in patients with cancer are a common cause of morbidity and mortality. Diagnosis of intracranial complications is challenging as clinical signs are usually nonspecific, and diagnosis is based on ancillary tests such as laboratory or imaging studies. Prompt recognition is essential to institute appropriate treatment and prevent dire outcomes.

Bleeding Complications

Tumor-related hemorrhage

Intracranial hemorrhage (IH) in patients with cancer is secondary to intratumoral hemorrhage (ITH) in 25% to 61% of cases.[2,3] Brain tumors bleed spontaneously (3.5–14%) depending on tumor type. ITH may be the initial presentation of cancer.[4,5] Malignant or highly vascular tumors pose a risk for ITH (Box 1).[2,3] Metastases and glioblastoma are the most prone to bleed.[3,4] Patients present acutely in 57% to 93% of cases.[3,4]

The cause of ITH is unclear, but it is likely due to presence of numerous thin-walled, poorly formed vessels, rapid tumor growth, vascular invasion, and tumor necrosis. Hemorrhage can mask an underlying malignancy. This is particularly important in large hemorrhagic lesions, where finding neoplastic cells is prone to sampling errors by the neurosurgeon and the pathologist. Therefore, information obtained in imaging studies helps achieve the correct diagnosis.

Imaging findings in tumor-related hemorrhage are like those in other benign causes of IH, such as hypertension or ruptured aneurysms and include a hyperdense parenchymal hematoma on CT, associated mass effect, and vasogenic edema. Subarachnoid hemorrhage (SAH) or intraventricular hemmorrhage (IVH) can also be seen.[2,3] Imaging features that suggest an underlying tumor include presence of disproportionate

---

> **Box 1**
> **Most common CNS tumors associated with ITH**
>
> Benign Tumors
> - Meningioma
> - Schwannoma
> - Hemangioblastoma
> - Pilocytic Astrocytoma
> - Pituitary Adenoma
> - Myxopapillary Ependymoma
>
> Malignant Tumors
> - Glioblastoma
> - Oligodendroglioma
> - Ependymoma
>
> Metastases
> - Melanoma
> - Lung
> - Breast
> - Germ Cell Tumor
> - Thyroid Carcinoma
> - Renal Cell Carcinoma
>
> *Abbreviation:* ITH, Intratumoral hemorrhage.
> *Data from* Refs.[1–4]

---

vasogenic edema, enhancement on MRI, unusual location for IH (gray-white matter interface or lobar location), or high relative cerebral blood volume (rCBV) within the lesion (Fig. 1). Review of clinical information shows that almost half of patients have a history of cancer at the time of IH.[3]

Hematologic disorders associated with cancer

The second most common cause of IH in the cancer population is coagulopathy, being the leading cause of IH in patients with hematologic malignancies and the second most common cause of IH in central nervous system (CNS) tumors after ITH.[3] Leukemia is the most common hematologic malignancy in patients with cancer and IH, followed by lymphoma and myeloma.[6] Conversely, in patients with intracranial disease involvement, lymphoma is more prone to cause IH than leukemia.[6]

Thrombocytopenia, sepsis, and prolongation of prothrombin time are major predisposing factors for IH in patients with hematologic malignancies.[6] Most hemorrhages associated with coagulopathy are intraparenchymal, but SAH, IVH, or multicompartmental IH also occur.[2,3] Parenchymal hematomas have a preference for the cerebral cortex,

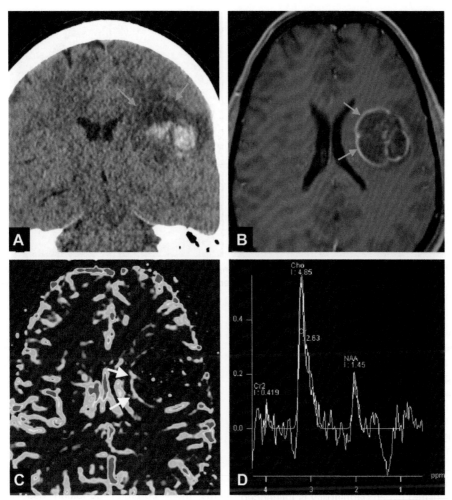

Fig. 1. Tumor-related hemorrhage. Coronal noncontrast CT (*A*) shows acute hematoma with vasogenic edema in the left frontal lobe. Vasogenic edema is slightly disproportionate relative to the size of the hematoma (*A, arrows*). MRI reveals associated peripheral ring enhancement (*arrows* in *B*) and increased CBV (*C, arrows*). Single-voxel spectroscopy from enhancing component (D) shows elevated Choline and low NAA. Final pathology revealed glioblastoma.

basal ganglia, and cerebellum.[6] Multifocal hemorrhages are seen in 46% of cases (**Fig. 2**).[6]

Mortality is high regardless of the type of hematologic malignancy, with a median survival of 1.5 months.[3] Also, prolonged prothrombin time, SAH, and multifocal cerebral hemorrhage are independent prognostic factors of poor outcome.[6]

Hypercoagulable States

Ischemic complications

Up to one-third of strokes have no clear underlying mechanism and are considered embolic strokes of undetermined source (ESUS).[7] Patients with active cancer represent 5% to 10% of ESUS, which increases as patients survive longer.[8,9]

Malignancies often associated with ESUS include breast, lung, prostate, and gastrointestinal tract cancers.[8,9]

Pathophysiology of stroke in patients with cancer is not elucidated but it is well established that cancer-mediated hypercoagulability plays an important role. Possible mechanisms include paradoxical embolism and nonbacterial thrombotic endocarditis. Additional mechanisms unrelated to hypercoagulability include atherosclerosis, radiation vasculitis, tumor embolism, and atrial fibrillation.[10]

Stroke can be the initial presentation of cancer. Up to 10% of ESUS patients are diagnosed with cancer within one year after stroke.[8,11] The actual rate and clinical indicators of occult cancer in

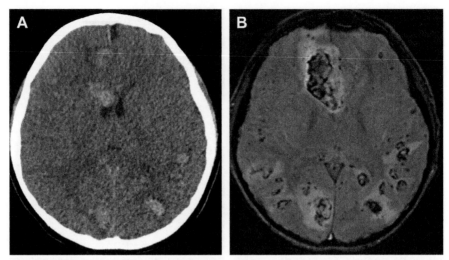

Fig. 2. Multifocal hemorrhage in a patient with acute lymphocytic leukemia. Axial noncontrast CT (A) shows multiple hyperdense parenchymal hemorrhages with intraventricular extension. MRI SWI sequence (B) reveals additional hemorrhages with surrounding edema.

patients with ESUS remain uncertain. Smoking, weight loss, increased C-reactive protein and D-dimer, and anemia can raise the suspicion of underlying malignancy in ESUS.[8,11]

On imaging, multiple acute infarcts involving more than one vascular territory are typical of cancer.[8,11] Patients with ESUS and cancer have worse long-term functional outcomes and survival rates than patients with ESUS and no cancer.

Thrombosis

Cancer-mediated hypercoagulability is influenced by tumor histology, which requires the interaction of different hypercoagulable promoters, such as procoagulant factors, neutrophil extracellular trap formation, and platelet dysfunction.[10] Adenocarcinoma, particularly from lung, is the most common cancer linked to hypercoagulability.[12]

The risk of cerebral venous thrombosis (CVT) is increased 5-fold in patients with cancer, particularly one year after diagnosis.[13] Hematological malignancies convey a higher risk of developing CVT than solid tumors.[13] Severe headaches, focal neurological deficits, and seizures should raise suspicion of CVT. Both CTV and contrast-enhanced MR venogram (CE-MRV) are appropriate studies and should be performed to confirm the diagnosis. Brain MRI is more sensitive than CT to exclude complications including hemorrhagic and nonhemorrhagic lesions (eg, infarction, cerebral edema) that affect one-third of patients with CVT and cancer.[13]

Cancer-mediated hypercoagulability also increases risk for arterial thromboembolism, which is associated with a threefold increased risk of

death in this population.[14] Although ischemic stroke and myocardial infarction are the main arterial thromboembolic events in patients with cancer,[14] other less known complications, such as free-floating thrombus (FFT), can be seen.

FFT is recognized as a string-like soft tissue density projecting into the arterial lumen on ultrasound or CTA, most commonly along the extracranial carotid system.[15] Presence of FFT increases the short-term risk of transient ischemic attach, stroke, or death up to 17%.[16] Atherosclerosis is the most common condition associated with FFT. However, hypercoagulability, thought to be the underlying mechanism in patients with cancer, also plays a role.[15]

Metabolic

Osmotic demyelination

Osmotic demyelination syndrome (ODS) is caused by rapid correction of an osmotic imbalance, most commonly hyponatremia that leads to demyelination.[17] In patients with cancer, ODS can occur without associated electrolyte imbalance and is thought to be secondary to the cancer itself or its treatment.[18]

ODS affects the pons and pontocerebellar fibers in the central variant or the basal ganglia, thalami, and cerebral white matter in the extrapontine type, although patients can present with overlapping findings. Clinical presentation correlates with site of involvement, including pseudobulbar palsy, tetraparesis, ophthalmoplegia, and cranial nerve palsy in pontine ODS, or seizures and extrapyramidal symptoms in extrapontine ODS.[17]

On MRI, high T2-WI/fluid attenuated inversion recovery (FLAIR) signal changes are seen in affected regions with or without restricted diffusion. Pontine ODS shows symmetric signal changes in the central pons with a characteristic trident-shape and sparing of the tegmentum and ventrolateral pons (**Fig. 3**). Extrapontine ODS usually involves the basal ganglia, thalami, cerebellum, or supratentorial white matter.

Wernicke encephalopathy

Wernicke encephalopathy is often under-recognized, given that a minority of patients present the classic triad of confusion, ataxia, and ophthalmoplegia. This syndrome caused by thiamine deficiency is more readily diagnosed in alcoholics. In the absence of this risk factor, such as in patients with cancer, the diagnosis is complex and often overlooked.[19]

In cancer, thiamine deficiency occurs due to decreased availability (eg, malabsorption in gastrointestinal malignancies, malnutrition); accelerated use (eg, high cell turnover); or inactivation by breakdown products of chemotherapy.[19,20] MRI is abnormal in 80% of patients showing areas of high T2-WI/FLAIR signal[19,20] that may show contrast enhancement.[20] Two-thirds of patients present high T2-WI/FLAIR signal involving the tectum, periaqueductal gray, thalamus, mammillary bodies, and surrounding the third ventricle (**Fig. 4**).[19,20] Atypical imaging findings include affection of the medulla, pons, frontal lobe, and cranial nerves.

Awareness of this syndrome in patients with cancer is needed to reduce treatment delays as only one-third of patients fully recover.[19]

Treatment-Related

Radiation necrosis

Radiation necrosis (RN) is the most severe late side effect of radiation therapy (RT). Our discussion focuses on a population where the diagnosis is usually not considered firsthand: temporal lobe RN following RT for head and neck tumors, particularly nasopharyngeal carcinoma (NPC).

It is well known that the higher the total radiation dose is, the higher the incidence of RN. The prescribed target volume is defined as the gross tumor volume plus a sub-clinical margin based on clinical experience, data inferred from pathology results, and patterns of failure from previous treatments. Thus, it is often inevitable to include the temporal lobes in the radiation field for tumors near or infiltrating the skull base. In cases of NPC, intensity-modulated radiotherapy (IMRT) has become mainstay given the lower 5-year incidence of temporal lobe RN (16%) compared with conventional RT (35%).[21]

Patients' symptoms in temporal lobe RN include seizures, cognitive decline, decline in verbal memory and language abilities (left temporal lesions), and impaired visual memory (right temporal lesions)[22]; whereas others could remain asymptomatic.

MRI findings are similar to those of RN following RT = radiation therapy for CNS malignancies and include a heterogenous intra-axial ring-enhancing lesion with thick irregular walls surrounded by vasogenic edema. Presence of a "Swiss-cheese" or "spreading wavefront" type of contrast enhancement, restricted diffusion in the non-enhancing central component, and low rCVB of

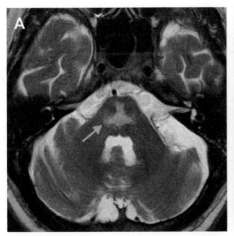
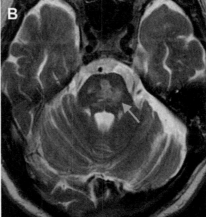

Fig. 3. Osmotic demyelination syndrome (ODS). Axial T2-WI images (*A, B*) show high signal in the central pons with sparing of the tegmentum and corticospinal tracts (*arrows*). Note the characteristic "trident-shaped" signal abnormality (*A*).

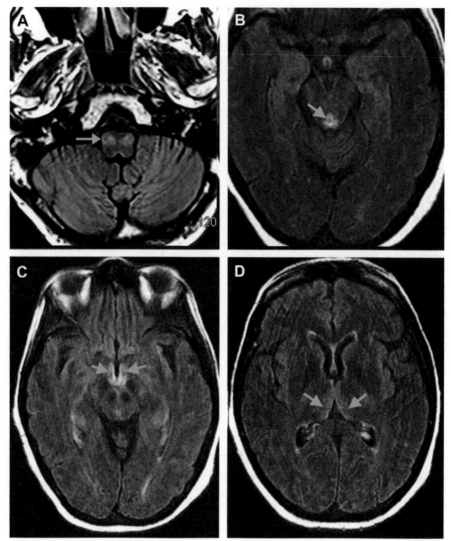

Fig. 4. Wernicke encephalopathy. Axial FLAIR images show abnormal symmetric high signal (*arrows*) in medulla, periaqueductal gray matter, hypothalami, and medial thalami.

the enhancing component are findings that favor RN (**Fig. 5**).

In RN following RT for NPC, other clues that may suggest the diagnosis are bilateral asymmetric temporal lobe involvement (seen in 70% of patients) and disproportionate symptoms relative to imaging findings.[23] RN develops with a median latency of 6 years (1–15 years) after initiation of RT.[23]

Hypophysitis

A therapy that has revolutionized cancer treatment is the use of immune checkpoint inhibitors (ICIs) for melanoma, renal, and lung cancers. One drawback is the unpredictable development of immune-related adverse events (irAEs), particularly endocrinopathies, given their long-lasting and irreversible side effects.

Hypophysitis is the second most common irAE after thyroid dysfunction, with an incidence of 14%.[24] Incidence of hypophysitis in combined ICI is more significant, likely to be symptomatic, and co-occurs with other irAEs (eg, skin, gastrointestinal, hepatic).[24]

Median time from therapy to hypophysitis is between 2 and 4 months, occurring earlier in combined regimens.[24] Patients present with headaches, nausea, hypopituitarism, and visual changes.[24]

MRI is abnormal in 47%.[24] Imaging findings include mild to moderate enlargement of the pituitary gland, loss of the posterior bright spot, and thickening and enhancement of the stalk (**Fig. 6**). Incidental pituitary enlargement on imaging in patients receiving ICI should prompt a clinical and

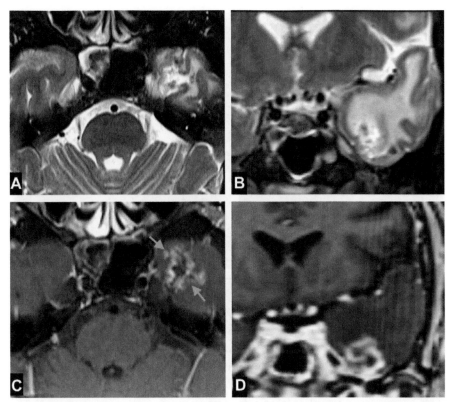

Fig. 5. Temporal lobe radiation necrosis in a patient with prior radiotherapy for nasopharyngeal carcinoma. There is a focal lesion with heterogeneous T2-WI signal (*A*, *B*) in the left temporal lobe, with surrounding vasogenic edema. On axial (*C*) and coronal (*D*) post gadolinium T1-WI, the lesion shows irregular ill-defined peripheral enhancement with Swiss-cheese appearance (*C*, *arrows*).

laboratory assessment as it could be the initial manifestation of hypophysitis.[24]

An emerging endocrine irAE related to ICI therapy that was recently described is a thyroid eye disease-like orbital inflammatory syndrome.[25] Patients present with diffuse symmetric enlargement of the extraocular muscles sparing the muscle tendons (**Fig. 7**).

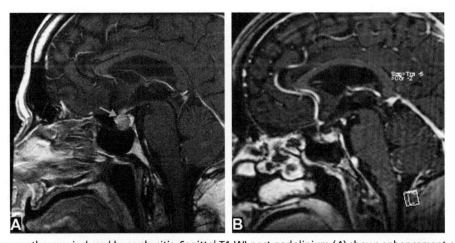

Fig. 6. Immunotherapy-induced hypophysitis. Sagittal T1-WI post gadolinium (*A*) shows enhancement of a thickened infundibulum and enlarged pituitary gland in a patient receiving immune checkpoint inhibitors for melanoma (*arrow*). Follow-up MRI (*B*) after immunotherapy discontinuation and steroid treatment shows the resolution of findings.

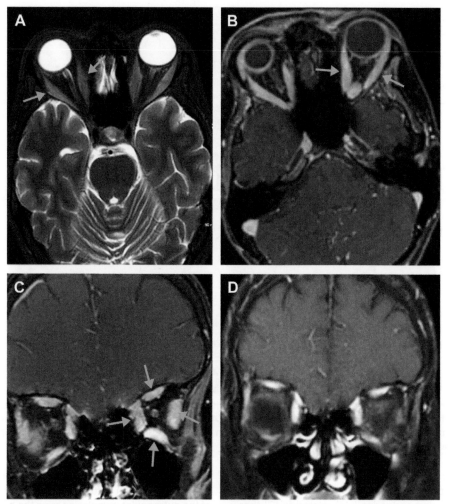

Fig. 7. Thyroid eye disease-like orbital inflammatory syndrome in a patient with immunotherapy for metastatic RCC. Axial T2-WI (A), axial (B), and coronal (C) T1-WI post gadolinium show symmetric diffuse enlargement of the extraocular muscles sparing the muscle tendons bilaterally (*arrows*). After steroid therapy, MRI shows interval resolution of abnormalities (D).

Posterior reversible encephalopathy syndrome

Posterior reversible encephalopathy syndrome (PRES) is typically seen in hypertension, preeclampsia/eclampsia, or autoimmune disorders but can also occur in patients receiving cytotoxic agents or targeted therapies. Patients present with confusion, seizure, visual disturbances, or headaches.[26] MRI findings include cortical or subcortical T2-WI/FLAIR hyperintensity in a "classic parieto-occipital pattern" (**Fig. 8**). However, 50% of cases show other imaging patterns including involvement of frontal or temporal lobes, thalami, basal ganglia, or brainstem. Restricted diffusion and contrast enhancement may be seen. IH can occur when associated with altered coagulation states.[27]

Patients have a good outcome and most recover fully.[26] Cancer treatment can be resumed successfully in most cases.

Acute leukoencephalopathy

Chemotherapy-induced toxic leukoencephalopathy is a progressive white matter disease due to myelin damage most commonly caused by methotrexate but also seen after cranial irradiation.[28]

Risk factors that increase the likelihood of developing leukoencephalopathy include intrathecal route of administration, dosage, associated irradiation, and patient-related risk factors, such as malnutrition or liver dysfunction.[29]

Clinical presentation is variable. Mild dizziness, headaches, and depression are seen when the toxic agent is taken in low doses. Seizures, stroke-like symptoms, and altered mental status occur with higher doses.[30]

On MRI, diffuse T2-WI/FLAIR hyperintensity of the deep white matter and corpus callosum are characteristic (**Fig. 9**). Signal changes are usually

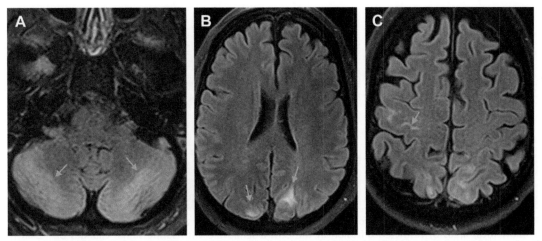

Fig. 8. Chemotherapy-induced PRES in a patient with confusion and visual disturbances. Axial FLAIR images (A–C) show high signal intensity in the cerebellum and in the subcortical parietooccipital regions (arrows in A, B). Subarachnoid hemorrhage (arrow in C) is noted in the right frontal region.

bilateral, but unilateral involvement can occur. Diffusion-weighted imaging (DWI) abnormalities can precede others.[29] This is particularly important in methotrexate-induced leukoencephalopathy, where areas of restricted diffusion in the centra semiovale occur first (Fig. 10).

MAXILLOFACIAL STRUCTURES AND ORBITS
Acute invasive fungal infection

Angioinvasive fungal species such as aspergillus, mucor, or less commonly fusarium, can cause a rapidly progressive sinonasal infection complicated by orbital and/or intracranial disease. Infection is usually seen in patients with neutropenia, poorly controlled diabetes, impaired humoral or cellular immunity, or receiving immunosuppressive treatments.[31] Acute invasive fungal infection has high mortality and requires prompt aggressive surgical debridement and antifungal therapy. Most infections originate in a sinonasal cavity and extend intracranially or into the orbits directly or through valveless emissary veins. Infection should be suspected in patients with cancer presenting with fever and sinonasal discharge, congestion, or pain, whereas patients with orbital involvement have periorbital edema, proptosis, and abnormal ocular motility.[31,32] Cranial neuropathies raise concern for cavernous sinus involvement, whereas altered mental status and focal neurologic deficits suggest brain extension.

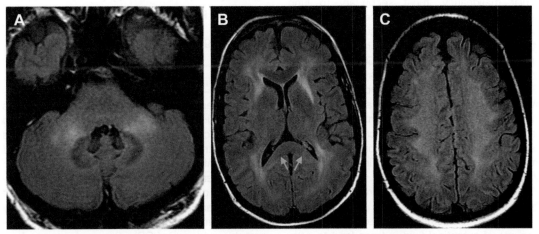

Fig. 9. Treatment-induced toxic leukoencephalopathy in a patient with acute myelogenous leukemia after intrathecal methotrexate administration. Axial FLAIR images (A–C) show symmetric high signal intensity in the middle cerebellar peduncles, corona radiata, and centrum semiovale. There is also a subtle increased signal in the splenium of the corpus callosum (B, arrows).

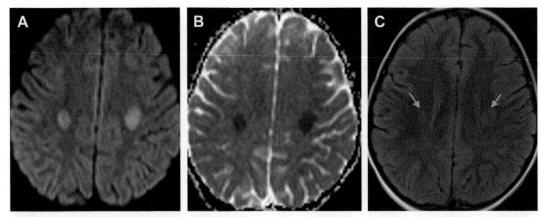

Fig. 10. Methotrexate neurotoxicity following intrathecal chemotherapy administration. DWI (*A*) and ADC map (*B*) show focal areas of restricted diffusion in the centra semiovale with subtle signal changes on FLAIR (*C, arrows*).

Contrast-enhanced CT or MRI are acceptable in patients with suspected acute invasive fungal infection. On CT, presence of sinonasal disease with periantral inflammatory changes is a concerning finding. Orbital fat should be scrutinized for inflammatory changes, particularly in patients with ethmoid sinus disease. On MRI, devitalized sinonasal mucosa can appear abnormally T2 dark with lack of contrast-enhancement ("black turbinate" sign) (**Fig. 11**).[32] Fungal elements can appear markedly T2 hypointense due to accumulation of iron and other paramagnetic metals such as manganese.

Hemorrhagic ocular malignancy and membranous detachments

The eye is a rare site for hematogenous metastases but metastases represent the most common ocular malignancy, most secondary to lung, breast, or gastrointestinal cancers.[33] In breast cancer, ocular metastases occur in advanced stages with almost all patients having systemic disease. In lung cancer, only 50% of patients with choroidal metastases have systemic disease (**Fig. 12**).[34] The choroid is the most affected site owing to its rich vasculature, but any ocular structure may be involved. Primary intraocular malignancies are less common but can present with hemorrhage. Most primary tumors in adults are melanomas (**Fig. 13**), whereas primary intraocular lymphomas are rare. In children, retinoblastomas (**Fig. 14**) are most common, whereas medulloepitheliomas are rare.[35]

Choroidal metastases present with large amounts of subretinal fluid but can lead to complete retinal detachment even when small. In contrast, melanomas need to grow larger before causing retinal detachment.[36] Intraocular

hemorrhage is present in approximately 3% of patients with uveal melanoma and may be secondary to vascular invasion by tumor or venous congestion with stasis.[37] Hemorrhagic ocular metastases are rare. A higher frequency of intraocular hemorrhage is reported in metastases from choriocarcinoma.[38]

Ophthalmologic examination including high-resolution imaging techniques such as optical coherence tomography and ultrasound are often utilized in non-emergent patients and suspected ocular metastases.[39] Tumor visualization may be obscured by hemorrhage. CT may be able to detect membranous detachments as areas of increased density due to hemorrhage. MRI is superior but requires fat-suppressed T2 and post-contrast T1 sequences. In patients with melanoma, tumors frequently have increased T1 and decreased T2 signal intensity due to the metal chelating properties of melanin (see **Fig. 13**).[40] However, signal intensity varies in presence of hemorrhage depending on the stage of blood products.

Osteoradionecrosis

Mandibular osteoradionecrosis (ORN) is a serious complication of radiation therapy for head and neck cancers and can occur months to years following treatment.[41] Its incidence has decreased and recently currently occurs in 4% to 9%.[41,42] Mandibular ORN is defined as exposed bone persisting for greater than 3 to 6 months in absence of local disease recurrence. A subset of patients may present with intact overlying mucosa and radiographic evidence of ORN. Severe cases can lead to hemorrhage, fracture, and infection with draining fistulae and sepsis. Septic ORN presents with severe pain.[43] Several risk factors associated

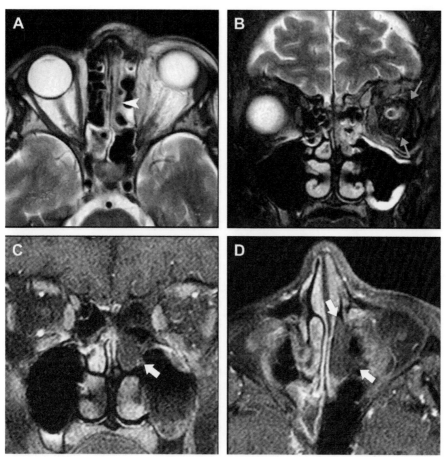

Fig. 11. Invasive fungal sinusitis. Axial (*A*) and coronal (*B*) T2 show opacification of ethmoid and sphenoid sinuses with areas of abnormally hypointense mucosa (*arrowhead*). Left retro-orbital stranding is seen on B indicating orbital extension (arrows). Coronal (*C*) and axial (*D*) postcontrast fat-suppressed T1 show devitalized non-enhancing mucosa ("black turbinate" sign, *arrows*).

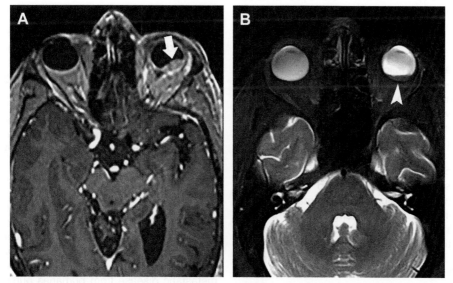

Fig. 12. Metastasis to the eye from lung cancer with acute hemorrhage. Axial postcontrast T1 (*A*) shows an enhancing mass in the left eye (*arrow*) with layering hemorrhage on T2 (*arrowhead, B*).

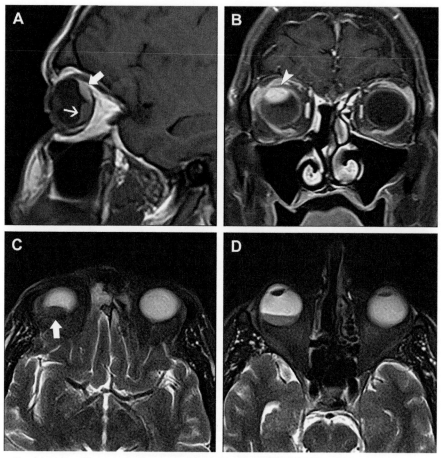

Fig. 13. Uveal melanoma with acute hemorrhage. MRI shows a T1-hyper, T2-hypointense mass in the right eye (*A* and *C, thick arrows*). Note subretinal hemorrhage (*thin arrow* in *A*). There is avid contrast enhancement (*B, arrowhead*) and layering hemorrhage on T2 (*D*).

with the development of ORN include pre- or post-radiotherapy tooth extraction, treatment of oral or oropharyngeal cancers, and greater than 14% volume of the mandible receiving a dose of 60 Gy.[41,44] In most patients, ORN affects the mandibular body, followed by the angle or ramus, and symphyseal or parasymphyseal regions.[44]

CT findings include osseous permeative changes with a mixed lytic/sclerotic appearance, loss of cortical and trabecular bone, and osseous sequestra typically involving the buccal or lingual surface.[45] Bicortical involvement is seen in severe cases and predisposes to fractures (Fig. 15). On MRI, fat-suppressed T2/STIR and post-contrast T1 sequences show abnormal bone marrow signal with edema and enhancement that may involve surrounding soft tissues and masticator space. In some patients, soft tissue enhancement can be masslike and indistinguishable from recurrent disease.[45] ORN can coexist with infection and cannot be differentiated by imaging unless there is an associated abscess.

NECK COMPLICATIONS
Airway Compromise

Respiratory compromise is common with advanced tumors of the base of tongue, larynx, and hypopharynx.[46] It can be the result of direct mechanical obstruction by tumor or may be secondary to hemorrhage or superimposed infection. In patients who receive chemoradiation, the tumor and surrounding tissues undergo acute inflammation and edema in the first 2 weeks that can result in new or worsened obstruction.[47] Advanced laryngeal cancers are likely to result in airway compromise requiring tracheostomy or tumor debulking and this can occur before, during, or after chemoradiation.[46] In addition, patients who undergo radiation have diminished salivary flow that affects mucosal integrity. Some patients have increased secretions due to impaired swallowing. Rarely, airway compromise can be secondary to metastatic disease from primaries outside of the head and neck. Contrast-enhanced CT is the

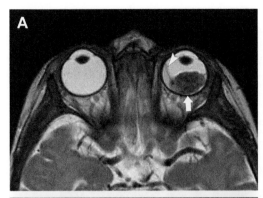

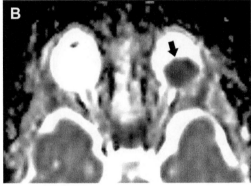

Fig. 14. Retinoblastoma and retinal detachment. Axial T2 (*A*) shows a hypointense mass in the left posterior globe (*white arrow*) with retinal detachment (*arrowhead*). ADC map (*B*) shows restricted diffusion due to high cellularity (*black arrow*).

imaging modality of choice in acute respiratory compromise as it can be done rapidly and is able to clearly depict the airway compared with MRI (**Fig. 16**).

Treatment Related

Post-radiation edema and mucositis. Acute oropharyngeal and laryngeal edema and mucositis are common in patients treated with radiation. Their prevalence is higher in those who received chemoradiation compared with radiation alone.[48] In addition, pharyngeal constrictor muscles become thickened and edematous following chemoradiation in patients receiving doses greater than 50 Gy.[49] These changes, along with iatrogenic anatomical alterations and nerve injury can lead to dysphagia and aspiration pneumonia. Likelihood of dysphagia and pneumonia is higher in patients undergoing chemoradiation than in those treated with surgery alone and the risk of stricture is higher after combined therapies.[50] On CT, pharyngeal and laryngeal structures appear thickened in a symmetric fashion. As opposed to tumor, soft tissue thickening related to radiation shows decreased attenuation due to edema.

Retropharyngeal effusion or edema is a common finding (**Fig. 17**). Contrast-enhanced CT shows areas of increased vascularity with prominent vessels due to hyperemia. Soft tissue thickening on MRI shows varying degrees of T2 signal intensity depending on presence of edema and inflammation that are best seen on fat-suppressed sequences. Post-contrast T1 shows varying degrees of enhancement.

Vascular injury. Several factors predispose patients with neck cancer to vascular injury, with carotid rupture being the most severe complication. The carotid arteries may have insufficient soft tissue covering following surgery that increases exposure, desiccation, and weakening of the vessel wall. There can also be enzymatic degradation of the carotid wall in patients with fistulas where the vessel is exposed to saliva. The carotid vessels can be directly infiltrated by metastatic cervical lymphadenopathy or primary tumor. Rapid tumor regression following chemoradiation can lead to weakening and rupture of the vessel wall. Patients present with imminent hemorrhage from a clinically exposed but unruptured vessel, contained sentinel hemorrhage, or full carotid blowout (**Figs. 18** and **19**). Mortality after carotid blowout is approximately 40%, whereas 60% of survivors sustain permanent neurological impairment.[51] Carotid blowout is rare after radiation but is more frequent in patients undergoing salvage reirradiation (3% of cases).[52] Radiation causes DNA damage in arteries leading to sustained upregulation of inflammatory transcription factors and production of free radicals and oxidative stress.[53] This results in vessel wall thickening with stenosis and atherosclerotic-like changes increasing the risk for cerebrovascular events.[53]

Chondronecrosis. Chondronecrosis is a severe complication of radiation that occurs months to years after treatment. Its incidence has decreased owing to improved radiotherapy techniques and is seen in 1% to 5% of patients.[54] Risk is increased in patients where cartilage has been subject to injury during surgery and infection. Inflammatory changes in irradiated tissue lead to obliterative endarteritis of cartilage vessels, edema, ischemia, fibrosis, and chondronecrosis.[54] Devitalized cartilage is predisposed to deformity and fracture and may collapse with resultant airway compromise. Patients present with hoarseness, severe pain, dysphagia, acute airway obstruction, and aspiration. CT shows lytic or permeative changes of the affected cartilage that may be accompanied by foci of gas, loss of normal architecture, or fracture (**Fig. 20**). MRI shows varying degrees of inflammatory changes with edema and enhancement of surrounding tissues.

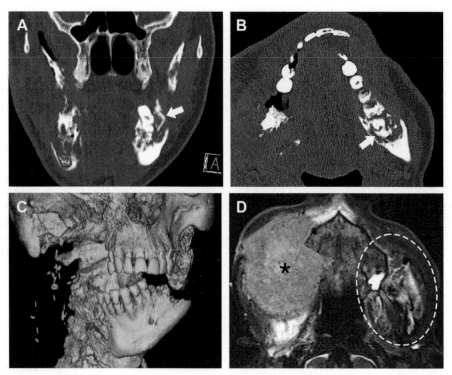

Fig. 15. Mandibular osteoradionecrosis in a patient with squamous cell carcinoma. Coronal (A) and axial (B) non-contrast CT shows extensive lytic and sclerotic changes in the mandible with osseous sequestra (*arrows*). Follow-up volume rendered 3D CT (C) after right hemimandibulectomy shows a pathologic left mandibular fracture. Fat-suppressed T2 MRI shows increased signal in left mandible and masticator space (*oval*). Note large recurrent tumor on the right (*asterisk*).

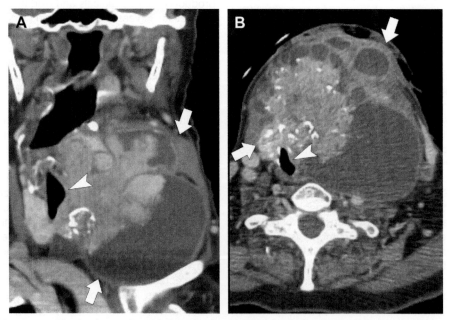

Fig. 16. Airway compromise due to thyroid gland tumor. Coronal (A) and axial (B) postcontrast CT show displacement and narrowing of the airway (*arrowheads*) due to a massive thyroid carcinoma (*arrows*).

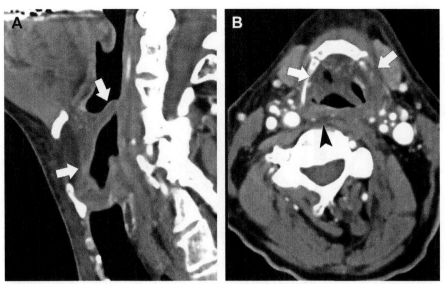

Fig. 17. Post-radiation mucositis and edema. Sagittal (*A*) and axial (*B*) postcontrast CT shows diffuse thickening of the posterior pharynx, pre-epiglottic space, and supraglottis (*white arrows*). Note small retropharyngeal effusion/edema (*black arrowhead*).

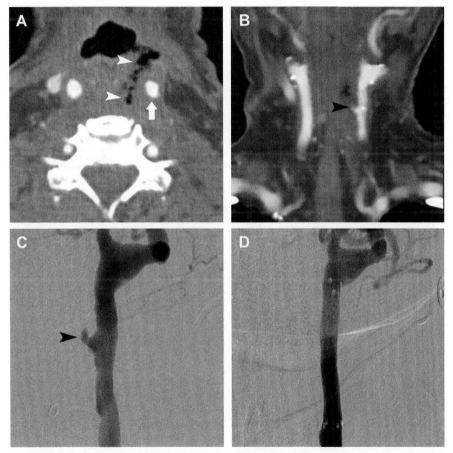

Fig. 18. Patient with laryngeal cancer post chemoradiation presenting with hemoptysis. Axial (*A*) and coronal (*B*) postcontrast CT and lateral view DSA (*C, D*). CT shows a hypopharyngeal-prevertebral fistula (*white arrowheads*) with an irregular contour of the common carotid artery (*arrow*). Note small focus of extravasation (*black arrowheads*) successfully treated with an endovascular stent (*D*). (*Courtesy of* Benjamin Y. Huang, MD, Chapel Hill, NC.)

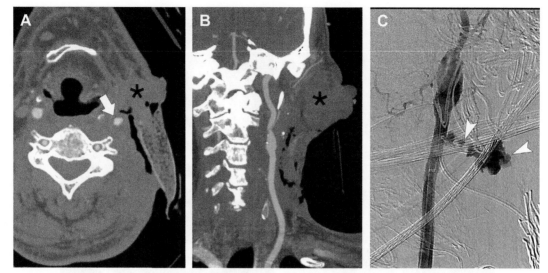

Fig. 19. Carotid blowout syndrome. Axial (*A*) and coronal (*B*) postcontrast CT shows large recurrent squamous cell carcinoma in the left neck (*asterisk*). Note irregular contour of the left common carotid artery (*arrow*). DSA (*C*) shows a large amount of active extravasation (*arrowheads*) that occurred during angiography. (*Courtesy of* Christine Glastonbury, MD, San Francisco, CA.)

Infection. Patients with neck malignancies may develop infection due to several causes. First, they have an inherent risk of infection associated with surgery that involves the aerodigestive tract. Second, extensive resections for neck malignancies alter anatomical barriers that normally protect against infection. Third, radiation-induced osteonecrosis predisposes bone to infection

(**Fig. 21**). Finally, indwelling devices represent another potential source of infection.

Contrast-enhanced CT is best for the initial assessment of patients with suspected infection. It depicts phlegmonous changes or abscess and can discriminate these against post-radiation edema/mucositis or recurrent tumor and can show gas along fascial planes in patients with

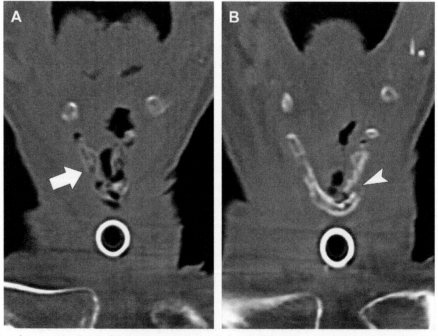

Fig. 20. Chondronecrosis. Coronal postcontrast CT (*A*, *B*) shows deformity of the thyroid cartilage with a mixed lytic/sclerotic appearance (*arrow*) and pathologic fracture (*arrowhead*).

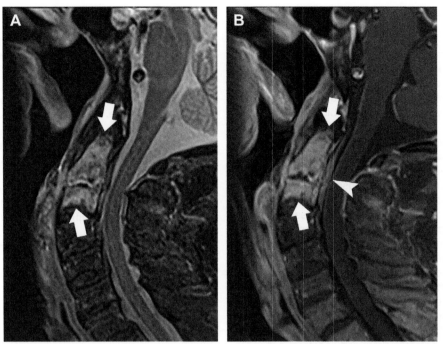

Fig. 21. Discitis-osteomyelitis in a patient with osteonecrosis of cervical spine following irradiation for nasopharyngeal carcinoma. Sagittal STIR (*A*) and fat-suppressed postcontrast T1 (*B*) show extensive edema and enhancement of the C2 and C3 vertebrae (*arrows*). There is fluid in the intervertebral disc with mild enhancement. Note thin epidural phlegmon (*arrowhead*).

necrotizing infections. However, differentiation from infection may be difficult in patients with infiltrative and necrotic malignancies. MRI may be helpful for additional characterization and requires fat-suppressed techniques to visualize edema and contrast enhancement. In abscesses, DWI shows restricted diffusion of pus, but restricted diffusion is also seen in the solid-enhancing components of necrotic tumors due to high cellularity.

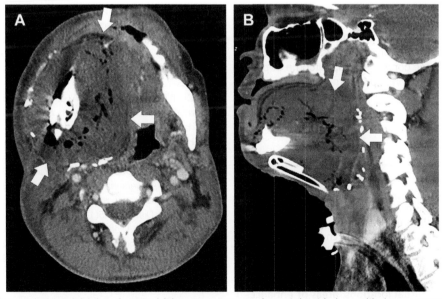

Fig. 22. Flap necrosis. Axial (*A*) and sagittal (*B*) post-contrast CT show right-sided mandibular reconstruction with a myocutaneous flap. The devitalized flap is abnormally hypodense (*arrows*) and contains intravascular gas.

Flap necrosis. Treatment of head and neck malignancies frequently requires extensive surgical resection to ensure negative margins. Several reconstruction techniques have been devised to regain function and for cosmetic purposes. As opposed to surgical grafts, whose vascular supply depends entirely on angiogenesis, flaps are reconstructed with a dedicated blood supply and achieve better soft tissue bulk and cosmesis. Local or regional flaps require anatomic rearrangement of surrounding tissues with preservation of their native blood supply. On the contrary, free flaps are created by transposing tissue from other sites and creating microvascular anastomoses.

Free flaps are standard in many head and neck reconstructions. Because their blood supply depends completely on the microvascular anastomosis until there is sufficient neovascularization, risk for necrosis and infection is greatest on days 2 to 5 after surgery and declines thereafter.[55] Smoking is a significant risk factor for flap necrosis.[56] Overall, necrosis with modern techniques is rare and flap survival is about 95%.[57] On CT and MRI, flaps normally show early contrast enhancement and edema after surgery, however, severe or progressive edema could indicate a devitalized flap and/or infection (**Fig. 22**).

SUMMARY

Patients with head and neck cancer experience a wide range of oncologic emergencies due to various mechanisms. Because of their anatomical location and potential involvement of critical structures, some of these are associated with high morbidity and mortality. Imaging plays a central role in evaluation and management and knowledge of their clinical context is important. For several of these complications, outcome depends on early recognition and treatment.

CLINICS CARE POINTS

- In general, computed tomography is the preferred modality for evaluation of acute complications in the head and neck, whereas MRI is reserved for further characterization.
- Intratumoral hemorrhage may be the first manifestation of cancer that should be suspected when there is disproportionate edema, unusual locations, areas of enhancement, or increased perfusion.

- Severe headaches, neurological deficits, and seizures in a patient with cancer should raise concern for cerebral venous thrombosis in addition to intracranial metastatic disease.
- Metabolic derangements are not always accompanied by electrolyte imbalances or the full spectrum of symptoms and are difficult to diagnose.
- Acute invasive fungal sinusitis has high mortality and should be suspected in patients with sinus disease who have adjacent inflammatory changes on imaging.
- Patients treated for neck cancer are subject to immediate life-threatening complications including airway compromise and carotid injuries.

DISCLOSURE

The authors have nothing to disclose.

REFERENCES

1. Head and neck cancer: statistics. cancer.net editorial board. 2022. Available at: https://www.cancer.net/cancer-types/head-and-neck-cancer/statistics. Accessed April/17/2022.
2. Graus F, Rogers LR, Posner JB. Cerebrovascular complications in patients with cancer. Medicine (Baltimore) 1985;64(1):16–35.
3. Navi BB, Reichman JS, Berlin D, et al. Intracerebral and subarachnoid hemorrhage in patients with cancer. Neurology 2010;74(6):494–501.
4. Kondziolka D, Bernstein M, Resch L, et al. Significance of hemorrhage into brain tumors: clinicopathological study. J Neurosurg 1987;67(6):852–7.
5. Lieu AS, Hwang SL, Howng SL, et al. Brain tumors with hemorrhage. J Formos Med Assoc 1999;98(5):365–7.
6. Chen CY, Tai CH, Cheng A, et al. Intracranial hemorrhage in adult patients with hematological malignancies. BMC Med 2012;10:97.
7. Hart RG, Catanese L, Perera KS, et al. Embolic stroke of undetermined source: a systematic review and clinical update. Stroke 2017;48(4):867–72.
8. Selvik HA, Bjerkreim AT, Thomassen L, et al. When to screen ischaemic stroke patients for cancer. Cerebrovasc Dis 2018;45(1–2):42–7.
9. Sanossian N, Djabiras C, Mack WJ, et al. Trends in cancer diagnoses among inpatients hospitalized with stroke. J Stroke Cerebrovasc Dis 2013;22(7):1146–50.
10. Navi BB, Kasner SE, Elkind MSV, et al. Cancer and embolic stroke of undetermined source. Stroke 2021;52(3):1121–30.

11. Gon Y, Sakaguchi M, Takasugi J, et al. Plasma D-dimer levels and ischaemic lesions in multiple vascular regions can predict occult cancer in patients with cryptogenic stroke. Eur J Neurol 2017; 24(3):503–8.

12. Chung JW, Cho YH, Ahn MJ, et al. Association of Cancer Cell Type and Extracellular Vesicles With Coagulopathy in Patients With Lung Cancer and Stroke. Stroke 2018;49(5):1282–5.

13. Silvis SM, Hiltunen S, Lindgren E, et al. Cancer and risk of cerebral venous thrombosis: a case-control study. J Thromb Haemost 2018;16(1):90–5.

14. Navi BB, Reiner AS, Kamel H, et al. Risk of arterial thromboembolism in patients with cancer. J Am Coll Cardiol 2017;70(8):926–38.

15. Torres C, Lum C, Puac-Polanco P, et al. Differentiating carotid free-floating thrombus from atheromatous plaque using intraluminal filling defect length on CTA: a validation study. Neurology 2021;97(8): e785–93.

16. Fridman S, Lownie SP, Mandzia J. Diagnosis and management of carotid free-floating thrombus: a systematic literature review. Int J Stroke 2019; 14(3):247–56.

17. Martin RJ. Central pontine and extrapontine myelinolysis: the osmotic demyelination syndromes. J Neurol Neurosurg Psychiatr 2004;75(Suppl 3): iii22–8.

18. Chung JH, Baik SK, Cho SH, et al. Reversible cerebellar ataxia related to extrapontine myelinolysis without hyponatremia after cisplatin-based chemotherapy for cholangiocarcinoma. Cancer Res Treat 2015;47(2):329–33.

19. Isenberg-Grzeda E, Rahane S, DeRosa AP, et al. Wernicke-Korsakoff syndrome in patients with cancer: a systematic review. Lancet Oncol 2016;17(4): e142–8.

20. Zuccoli G, Santa Cruz D, Bertolini M, et al. MR imaging findings in 56 patients with Wernicke encephalopathy: nonalcoholics may differ from alcoholics. AJNR Am J Neuroradiol 2009;30(1):171–6.

21. Zhou GQ, Yu XL, Chen M, et al. Radiation-induced temporal lobe injury for nasopharyngeal carcinoma: a comparison of intensity-modulated radiotherapy and conventional two-dimensional radiotherapy. PLoS One 2013;8(7):e67488.

22. Cheung MC, Chan AS, Law SC, et al. Impact of radionecrosis on cognitive dysfunction in patients after radiotherapy for nasopharyngeal carcinoma. Cancer 2003;97(8):2019–26.

23. Lee AW, Foo W, Chappell R, et al. Effect of time, dose, and fractionation on temporal lobe necrosis following radiotherapy for nasopharyngeal carcinoma. Int J Radiat Oncol Biol Phys 1998;40(1):35–42.

24. Jessel S, Weiss SA, Austin M, et al. Immune checkpoint inhibitor-induced hypophysitis and patterns of loss of pituitary function. Front Oncol 2022;12: 836859.

25. Sagiv O, Kandl TJ, Thakar SD, et al. Extraocular muscle enlargement and thyroid eye disease-like orbital inflammation associated with immune checkpoint inhibitor therapy in cancer patients. Ophthal Plast Reconstr Surg 2019;35(1):50–2.

26. Singer S, Grommes C, Reiner AS, et al. Posterior Reversible encephalopathy syndrome in patients with cancer. Oncologist 2015;20(7):806–11.

27. Liman TG, Bohner G, Heuschmann PU, et al. The clinical and radiological spectrum of posterior reversible encephalopathy syndrome: the retrospective Berlin PRES study. J Neurol 2012;259(1): 155–64.

28. Crossen JR, Garwood D, Glatstein E, et al. Neurobehavioral sequelae of cranial irradiation in adults: a review of radiation-induced encephalopathy. J Clin Oncol 1994;12(3):627–42.

29. Sindhwani G, Arora M, Thakker VD, et al. MRI in Chemotherapy induced leukoencephalopathy: report of two cases and radiologist's perspective. J Clin Diagn Res 2017;11(7):TD08–9.

30. Moore-Maxwell CA, Datto MB, Hulette CM. Chemotherapy-induced toxic leukoencephalopathy causes a wide range of symptoms: a series of four autopsies. Mod Pathol 2004;17(2):241–7.

31. Trief D, Gray ST, Jakobiec FA, et al. Invasive fungal disease of the sinus and orbit: a comparison between mucormycosis and Aspergillus. Br J Ophthalmol 2016;100(2):184–8.

32. Safder S, Carpenter JS, Roberts TD, et al. The "black turbinate" sign: an early MR imaging finding of nasal mucormycosis. AJNR Am J Neuroradiol 2010;31(4): 771–4.

33. Shields CL, Shields JA, Gross NE, et al. Survey of 520 eyes with uveal metastases. Ophthalmology 1997;104(8):1265–76.

34. Blasi MA, Maceroni M, Caputo CG, et al. Clinical and ultrasonographic features of choroidal metastases based on primary cancer site: Long-term experience in a single center. PLoS One 2021;16(3): e0249210.

35. Lee J, Choung HK, Kim YA, et al. Intraocular medulloepithelioma in children: clinicopathologic features itself hardly differentiate it from retinoblastoma. Int J Ophthalmol 2019;12(7):1227–30.

36. Cohen VM. Ocular metastases. Eye (Lond). 2013; 27(2):137–41.

37. Chee YE, Mudumbai R, Saraf SS, et al. Hemorrhagic choroidal detachment as the presenting sign of uveal melanoma. Am J Ophthalmol Case Rep 2021;23:101173.

38. Kavanagh MC, Pakala SR, Hollander DA, et al. Choriocarcinoma metastatic to the choroid. Br J Ophthalmol 2006;90(5):650–2.

39. Cennamo G, Montorio D, Carosielli M, et al. Multi-modal Imaging in Choroidal Metastasis. Ophthalmic Res 2021;64(3):411–6.

40. Enochs WS, Petherick P, Bogdanova A, et al. Para-magnetic metal scavenging by melanin: MR imaging. Radiology 1997;204(2):417–23.

41. Lang K, Held T, Meixner E, et al. Frequency of osteoradionecrosis of the lower jaw after radiotherapy of oral cancer patients correlated with dosimetric parameters and other risk factors. Head Face Med 2022;18(1):7.

42. Owosho AA, Tsai CJ, Lee RS, et al. The prevalence and risk factors associated with osteoradionecrosis of the jaw in oral and oropharyngeal cancer patients treated with intensity-modulated radiation therapy (IMRT): The Memorial Sloan Kettering Cancer Center experience. Oral Oncol 2017;64:44–51.

43. Chronopoulos A, Zarra T, Ehrenfeld M, et al. Osteoradionecrosis of the jaws: definition, epidemiology, staging and clinical and radiological findings. A concise review. Int Dent J 2018;68(1):22–30.

44. Kubota H, Miyawaki D, Mukumoto N, et al. Risk factors for osteoradionecrosis of the jaw in patients with head and neck squamous cell carcinoma. Radiat Oncol 2021;16(1):1.

45. Deshpande SS, Thakur MH, Dholam K, et al. Osteoradionecrosis of the mandible: through a radiologist's eyes. Clin Radiol 2015;70(2):197–205.

46. Langerman A, Patel RM, Cohen EE, et al. Airway management before chemoradiation for advanced head and neck cancer. Head Neck 2012;34(2): 254–9.

47. Hermans R. Post-treatment imaging of head and neck cancer. Cancer Imaging 2004;4. Spec No A: S6-S15.

48. Kawashita Y, Kitamura M, Soutome S, et al. Association of neutrophil-to-lymphocyte ratio with severe radiation-induced mucositis in pharyngeal or laryngeal cancer patients: a retrospective study. BMC Cancer 2021;21(1):1064.

49. Popovtzer A, Cao Y, Feng FY, et al. Anatomical changes in the pharyngeal constrictors after chemo-irradiation of head and neck cancer and their dose-effect relationships: MRI-based study. Radiother Oncol 2009;93(3):510–5.

50. Francis DO, Weymuller EA Jr, Parvathaneni U, et al. Dysphagia, stricture, and pneumonia in head and neck cancer patients: does treatment modality matter? Ann Otol Rhinol Laryngol 2010;119(6):391–7.

51. Rimmer J, Giddings CE, Vaz F, et al. Management of vascular complications of head and neck cancer. J Laryngol Otol 2012;126(2):111–5.

52. McDonald MW, Moore MG, Johnstone PA. Risk of carotid blowout after reirradiation of the head and neck: a systematic review. Int J Radiat Oncol Biol Phys 2012;82(3):1083–9.

53. Weintraub NL, Jones WK, Manka D. Understanding radiation-induced vascular disease. J Am Coll Cardiol 2010;55(12):1237–9.

54. Gessert TG, Britt CJ, Maas AMW, et al. Chondroradionecrosis of the larynx: 24-year University of Wisconsin experience. Head Neck 2017;39(6):1189–94.

55. Yoon AP, Jones NF. Critical time for neovascularization/angiogenesis to allow free flap survival after delayed postoperative anastomotic compromise without surgical intervention: a review of the literature. Microsurgery 2016;36(7):604–12.

56. Hwang K, Son JS, Ryu WK. Smoking and Flap Survival. Plast Surg (Oakv) 2018;26(4):280–5.

57. Haughey BH, Wilson E, Kluwe L, et al. Free flap reconstruction of the head and neck: analysis of 241 cases. Otolaryngol Head Neck Surg 2001; 125(1):10–7.

Oncologic Emergencies in the Chest, Abdomen, and Pelvis

Lokesh Khanna, MD[a], Daniel Vargas, MD[a], Christine 'Cooky' Menias, MD[b], Venkat Katabathina, MD[a],*

KEYWORDS

• Oncologic emergencies • Chest • Abdomen • Hepatobiliary • Intestinal • Urinary • Vascular

KEY POINTS

• Oncology patients can present with acute, life-threatening conditions that may arise either due to underlying malignancy or secondary to cancer therapy.
• Select oncologic emergencies demonstrate characteristic imaging findings on radiographs, ultrasound, CT, and MRI that helps in timely diagnosis.
• Radiologists need to be aware of typical imaging findings in such patients in an emergency setting and should be able to guide the clinicians for proper patient management.
• Appropriate knowledge of the treatment and its timing is pivotal in diagnosing treatment-related complications.

INTRODUCTION

Cancer is the second leading cause of death worldwide, accounting for almost 10 million cancer-related deaths in 2020.[1] Select acute life-threatening emergencies can develop in patients with cancer either due to underlying malignancy or could be treatment-related.[2,3] Although clinical and laboratory findings are the basis for diagnosing metabolic and hematologic emergencies, structural pathologies resulting in mechanical compression, hollow organ obstruction, or bleeding need imaging studies for timely diagnosis and management. In the appropriate clinical scenarios, select oncologic emergencies involving the chest, abdomen, and pelvis can be confidently diagnosed based on imaging findings that can help to provide timely treatment (Box 1). The most common thoracic emergencies encountered in patients with cancer include airway obstruction, esophago-respiratory fistula, superior vena cava (SVC) syndrome, massive hemoptysis, pulmonary thromboembolism (PE), cardiac tamponade, and spinal cord compression (Table 1).[2,4] The common abdominopelvic oncologic emergencies include uncontrolled bleeding, intestinal obstruction/ischemia/perforation, intussusception, urinary tract obstruction, biliary obstruction, acute cholecystitis, and acute cholangitis (Table 2).[5] Targeted chemotherapy agents can cause acute complications such as thromboembolism, hepatic veno-occlusive disease, gastrointestinal necrosis/perforation due to microvascular injury, and inflammation of the bowel and pancreas.[6] Radiotherapy can result in bowel ischemia and distal ureteric narrowing with subsequent urinary tract obstruction. Iatrogenic emergencies may result from surgery, interventional treatment procedures, and central venous catheter placement in patients with cancer. In this article, we discuss select emergencies involving the chest, abdomen, and pelvis in oncologic patients and the pertinent imaging

The authors have nothing to disclose.
a Department of Radiology, Body Imaging, University of Texas Health Science Center at San Antonio, 7703 Floyd Curl Drive, MC 7790, San Antonio, TX 78229-3900, USA; b Mayo Clinic Radiology, 13400 E. Shea Boulevard, Scottsdale, AZ 85259, USA
* Corresponding author.
E-mail address: katabathina@uthscsa.edu

Radiol Clin N Am 61 (2023) 91–110
https://doi.org/10.1016/j.rcl.2022.09.003

findings, which can be helpful in early diagnosis and guide management.

ROLE OF IMAGING

Imaging plays a critical role in diagnosis and guiding the management when oncology patients present to the emergency room (ER) with acute symptoms.[2] Radiography, ultrasound (US), computed tomography (CT), and MRI are the commonly used imaging techniques in suspected oncologic emergencies.[2] Plain radiographs help screen for potential catastrophes that need an urgent response, such as tension pneumothorax, large malignant pleural effusion, mediastinal shift, bowel obstruction, pneumoperitoneum, pneumatosis, and toxic colitis (Fig. 1).[3] Fluoroscopy is used to evaluate bowel leaks and fistula. US is beneficial in assessing suspected biliary obstruction, acute cholecystitis/cholangitis, a large volume of ascites, and urinary obstruction (Fig. 2). CT is readily accessible and serves as the workhorse in evaluating patients with cancer with acute chest or abdominal pain; most oncologic emergencies are diagnosed on CT[5] (Fig. 3). MRI has limited utility in the evaluation of patients

presenting with oncologic emergencies and is often used as a problem-solving tool in patients with suspected biliary obstruction/sepsis and acute cholecystitis (Fig. 4). Interventional radiologists play a critical role in treating massive pleural/pericardial effusions, severe ascites, hemoptysis, SVC obstruction, bleeding, biliary obstruction, and urinary tract obstruction (see Fig. 3).[7]

Thoracic Emergencies

Airway obstruction

Airway obstruction from primary or secondary thoracic malignancies can result in decreased luminal diameter at any point of the airway from external compression or endoluminal lesion growth.[8,9] Lung cancer is the most common malignancy to result in airway obstruction, followed by lymphoma, metastatic lymphadenopathy, endobronchial carcinoid, or primary tracheal tumors.[9] Patients can present with progressive dyspnea, recurrent infections, hemoptysis, or respiratory failure.[10]

Chest radiography is often initially ordered in chest emergencies. Abnormal findings include tracheal deviation, compression, abrupt airway cutoff, post-obstructive atelectasis, or consolidation.[4,8] CT with coronal and sagittal reformations is the modality of choice and clearly depicts the site, etiology, and severity of airway obstruction and can triage for appropriate management (Fig. 5). Virtual CT bronchoscopy is another novel CT option that allows for detailed visualization of the tracheobronchial tree.[11]

Aerodigestive fistula

Aerodigestive fistula (ADF) refers to abnormal fistulous communication between the esophagus/stomach and respiratory system either due to a primary tumor infiltrating into the esophagorespiratory space or may be treatment-related. It can result in potentially life-threatening complications due to the aspiration of esophageal contents into the respiratory system.[12] Trachea (52% to 57%), bronchial airways (37% to 40%), or lung parenchyma (3% to 11%) can be involved.[13] A fistula may also develop following radiation therapy for tumors involving either the esophagus or central airways.[4] Esophageal and lung carcinomas, lymphoma, tracheal, laryngeal, or thyroid malignancy, and mediastinal metastases are the most common malignant causes of ADF.[14,15] Large necrotic tumors with poor differentiation have a greater incidence of ADF development[16]; often fistulizing to the adjacent airway. Patient symptoms are related to aspiration, including pneumonitis, increased secretions, and choking spells.[4]

Table 1
Oncologic emergencies in the chest: spectrum of imaging findings

Clinical Diagnosis	Imaging Findings
Airway obstruction	Chest radiograph/CT: A large mediastinal mass may be seen causing tracheal compression or deviation. Bronchus cutoff sign that refers to abrupt termination of bronchus due to obstructing tumor is seen with collapse/atelectasis of distal lung.
Aerodigestive fistula	Chest radiograph/CT: Recurrent pulmonary opacities can be seen due to infection. Round opacity with air-fluid level suggests lung abscesses. CT is highly sensitive in showing abnormal communication between esophagus and airway.
Superior vena cava syndrome	Chest radiograph may show superior mediational widening. CECT can show SVC obstruction due to direct infiltration from mediastinal/bronchogenic tumor or luminal thrombus within the IVC from distant primary cancer, and multiple collateral vessels over the chest wall.
Massive hemoptysis	Chest radiograph can show nonspecific acinar opacities due hemorrhagic mass. CECT will show mass lesion and CT angiogram may also show site of active bleed (pseudoaneurysm).
Pulmonary thromboembolism	CT angiogram will show filling defects in main pulmonary artery and branches, with peripheral contrast, "tram track appearance."
Cardiac tamponade	Chest radiograph will show enlarged cardiac silhouette, "water bottle" appearance. CT show high-density pericardial effusion with compression of cardiac chambers.
Spinal cord compression	CT/MRI shows soft-tissue mass causing collapse of vertebral body with epidural extension and compression of thecal sac/cord. MRI is more sensitive in showing marrow infiltration and showing extent of tumor infiltration into the spinal canal

CT is beneficial for identifying ADF as it can show areas of esophageal thickening and associated loss of fat planes with the adjacent airways. Direct communication may be seen as linear air density tracts that traverse between the trachea and esophagus (Fig. 6). Virtual CT endoscopy can help detect the site and size of the fistulae.[4] On chest radiographs, recurrent pulmonary opacities, lung abscess, and pleural effusions may point to ADF.[17] Fluoroscopy can show the passage of ingested contrast material into the airways. Although iso-osmolar water-soluble contrast can be used, high osmolar water-soluble contrast material should not be administered, given the substantial risk of developing bronchial irritation and pulmonary edema.[18]

The presence of ADF in oncologic patients carries a worse prognosis, even following treatment, which in most cases is limited to palliative care.[16] Metallic stents placed by interventional gastroenterology (GI) service may provide a safe and effective palliative option. Other options include esophageal bypass or exclusion, chemoradiation therapy, and in exceptional cases, fistula resection.[12,13] CT is the best imaging technique to assess potential post-treatment complications such as stent migration, fracture, or tracheal stenosis.[4]

Superior vena cava syndrome SVC syndrome refers to increased retrograde pressure in the venous system draining into the SVC from the head, neck, and upper extremities, due to external compression or invasion of the SVC, with a majority of cases due to malignancy, lung cancer being most common (50% to 80%), followed by non-Hodgkin's lymphoma (20%).[19,20] Mediastinal lymphadenopathy, germ cell tumors, and malignant thymomas are other potential causes.[19] The most common symptoms are facial flushing,

Table 2
Oncologic emergencies in the abdomen and pelvis: spectrum of imaging findings

Uncontrolled intraabdominal hemorrhage	CT can show ruptured tumor with perilesional hematoma (sentinel clot) and high-density ascites. CT angiography is excellent to show active extravasation of contrast (active hemorrhage) on arterial phase and blush on delayed phase.
Intestinal emergencies (bowel obstruction, ischemia, perforation, and intussusception)	Abdominal radiograph/CT show dilated bowel loops with air-fluid levels and may show related complications including pneumatosis and pneumoperitoneum, in severe cases. CT shows sight of obstruction and the obstructing mass.
Hepatobiliary emergencies	Ultrasound/CT/MRI show dilated intra and or extrahepatic biliary ducts and may reveal the obstructing mass. Thickened enhancing ductal walls suggest cholangitis, from superimposed infection. Multiple rim-enhancing liver lesions suggest hepatic abscesses, showing diffusion restriction on MRI.
Urinary tract obstruction	Ultrasound/CT shows hydronephrosis ± hydroureter and obstructing pelvic mass. Urothelial thickening from infiltrating tumors or a intraluminal polypoid lesion along the urinary tract can be seen on CT Urogram.
Torsion	Ultrasound and CT can show a large mass, most commonly arising in pelvis, with twisting at the vascular pedicle. The mass may appear heterogeneous due to hemorrhage and necrosis.

erythema, edema of the head, neck, and thorax, and engorgement of draining veins.[20]

CT allows precise identification of the site and severity of obstruction, the obstructing lesion, and the presence of thrombus and collateral vessels.[2,20] On imaging, ill-defined soft-tissue thickening/mass compressing or invading the SVC is usually appreciated; tumor thrombus in the SVC may also be seen (Fig. 7).[19] Large chest and abdominal wall collaterals are well depicted at CT, with the most common collateral pathways, including the azygos-hemiazygos system, which then drain through the paraumbilical venous system and results in the "hot quadrate sign," with an arterial enhancement of segment 4A of the liver (Quadrate lobe) (see Fig. 7). Venography with subsequent venous stent placement by vascular interventional radiology is often helpful to decompress the venous collaterals.

Management with SVC angioplasty with or without stent placement is the treatment choice, especially in critical clinical conditions (Fig. 8).[19] Depending on the severity, surgical bypass or anticoagulation might also be used. The SVC syndrome classification system developed by Yu and colleagues[21] incorporates factors such as the severity of symptoms, likelihood of response to a particular treatment, and treatment of the primary lesion and is helpful in management.

Massive hemoptysis Massive hemoptysis is a life-threatening condition, arbitrarily defined as the expectoration of 300 to 600 mL of blood in 24 h; the majority (90%) are due to invasion of bronchial arteries, and a few (5%) due to invasion of pulmonary arteries, although both may coexist.[22,23] When associated with malignancy, there is increased mortality ranging from 60%, primarily due to asphyxiation rather than hypovolemia.[3,24–26] The most common cause is bronchogenic carcinoma, followed by bronchial carcinoid and endobronchial metastatic lesions from colon, breast, or renal carcinoma.[26] Another important cause is angio-invasive pulmonary aspergillosis, common in immunocompromised patients with cancer.[27]

CT helps identify the cause of the bleeding and parenchymal abnormalities, including ground

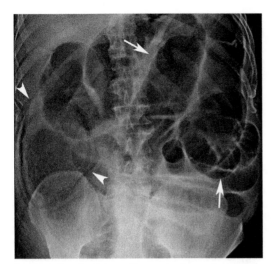

Fig. 1. Role of plain radiographs in evaluating patients with oncologic emergencies. A 63-year-old man with invasive sigmoid neoplasm presenting with bowel obstruction with pneumatosis. Plain abdominal radiograph shows dilated small and large bowel loops (*arrows*) with pneumatosis in the cecal wall (*arrowheads*), consistent with bowel ischemia, which was confirmed at surgical pathology.

glass opacities or focal consolidation. CT angiography can show contrast extravasation and pseudoaneurysm; identifying the source of bleeding is valuable to guide therapeutic angioembolization (**Fig. 9**). Chest radiograph shows focal airspace opacities at the bleeding site and underlying lung mass.[3,22,28] Unstable patients with rapid clinical deterioration require initial supportive and resuscitation measures followed by emergent bronchoscopy and bronchial artery embolization.[3,25]

Pulmonary thromboembolism PE can be seen in oncologic patients with an incidence of 1% to 2.5%, usually due to underlying hypercoagulability,

local tumor, or treatment (chemotherapy/radiotherapy) effects.[3,29] Gynecologic malignancies and melanoma are the two most common cancers associated with PE.[3] Tumor emboli can obstruct pulmonary capillaries leading to pulmonary artery medial hypertrophy and intimal fibrosis and resulting in irreversible obstruction.[30,31] Patients often present with pleuritic chest pain, dyspnea, tachycardia, and hemoptysis.[32]

CT chest with a special protocol for adequate contrast opacification of pulmonary arteries, two-dimensional multiplanar, and Maximum intensity projection reformats, is the gold standard for PE assessment.[33] Characteristic CT findings include acute angle formation between the thrombus and vessel wall, or "tram-track" appearance, referring to the presence of filling defects with peripheral contrast (**Fig. 10**).[32] The presence of multifocal dilatation and beading of the peripheral pulmonary arteries due to multiple small emboli, mainly in a subsegmental distribution with multilobar involvement, is a highly specific finding for tumor emboli.[34]

Anticoagulation is the mainstay of treatment. However, for patients with hemodynamic instability after fibrinolysis or contraindications for it or massive PE, thrombectomy and thrombus fragmentation are adequate options to decrease the overall burden.[35]

Cardiac tamponade Cardiac tamponade is a critical condition due to rapid fluid accumulation within the pericardial space causing increased intrapericardial pressures leading to decreased venous return and hemodynamic compromise.[36] A malignant etiology is present in up to 30% of cases, usually due to primary tumors infiltrating into the pericardium and pericardial malignancies such as mesothelioma or rhabdomyosarcoma,

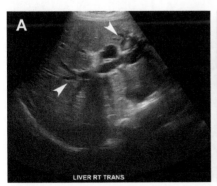

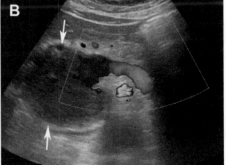

Fig. 2. Role of ultrasound in evaluating patients with oncologic emergencies. Axial grayscale ultrasound (*A*) and color Doppler (*B*) images of the right upper quadrant show dilated intrahepatic biliary ducts (*arrowheads*) and an enlarged porta hepatis lymph nodal mass, confirmed to be non-Hodgkin's lymphoma, which is the cause of biliary obstruction (*arrows*).

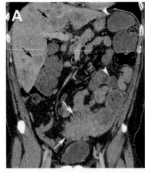
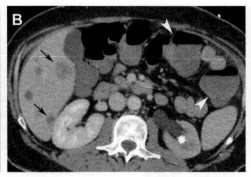
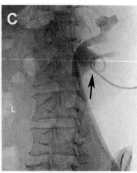

Fig. 3. Role of CT and interventional radiologist in evaluating patients with oncologic emergencies. A 40-year-old man with metastatic colon cancer present with bowel and urinary tract obstruction. (*A, B*) Coronal (*A*) and axial (*B*) contrast-enhanced CT images of abdomen and pelvis show an obstructing sigmoid colon cancer (*white arrows*) with dilated proximal small and large bowel (*arrowheads*), multiple liver metastases (*black arrows*), and left hydroureteronephrosis (star) due to ureteric obstruction. (*C*) Fluoroscopic image shows the placement of the nephrostomy tube (*black arrow*) by interventional radiology to decompress left hydroureteronephrosis.

metastatic disease commonly from lung, breast, and hematologic malignancies.[2,37,38] It may be secondary to radiation therapy or opportunistic infections due to the immunocompromised status of such patients.[2,39]

Echocardiography is the modality of choice for initial assessment and is excellent in assessing the cardiac tamponade's volume, location, and hemodynamic implications.[36,40] CT shows the extent of pericardial effusion and secondary changes, including narrowing and compression of the cardiac chambers (**Fig. 11**).[2,32,36,40] Intrinsic fluid characteristics such as thickening, septations, bleeding, or debris suggests malignant etiology. Enlargement of the cardiac silhouette with the classic "water bottle" appearance and mediastinal widening can be seen on plain chest radiographs.[39] Pericardiocentesis is the mainstay of

treatment, where pericardial fluid is promptly evacuated to decrease the pressure and avoid circulatory collapse.[2,4]

Spinal cord compression Malignant spinal cord compression (MSCC) is a dreadful complication in patients with cancer. It is characterized by compression of the spinal cord or cauda equina due to metastases or direct tumor spread, resulting in neurologic deficits.[41] It is seen in up to 10% of patients with advanced disease, most commonly involving the thoracic spine, followed by the lumbosacral spine.[2] MSCC is either due to spinal epidural metastases, most commonly from breast, lung, and prostate tumors, or to contiguous spread from tumors originating in the spine or extending from the paraspinal region, such as lymphoma, sarcoma, and lung cancer.[38] Back pain is the most common

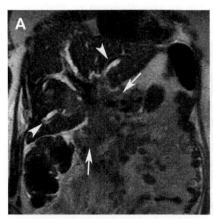
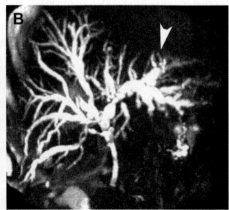

Fig. 4. Role of MRI in evaluating patients with oncologic emergencies. A 65-year-old woman with metastatic breast cancer causing biliary obstruction. (*A, B*) Coronal T2-weighted MRI (*A*) and 3D MRCP (*B*) images show a heterogeneous, moderately T2 hyperintense infiltrating hilar mass (*arrows*) causing biliary obstruction with dilated biliary ducts (*arrowheads*), confirmed to be metastatic breast carcinoma on cytology.

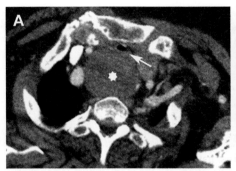
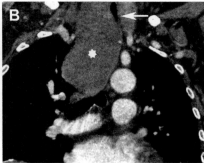

Fig. 5. A 57-year-old woman with metastatic poorly differentiated carcinoma of unknown primary resulting in airway obstruction. (*A, B*) Axial (*A*) and coronal (*B*) contrast-enhanced CT images of the chest show the large mediastinal mass (star) causing severe narrowing of trachea (*arrows*) resulting in central airway obstruction.

symptom to appear. Sensory deficits, focal motor deficits, and bowel and bladder dysfunction are other common symptoms.[38]

MRI is the gold standard for imaging patients with MSCC. It should include imaging the whole spine due to lesions at multiple levels with T1- and T2-weighted images acquired in the axial, coronal, and sagittal plane.[38] The use of intravenous (IV) contrast may improve the detection of leptomeningeal and intramedullary metastases; however, its use is optional. At CT/MRI, the most common finding is that collapsed vertebral bodies with associated soft-tissue spinal/paraspinal mass cause compression of the spinal cord/thecal sac (**Fig. 12**).[3,38]

Emergent treatment with IV corticosteroids can help improve symptoms by decreasing vasogenic edema and is indicated in all patients with suspected or diagnosed MSCC.[42] Radiotherapy and surgical decompression are valuable options for local management.[42]

Abdominal and Pelvic Emergencies

Uncontrolled intraabdominal hemorrhage

Severe intraabdominal hemorrhage is a rare, life-threatening complication, predominantly with hypervascular malignancies such as hepatocellular carcinoma (HCC), renal cell carcinoma, and melanoma.[43] A ruptured HCC is the third most common cause of death due to HCC after tumor progression and liver failure.[44] Tumors located in subcapsular locations, left lateral segments, right posterior segment, and caudate lobe have a higher risk of spontaneous rupture. Size of the tumor (HCC > 5 cm), increased tumor vascularity, vascular invasion, portal, and hepatic vein thrombosis, systemic hypertension, and intraarterial chemoembolization therapy are other factors that increase the risk of rupture (**Fig. 13**).[45] Spontaneous splenic rupture is a rare complication in patients with massive splenomegaly, with hematologic malignancies including leukemia

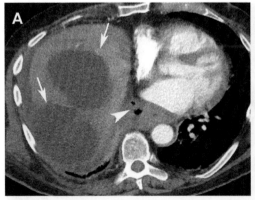
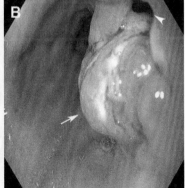

Fig. 6. Aerodigestive fistula (ADF) in a 76-year-old man with metastatic melanoma after pembrolizumab therapy. (*A*) Axial contrast-enhanced CT image of the chest shows multiple necrotic liver metastases (*arrows*) and suspected fistulous communication between the esophagus and right bronchial tree, (*arrowhead*). (*B*) Endoscopic image shows a large esophageal mass (*arrow*) fistulizing into the right bronchus (*arrowhead*), which confirmed metastatic melanoma.

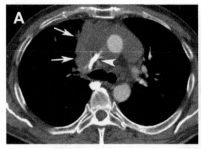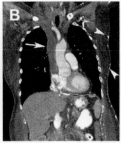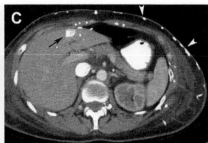

Fig. 7. Superior vena cava (SVC) syndrome in two different patients. (*A*) A 63-year-old man with lung cancer. Axial contrast-enhanced CT image shows a right lung mass infiltrating into the mediastinum (*arrows*) causing significant SVC compression (*arrowheads*) resulting in SVC syndrome (*arrow*), confirmed to be a primary lung carcinoma. (*B, C*) A 56-year-old woman with metastatic ovarian cancer and SVC syndrome. Coronal (*B*) and axial (*C*) contrast-enhanced CT images of the chest show bland thrombus obstructing SVC (*white arrow*) and resulting in multiple chest/abdominal wall collaterals (*arrowheads*) and focal hyperenhancement of quadrate lobe of the liver (*black arrow*) known as "hot quadrate lobe," features of SVC syndrome.

and lymphoma.[46] Acute tumoral bleeding can result from primary GI malignancies, such as adenocarcinoma, gastrointestinal stromal tumor (GIST), lymphoma, or direct infiltration of the GI tract from other primary malignancies or metastases.[47]

Multiphasic CT angiography is the diagnostic modality of choice to detect active bleeding and ascertain the source, type of bleed (arterial or venous), and its severity.[3] Acute hemoperitoneum is seen as high-density fluid on non-contrast CT, due to the high protein content of unclotted blood, with attenuation values ranging from 30 to 45 HU (see **Fig. 13**). "Sentinel clot," which refers to a hyperdense clot, provides valuable information about the source of the bleed (see **Fig. 13**).[2] Active extravasation of contrast, best seen as swirly/wiggly hyperdense contrast in the arterial phase, indicates active hemorrhage and may necessitate

urgent transcatheter embolization or surgical intervention (**Fig. 14**). Delayed phases may show a blush of contrast at the site of active bleed.[48]

Intestinal emergencies

Patients with abdominal/pelvic malignancies can present with acute abdominal pain and vomiting due to mechanical bowel obstruction, which may result in ischemic bowel or bowel perforation.[49] Malignant bowel obstruction is seen in approximately 3-15% of all patients with cancer with incurable primary abdominal cancer, the most common being ovarian and colon cancer, followed by stomach, pancreas, urinary bladder, and endometrium; or peritoneal carcinomatosis from the extra-abdominal primary.[49,50] It can be due to mechanical obstruction due to intraluminal masses or direct bowel invasion from adjacent tumoral masses. Abdominal or pelvic adhesions and

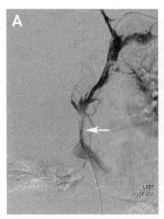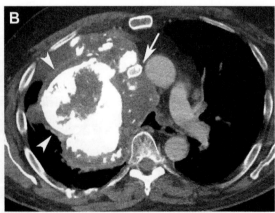

Fig. 8. A 58-year-old man with metastatic osteosarcoma resulting in superior vena cava (SVC) obstruction, requiring vascular stent decompression. (*A*) Venogram shows narrowed SVC (*arrow*) with multiple adjacent venous collaterals. (*B*) Axial contrast-enhanced CT image of the chest shows a large, calcified metastatic osteosarcomatous mediastinal mass (*arrowheads*) and the vascular wall stent within the SVC (*arrow*).

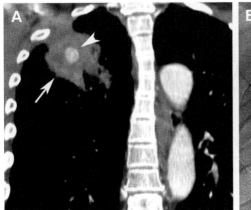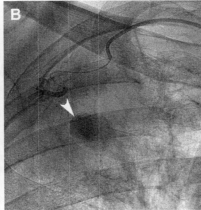

Fig. 9. Massive hemoptysis in a 54-year-old man with lung cancer. (*A*) Coronal contrast-enhanced CT image of the chest shows a right upper lobe lung cancer (*arrow*) with a pseudoaneurysm (*arrowhead*). (*B*) Conventional angiogram image shows the pseudoaneurysm within the right upper lobe mass (*arrowhead*), which was subsequently embolized.

post-irradiation fibrosis can cause bowel compression and resultant obstruction. A plain abdominal radiograph shows dilated bowel loops with air-fluid levels. CT is the modality of choice to characterize the level and severity of obstruction and identify the cause of obstruction (**Fig. 15**).[51] Bowel wall thickening, mesenteric fat stranding, and free fluid indicate increased severity of obstruction. Bowel wall hypoenhancement and pneumatosis suggest ischemia.[52] Mechanical small bowel obstruction may be treated by endoscopic placement of a self-expanding metal stent or enteric tube placement or may require surgical intervention.[53] Functional obstruction due to myenteric plexus involvement can be

seen in patients with peritoneal carcinomatosis, most commonly from breast cancer, melanoma, and lung cancer.[54] Paraneoplastic neuropathy in patients with lung cancer, chronic intestinal pseudo-obstruction (CIP), and paraneoplastic pseudo-obstruction are other causes of functional obstruction.

Bowel perforation is a life-threatening complication in patients with cancer due to acute bowel obstruction, tumor necrosis due to rapid growth, or after chemotherapy or radiation.[55] Spontaneous perforation is commonly seen with colorectal carcinomas and gastrointestinal lymphomas.[2] Abdominal radiographs, including upright chest and abdominal radiographs, are sensitive in

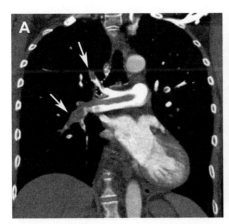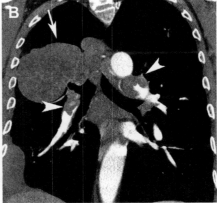

Fig. 10. Pulmonary embolism (PE) in two different patients with cancer. (*A*) A 45-year-old woman with pancreatic ductal adenocarcinoma. Coronal contrast-enhanced CT image of the chest shows PE in the right pulmonary arteries (*arrows*). (*B*) A 61-year-old man with metastatic neuroendocrine carcinoma. Coronal contrast-enhanced CT image of the chest shows multiple, large soft-tissue masses in the right lung infiltrating into mediastinum (*arrow*) with multiple thrombi (*arrowheads*) in bilateral pulmonary arteries.

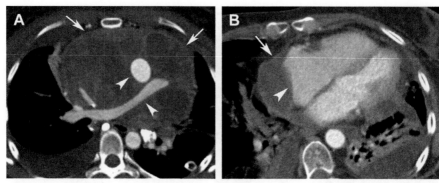

Fig. 11. A 38-year-old man with pericardial mesothelioma causing pericardial tamponade. (A, B) Axial contrast-enhanced CT images of the chest show a large heterogeneously enhancing pericardial mass (arrows) causing significant compression on cardiac chambers, pulmonary arteries, and aorta (arrowheads) consistent with pericardial tamponade.

detecting pneumoperitoneum.[56] CT is excellent in demonstrating small amounts of free air, site of perforation, and can suggest the underlying cause. Imaging findings include extraluminal air locules adjacent to the bowel wall, gas locules within the necrotic tumor, segmental bowel-wall thickening, adjacent fat stranding, extraluminal fluid, and leakage of orally administered enteric contrast (Fig. 16).[57] Rarely tumoral entero-enteric fistulas may be seen, in particular after targeted therapy.[2] Loculated fluid collections and possible abscesses can be identified, which may require CT-guided drainage.[55,57]

Bowel ischemia is a serious complication in oncologic patients, seen in 1% to 7% of colon patients with cancer, and can result in perforation.[58] Severe colonic distension from mechanical obstruction, thromboembolism, and chemoradiation are some of the mechanisms which can compromise bowel vascularity.[58] Plain radiographs may show bowel distension, gasless abdomen due to fluid-filled bowel, pneumatosis,

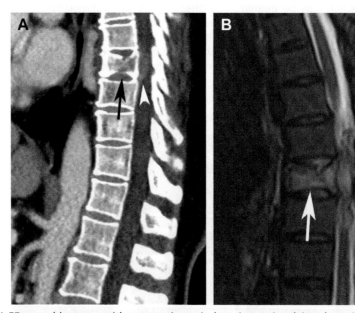

Fig. 12. A 55-year-old woman with metastatic cervical carcinoma involving thoracic vertebra causing spinal cord compression. (A) Sagittal contrast-enhanced CT image of the chest shows compression deformity of the T9 vertebral body (arrow), with epidural soft-tissue mass (arrowhead) causing thecal sac compression. (B) Sagittal T2-weighted MR image of the thoracic spine depicts compression deformity of the T9 vertebral body with heterogeneous mildly hyperintense marrow signal (arrow) and moderately hyperintense mass (arrowhead) in anterior epidural space causing thecal sac/spinal cord compression.

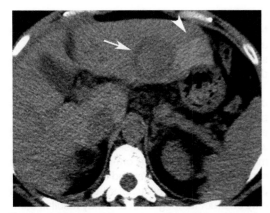

Fig. 13. A 63-year-old woman with combined hepatocellular carcinoma/intrahepatic cholangiocarcinoma presenting with spontaneous tumor rupture. Axial unenhanced CT image of the liver shows a hypodense mass in the left hepatic lobe (*arrow*) with an adjacent perihepatic hematoma (*arrowhead*) suggestive a "sentinel clot."

and portal venous gas. CT provides high diagnostic accuracy, detecting the intra-abdominal mass, demonstrating arterial or venous occlusion, bowel dilatation, mesenteric fat stranding, intramural gas (pneumatosis), mesenteric or portal venous gas, hypoenhancement of bowel wall (**Fig. 17**).[58] The ischemic segment can show thumbprinting, loss of abrupt transition, or prominent transverse ridging at the proximal end of the tumoral segment and may be better evaluated on CT.[58,59] Invasion of the mesenteric root by primary tumors such as pancreatic adenocarcinoma or metastases from neuroendocrine tumors or colon, breast, ovarian, and lung carcinoma can compromise mesenteric vessels and result in bowel ischemia.[2,58]

Oncologic patients can present with recurrent episodes of colicky abdominal pain and acute obstruction due to intussusception caused by the primary or secondary neoplasms of the GI tract acting as lead points.[60] Polyposis syndromes, including familial adenomatous polyposis and Peutz-Jeghers syndrome, can present with recurrent pain due to intermittent intussusception from multiple polyps affecting part or all of the gastrointestinal tract and are well characterized by CT or MR enterography.[61] Malignant intussusceptions with a lead point due to neoplasms such as adenocarcinoma, lymphoma, and metastases are more common in the colon than in the small bowel.[62,63] CT shows a target or sausage-like mass telescoping a bowel segment into the adjacent segment, with alternating low- and high-attenuation layers of intussusceptum surrounded by a thin rim of intussuscipiens, with or without mesenteric vessels and fat (**Fig. 18**).[64] Bowel wall thickening, fat stranding, and free fluid suggest increased congestion, ischemia, and developing bowel obstruction.

Hepatobiliary complications
Primary or secondary malignancies can cause biliary obstruction, which can be intra- or extrahepatic, and is a poor prognostic sign in such patients.[65] Pancreatic ductal and duodenal adenocarcinoma, pancreatic neuroendocrine carcinoma, and cholangiocarcinoma can cause extrahepatic biliary and pancreatic ductal obstruction near the ampulla.[43,65] Intrahepatic masses can cause biliary ductal dilation and include primary malignancies such as infiltrative HCC, cholangiocarcinoma, and widespread metastases from primary tumors of the colon, pancreas, breast, and lung (**Fig. 19**).[43] Biliary stasis from

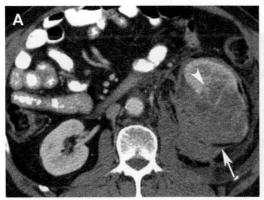
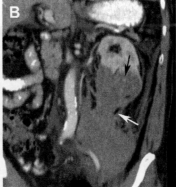

Fig. 14. A 60-year-old man with spontaneous rupture of the left renal cell carcinoma. (*A, B*) Axial (*A*) and coronal (*B*) contrast-enhanced CT images of the abdomen show a large left perinephric/retroperitoneal hematoma (*white arrow*) secondary to spontaneous rupture of the clear cell renal cell carcinoma of the left kidney (*arrowhead*). A focus of contrast extravasation is seen on coronal image (*black arrow*).

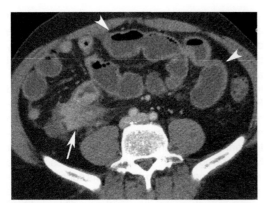

Fig. 15. A 54-year-old man with small bowel adeno-carcinoma presenting with small bowel obstruction. Axial contrast-enhanced CT image of abdomen shows a heterogeneously enhancing infiltrating soft-tissue mass (*arrows*) of the terminal ileum, causing small bowel obstruction with dilated loops (*arrowheads*).

chronic obstruction can cause superimposed infection and cholangitis.

Gallbladder cancer can masquerade as chole-cystitis and maybe with or without cholelithiasis or choledocholithiasis.[65,66] In advanced cases, infiltration into the adjacent liver parenchyma with biliary obstruction and gallbladder perforation may be seen.[65] On US, gallbladder cancer can present as a focal or diffuse mural thickening, non-shadowing polypoid mass, or a diffuse infil-trating mass of variable echogenicity.[67] On CT/MRI, a small gallbladder with diffuse wall thick-ening in patients with clinical signs of acute chole-cystitis, heterogeneously enhancing thickened single-layered gallbladder wall or a double-layered pattern with hyperenhancing inner layer and hypoenhancing outer layer can indicate un-derlying gallbladder malignancy (**Fig. 20**).[68,69] Immunosuppressive drugs and malnutrition can

predispose to acalculous cholecystitis.[3,65] In addi-tion, acute cholecystitis may be seen in patients after radio-/chemoembolization of liver tumors or stent placement or after select chemotherapy drugs.[3,65]

Patients with malignant bile duct strictures may develop secondary cholangitis that appears as biliary ductal wall enhancement on contrast-enhanced CT/MRI studies and may be complicated with cholangitic abscesses.[65] Self-expanding metallic biliary stents are often used for palliative care in patients with advanced cancer, obstructing the extrahepatic biliary ductal system. These stents may obstruct tumor growth and may result in com-plications such as cholangitis, pancreatitis, chole-cystitis, biloma, or abscesses (**Fig. 21**).[70] The presence of patchy parenchymal enhancement, arterial rim enhancement that persists through the portal venous phase, and perilesional hyperemia are some of the features of dynamic contrast-enhanced CT and MRI that strongly favor hepatic abscesses over metastatic disease.[71] Arterial rim enhancement may be absent in metastases, and when present, it shows fuzzy outer and inner margin, which disappears during the portal venous phase.[71] Metastatic lesions may show persistent rim enhancement on the transitional phase and appear hypointense on the hepatobiliary phase (HBP) when imaged with hepatobiliary specific gadolinium agents.[72] Ill-defined margin, absence of perilesional low signal intensity rim on HBP, and central hyperintensity in diffusion-weighted im-aging are more frequent with abscesses than metastases.[72]

Urinary tract obstruction

Urinary tract obstruction due to pelvic malig-nancies can cause acute renal failure and may require urgent decompression with nephrostomy tube placement.[73,74] Acute urinary tract

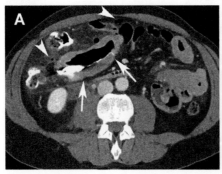
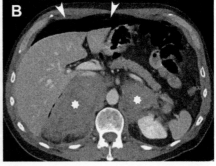

Fig. 16. A 46-year-old man with lymphoma presenting with small bowel perforation. (*A, B*) Axial contrast-enhanced CT images of the abdomen show a dilated small bowel loop with diffuse wall thickening (*arrows*) and pneumoperitoneum (*arrowheads*) due to spontaneous perforation of the small bowel lymphoma. Also note bilateral adrenal masses due to lymphomatous involvement of the adrenal glands (*stars*).

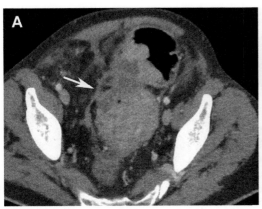
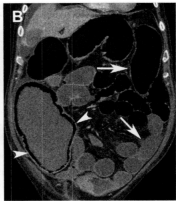

Fig. 17. A 63-year-old man with sigmoid colon malignancy presenting with bowel obstruction, and bowel ischemia. (*A, B*) Axial (*A*) and coronal (*B*) contrast-enhanced CT images of the abdomen show an enhancing bulky soft-tissue mass (*arrows*) involving sigmoid colon, causing small and large bowel obstruction with dilated loops (*arrows* in *B*), and pneumatosis of the cecal wall (*arrowheads*), consistent with bowel ischemia, which was confirmed at surgical pathology.

obstruction is one of the important treatable causes of acute renal injury in patients with cancer, most commonly seen with primary neoplasms of the prostate, bladder, uterus, and cervix.[73] Retroperitoneal metastases from the above primary malignancies, rectal, ovarian, and testicular cancers; lymphoma, and sarcoma can also cause ureteral obstruction.[73] Postsurgical fibrosis, radiation-induced strictures, and clots in the urinary tract, as seen with hemorrhagic cystitis, are other important causes of obstructive uropathy in these patients. Patients may present with complete or partial obstruction, unilateral or bilateral. Depending upon the tumor site, obstruction can be seen at the level of the renal pelvis, ureter, and bladder outlet. Ureters are commonly involved distal to the level of common iliac vessels.[74] Ureteral

obstruction can cause hydronephrosis, acute renal failure, and superimposed infection.

US is sensitive in detecting hydronephrosis and is often used as a screening modality. It may also show the retroperitoneal or pelvic mass lesion causing obstruction.[2] CT is highly sensitive and specific in patients with urinary tract neoplasms.[75] Noncontrast CT is often used in acute renal failure and can readily establish soft-tissue tumoral source of obstructive uropathy. If the patient can receive IV contrast, a CT urogram protocol with a 10-minute delayed urographic phase may show signs of obstructive uropathy, including asymmetrically enlarged hypoenhancing kidney, hydronephrosis with or without hydroureter, delayed excretion of contrast, and perinephric fat stranding (**Fig. 22**).[2] It also shows the level and severity of

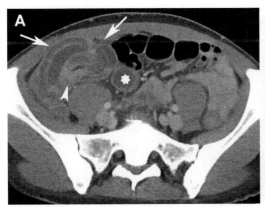
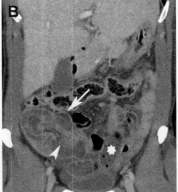

Fig. 18. A 41-year-old man with intussuscepting melanoma presenting with bowel obstruction (*A, B*) Axial (*A*) and coronal (*B*) contrast-enhanced CT images of the abdomen show ileocolic intussusception (*arrows*), multiple dilated small bowel loops (*star*), and enhancing soft-tissue mass in the ileum (*arrowheads*) confirmed to be melanoma as the lead point for the intussusception at surgery.

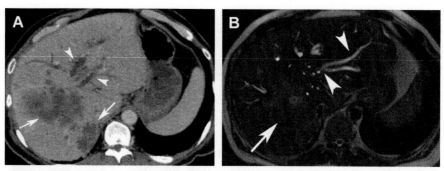

Fig. 19. A 50-year-old man with hepatic metastases from colon cancer-causing biliary obstruction. (A) Axial contrast-enhanced CT image of the liver shows heterogeneous hypoenhancing liver metastases (*arrows*) resulting in dilated intrahepatic bile ducts (*arrowheads*). (B) Axial T2-weighted MR image of the liver shows moderately T2 hyperintense hepatic parenchymal masses (*arrows*) and dilated intrahepatic biliary ducts (*arrowheads*).

obstruction and its cause. MR urography (MRU) is performed in some patients where high-resolution T2-weighted images, along with post-contrast images of the urinary tract in the excretory phase, can provide high-quality images to detect an obstruction and culprit tumor (**Fig. 23**).[76] MR is limited due to increased susceptibility to motion artifacts, low spatial resolution, and lack of widespread availability.[76] Most of these patients have advanced disease with poor prognosis and undergo palliative decompression with a percutaneous nephrostomy tube or a ureteric stent.[77]

Torsion

Tumors can potentially twist along their axis, resulting in acute pain, ischemia, hemorrhage, or rupture. Torsion is often seen with large pedunculated gynecological malignancies; the most common among those are benign ovarian teratomas, although it can also be seen with other benign and malignant neoplasms.[78,79] There have been cases of pedunculated GISTs undergoing torsion. US can show decreased Doppler flow in cases of ischemia.[80] CT will show a sizeable

hypoenhancing mass and twisted pedicle with inflammatory fat stranding and free fluid. Intratumoral edema with hemorrhagic infarction and tumor rupture can be seen.[80]

Treatment-related emergencies

Surgery, chemotherapy, and radiotherapy are the commonly used treatment options in patients with cancer and may result in select complications. Acute pancreatitis can be seen in patients treated with L-asparaginase for acute leukemia.[6] Multitargeted protein kinase inhibitors can cause pneumatosis (**Fig. 24**). Hepatic veno-occlusive disease, sinusoidal obstruction syndrome, can develop in patients treated with oxaliplatin therapy for colorectal cancer, presenting with hepatosplenomegaly and ascites.[81] Platinum-based chemotherapeutic agents used for gynecologic and genitourinary tumors are associated with thromboembolic events.[82] Patients receiving long-term chemotherapeutic drugs for leukemia or lymphoma and immunosuppressive agents for graft rejection can cause spontaneous gastrointestinal necrosis and perforation.[83] Spontaneous gastrointestinal perforation

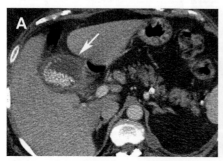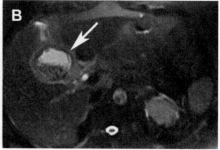

Fig. 20. A 72-year-old woman with gallbladder cancer presenting with acute cholecystitis. (A, B) Axial contrast-enhanced CT (A) and axial T2-weighted MR images (B) of the liver show dilated gallbladder with calculi and thick wall and pericholecystic fat stranding (*arrows*). Surgical pathology confirmed acute on chronic calculus cholecystitis with focal invasive, moderately differentiated adenocarcinoma.

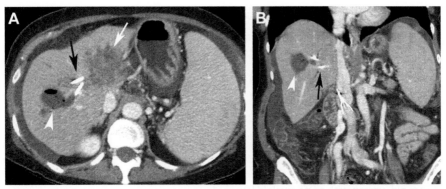

Fig. 21. A 66-year-old woman with intrahepatic cholangiocarcinoma, status post bile duct stents placement, presenting with acute cholangitis and cholangitic abscess. (*A, B*) Axial (*A*) and coronal (*B*) contrast-enhanced CT images of the liver show a left hepatic lobe mass (*white arrow*) with biliary stents (*black arrows*), and a cholangitic abscess in the right hepatic lobe (*arrowheads*).

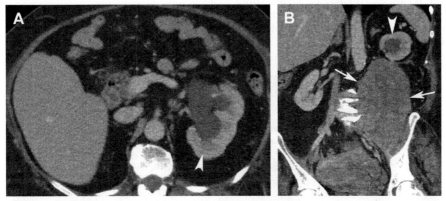

Fig. 22. A 65-year-old woman with retroperitoneal lymph nodal metastases from adenocarcinoma from unknown primary causing urinary obstruction. (*A, B*) Axial (*A*) and coronal (*B*) contrast-enhanced CT images of the abdomen and pelvis show a large left retroperitoneal lymph nodal mass (*arrows*) obstructing left ureter and causing moderate left hydronephrosis and decreased enhancement of the left renal parenchyma (*arrowheads*).

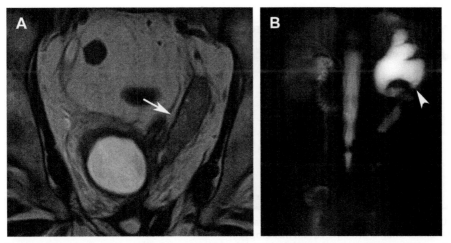

Fig. 23. A 67-year-old woman with urothelial carcinoma of the left distal ureter resulting in urinary obstruction. (*A*) Coronal T2-weighted image of pelvis shows a heterogeneously T2 hyperintense mass (*arrow*) in distal left ureter (*B*), confirmed to be poorly differentiated urothelial carcinoma on cytology. Coronal 3D MR urogram image shows moderate left hydroureteronephrosis (*arrowhead*).

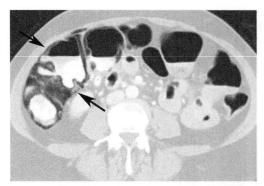

Fig. 24. A 64-year-old woman with acute myeloid leukemia treated with Midostaurin, a multi-targeted protein kinase inhibitor, presenting with abdominal pain. Axial contrast-enhanced CT image of abdomen shows air within the wall of ascending and transverse colon (*arrows*), with no associated mesocolic inflammatory change, features of benign pneumatosis, which subsequently resolved on follow-up imaging after stopping use of targeted therapy.

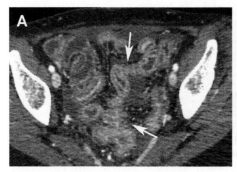 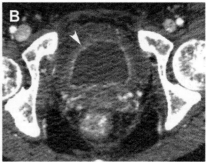

Fig. 25. A 25-year-old man with Ewing's sarcoma, undergoing radiation. (*A, B*) Axial contrast-enhanced CT of the pelvis shows diffuse mural stratification of pelvic ileal small bowel (*arrows*) as well as diffuse mural edema of the urinary bladder wall (*arrowhead*) consistent with acute radiation changes.

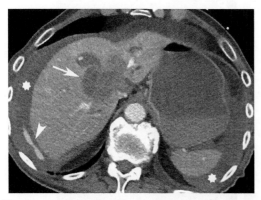

Fig. 26. Iatrogenic bleeding in a patient with intrahepatic cholangiocarcinoma after percutaneous biopsy. Axial contrast-enhanced CT image of the abdomen shows a left liver mass (*arrow*), active contrast extravasation in the perihepatic space and moderate amount of hemoperitoneum (star).

can also be seen in patients undergoing treatment for advanced colorectal cancer with Bevacizumab, a monoclonal antibody targeting vascular endothelial growth factor.[6] Antiangiogenic drugs may cause delayed anastomotic leaks, mainly if there is concomitant radiation therapy.[84] Patients receiving radiotherapy may develop various complications depending upon the area of exposure. Acute complications in patients receiving radiotherapy may include pneumonia, pleural or pericardial effusion, esophageal perforation or fistula, gastrointestinal hemorrhage, acute enteritis, mechanical bowel obstruction secondary to strictures, from bowel ischemia, and necrosis (**Fig. 25**).[85,86] Iatrogenic complications may develop after interventional treatment procedures, surgery, and central venous catheters placement for chemotherapy, including arterial injury with active bleeding, venous thrombosis, hematomas, and pneumothorax (**Fig. 26**).

SUMMARY

Patients with cancer can present with a variety of acute life-threatening conditions, which may be related to underlying malignancy or treatment-related. Select oncologic emergencies of the thorax, abdomen, and pelvis show characteristic imaging findings. It is essential for radiologists to be aware of such complications, be able to recognize them, and provide essential information to clinicians, which will guide them for appropriate clinical management.

CLINICS CARE POINTS

- CT is beneficial for identifying Aerodigestive fistula (ADF) as it can show areas of esophageal thickening and associated loss of fat planes with the adjacent airways. Direct communication may be seen as linear air density tracts that traverse between the trachea and esophagus. Virtual CT endoscopy can help detect the site and size of the fistulae.
- High osmolar water-soluble contrast material should not be administered during fluoroscopy to evaluate for ADF, given the substantial risk of developing bronchial irritation and pulmonary edema.
- "Hot quadrate sign," with an arterial enhancement of segment 4A of the liver (Quadrate lobe), is a sensitive and specific sign of SVC obstruction.
- Pseudoaneurysm in a lung mass suggest active bleed and cause of massive hemoptysis.

- The presence of multifocal dilatation and beading of the peripheral pulmonary arteries due to multiple small emboli, mainly in a sub-segmental distribution with multilobar involvement, is a highly specific finding for tumor emboli in pulmoary thromboembolism.
- Intrinsic fluid characteristics such as thickening, septations, bleeding, or debris suggests malignant etiology in patients with cardiac tamponade.
- Collapsed vertebral body with associated soft tissue spinal/paraspinal mass causing compression of the spinal cord/thecal sac, is highly suggestive of pathological fracture vs oestoportic fracture.
- Hepatic tumors located in subcapsular locations, left lateral segments, right posterior segment, and caudate lobe have a higher risk of spontaneous rupture. Size of the tumor (HCC > 5 cm), increased tumor vascularity, vascular invasion, portal, and hepatic vein thrombosis, systemic hypertension, and intraarterial chemoembolization therapy are other factors that increase the risk of rupture.
- "Sentinel clot," which refers to a hyperdense clot, provides valuable information about the source of the bleed. Active extravasation of contrast, best seen as swirly/wiggly hyperdense contrast in the arterial phase, indicates active hemorrhage and may necessitate urgent transcatheter embolization or surgical intervention.
- CT provides high diagnostic accuracy in bwel ischemia, detecting the intra-abdominal mass, demonstrating arterial or venous occlusion, bowel dilatation, mesenteric fat stranding, intramural gas (pneumatosis), mesenteric or portal venous gas, hypoenhancement of bowel wal.
- The presence of patchy parenchymal enhancement, arterial rim enhancement that persists through the portal venous phase, and perilesional hyperemia are some of the features of dynamic contrast-enhanced CT and MRI that strongly favor hepatic abscesses over metastatic disease.
- Spontaneous gastrointestinal perforation can also be seen in patients undergoing treatment for advanced colorectal cancer with Bevacizumab, a monoclonal antibody targeting vascular endothelial growth factor.

REFERENCES

1. Sung H, Ferlay J, Siegel RL, et al. Global cancer statistics 2020: GLOBOCAN estimates of incidence and mortality worldwide for 36 cancers in 185 countries. CA: a Cancer J Clinicians 2021;71(3):209–49.

2. Katabathina VS, Restrepo CS, Cuellar SLB, et al. Imaging of oncologic emergencies: what every radiologist should know. RadioGraphics 2013;33(6):1533–53.

3. Iacobellis F, Perillo A, Iadevito I, et al. Imaging of Oncologic Emergencies. Semin Ultrasound CT MR 2018;39(2):151–66.

4. Quint LE. Thoracic complications and emergencies in oncologic patients. Cancer Imaging 2009; 9(Special Issue A):S75–82.

5. Tirumani SH, Ojili V, Gunabushanam G, et al. MDCT of abdominopelvic oncologic emergencies. Cancer Imaging 2013;13(2):238–52.

6. Torrisi JM, Schwartz LH, Gollub MJ, et al. CT findings of chemotherapy-induced toxicity: what radiologists need to know about the clinical and radiologic manifestations of chemotherapy toxicity. Radiology 2011;258(1):41–56.

7. O'Neill SB, O'Connor OJ, Ryan MF, et al. Interventional radiology and the care of the oncology patient. Radiol Res Pract 2011;2011:160867.

8. Kohek PH, Pakisch B, Glanzer H. Intraluminal irradiation in the treatment of malignant airway obstruction. Eur J Surg Oncol 1994;20(6):674–80.

9. Zhao W, Yang Z, Chen L-A. [Etiological diagnosis and treatment of central airway obstruction: report of 40 cases and review of the literature]. Zhonghua jie he he hu xi za zhi 2011;34(8):590–4.

10. Chen K, Varon J, Wenker OC. Malignant airway obstruction: recognition and management. J Emerg Med 1998;16(1):83–92.

11. Hoppe H, Dinkel HP, Thoeny H, et al. Virtuelle Endoskopie der oberen, zentralen und peripheren Atemwege mit Mehrzeilen-Spiral-CT. Der Radiologe 2002; 42(9):703–11.

12. Reed MF, Mathisen DJ. Tracheoesophageal fistula. Chest Surg Clin N Am 2003;13(2):271–89.

13. Shin JH, Kim J-H, Song H-Y. Interventional management of esophagorespiratory fistula. Korean J Radiol 2010;11(2):133.

14. Giménez A, Franquet T, Erasmus JJ, et al. Thoracic complications of esophageal disorders. RadioGraphics 2002;22(suppl_1):S247–58.

15. Moree JS, Bhakta MG, Ledbetter J. Complication of mediastinal mass: acquired tracheoesophageal fistula associated with T-cell lymphoblastic lymphoma. Pediatr Pulmonol 2006;41(7):688–9.

16. Balazs A, Galambos Z, Kupcsulik PK. Characteristics of esophagorespiratory fistulas resulting from esophageal cancers: a single-center study on 243 cases in a 20-year period. World J Surg 2009; 33(5):994–1001.

17. Katabathina VS, Restrepo CS, Martinez-Jimenez S, et al. Nonvascular, nontrau-matic mediastinal emergencies in adults: a comprehensive review of imaging findings. Radiographics 2011;31(4):1141–60.

18. Morcos SK. Effects of radiographic contrast media on the lung. Br J Radiol 2003;76(905):290–5.

19. Eren S, Karaman A, Okur A. The superior vena cava syndrome caused by malignant disease. Eur J Radiol 2006;59(1):93–103.

20. Wilson LD, Detterbeck FC, Yahalom J. Superior vena cava syndrome with malignant causes. N Engl J Med 2007;356(18):1862–9.

21. Yu JB, Wilson LD, Detterbeck FC. Superior vena cava syndrome—a proposed classification system and algorithm for management. J Thorac Oncol 2008;3(8):811–4.

22. Noë GD, Jaffé SM, Molan MP. CT and CT angiography in massive haemoptysis with emphasis on pre-embolization assessment. Clin Radiol 2011; 66(9):869–75.

23. McCaughan BC, Martini N, Bains MS. Bronchial carcinoids. Review of 124 cases. J Thorac Cardiovasc Surg 1985;89(1):8–17.

24. Lordan JL. The pulmonary physician in critical care * Illustrative case 7: assessment and management of massive haemoptysis. Thorax 2003;58(9):814–9.

25. Jean-Baptiste E. Clinical assessment and management of massive hemoptysis. Crit Care Med 2000; 28(5):1642–7.

26. Wang GR, Ensor JE, Gupta S, et al. Bronchial artery embolization for the management of hemoptysis in oncology patients: utility and prognostic factors. J Vasc Interv Radiol 2009;20(6):722–9.

27. Rolston KVI. The spectrum of pulmonary infections in patients with cancer. Curr Opin Oncol 2001; 13(4):218–23.

28. Camargo JdJ, Camargo SM, Machuca TN, et al. Large pulmonary artery pseudoaneurysm due to lung carcinoma. J Thorac Imaging 2010;25(1): W4–5.

29. Storto ML, Di Credico A, Guido F, et al. Incidental detection of pulmonary emboli on routine MDCT of the chest. Am J Roentgenol 2005;184(1):264–7.

30. Bassiri AG, Haghighi B, Doyle RL, et al. Pulmonary tumor embolism. Am J Respir Crit Care Med 1997; 155(6):2089–95.

31. Roberts KE, Hamele-Bena D, Saqi A, et al. Pulmonary tumor embolism: a review of the literature. Am J Med 2003;115(3):228–32.

32. Carter BW, Erasmus JJ. Acute thoracic findings in oncologic patients. J Thorac Imaging 2015;30(4): 233–46.

33. Hui GC, Legasto A, Wittram C. The prevalence of symptomatic and coincidental pulmonary embolism on computed tomography. J Comput Assist Tomogr 2008;32(5):783–7.

34. Shepard JA, Moore EH, Templeton PA, et al. Pulmonary intravascular tumor emboli: dilated and beaded peripheral pulmonary arteries at CT. Radiology 1993;187(3):797–801.

35. Jaff MR, McMurtry MS, Archer SL, et al. Management of massive and submassive pulmonary embolism, iliofemoral deep vein thrombosis, and chronic

thromboembolic pulmonary hypertension. Circulation 2011;123(16):1788–830.

36. Spodick DH. Acute cardiac tamponade. N Engl J Med 2003;349(7):684–90.

37. Imazio M, Demichelis B, Parrini I, et al. Relation of acute pericardial disease to malignancy. Am J Cardiol 2005;95(11):1393–4.

38. McCurdy MT, Shanholtz CB. Oncologic emergencies. Crit Care Med 2012;40(7):2212–22.

39. Refaat MM, Katz WE. Neoplastic pericardial effusion. Clin Cardiol 2011;34(10):593–8.

40. Khan UA, Shanholtz CB, McCurdy MT. Oncologic mechanical emergencies. Hematology/Oncology Clin North America 2017;31(6):927–40.

41. Drudge-Coates L, Rajbabu K. Diagnosis and management of malignant spinal cord compression: part 1. Int J Palliat Nurs 2008;14(3):110–6.

42. Boussios S, Cooke D, Hayward C, et al. Metastatic spinal cord compression: unraveling the diagnostic and therapeutic challenges. Anticancer Res 2018; 38(9):4987–97.

43. Heller MT, Khanna V. Cross-sectional imaging of acute abdominal conditions in the oncologic patient. Emerg Radiol 2011;18(5):417–28.

44. Bassi N, Caratozzolo E, Bonariol L, et al. Management of ruptured hepatocellular carcinoma: implications for therapy. World J Gastroenterol 2010;16(10): 1221.

45. Sahu SK, Chawla YK, Dhiman RK, et al. Rupture of hepatocellular carcinoma: a review of literature. J Clin Exp Hepatol 2019;9(2):245–56.

46. Renzulli P, Hostettler A, Schoepfer A, et al. Systematic review of atraumatic splenic rupture. J Br Surg 2009;96(10):1114–21.

47. Zandrino F, Tettoni S, Gallesio I, et al. Emergency arterial embolization of upper gastrointestinal and jejunal tumors: an analysis of 12 patients with severe bleeding. Diagn Interv Imaging 2017;98(1): 51–6.

48. Artigas JM, Martí M, Soto JA, et al. Multidetector CT angiography for acute gastrointestinal bleeding: technique and findings. RadioGraphics 2013;33(5): 1453–70.

49. Tuca A, Guell E, Martinez-Losada E, et al. Malignant bowel obstruction in advanced patients with cancer: epidemiology, management, and factors influencing spontaneous resolution. Cancer Manag Res 2012;4: 159.

50. Anthony T, Baron T, Mercadante S, et al. Report of the clinical protocol committee: development of randomized trials for malignant bowel obstruction. J Pain Symptom Manage 2007;34(1):S49–59.

51. Li Z, Zhang L, Liu X, et al. Diagnostic utility of CT for small bowel obstruction: systematic review and meta-analysis. PloS one 2019;14(12):e0226740.

52. Millet I, Taourel P, Ruyer A, et al. Value of CT findings to predict surgical ischemia in small bowel obstruction: a systematic review and meta-analysis. Eur Radiol 2015;25(6):1823–35.

53. Ripamonti C, Bruera E. Palliative management of malignant bowel obstruction. Int J Gynecol Cancer 2002;12(2).

54. Campagna M-C, George M, Halm J, et al. Gastrointestinal emergencies in the oncology patient. In: Manzullo EF, Gonzalez CE, Escalante CP, et al, editors. Oncologic emergencies. New York, NY: Springer New York; 2016. p. 113–41.

55. Romano L, Fulciniti S, Silva M, et al. Imaging of Gastrointestinal Tract Perforation in the Oncologic Patients, . Imaging of alimentary tract perforation. Springer; 2015. p. 115–32.

56. Sureka B, Bansal K, Arora A. Pneumoperitoneum: what to look for in a radiograph? J Fam Med Prim Care 2015;4(3):477–8.

57. Hainaux B, Agneessens E, Bertinotti R, et al. Accuracy of MDCT in predicting site of gastrointestinal tract perforation. Am J Roentgenol 2006;187(5): 1179–83.

58. Rha SE, Ha HK, Lee S-H, et al. CT and MR imaging findings of bowel ischemia from various primary causes. Radiographics 2000;20(1):29–42.

59. Ko G, Ha HK, Lee H, et al. Usefulness of CT in patients with ischemic colitis proximal to colonic cancer. AJR Am J Roentgenol 1997;168(4):951–6.

60. Jasti R, Carucci LR. Small bowel neoplasms: a pictorial review. RadioGraphics 2020;40(4):1020–38.

61. Katabathina VS, Menias CO, Khanna L, et al. Hereditary gastrointestinal cancer syndromes: role of imaging in screening, diagnosis, and management. Radiographics 2019;39(5):1280–301.

62. Kim YH, Blake MA, Harisinghani MG, et al. Adult intestinal intussusception: CT appearances and identification of a causative lead point. Radiographics 2006;26(3):733–44.

63. Chiang JM, Lin YS. Tumor spectrum of adult intussusception. J Surg Oncol 2008;98(6):444–7.

64. Choi SH, Han JK, Kim SH, et al. Intussusception in adults: from stomach to rectum. AJR Am J Roentgenol 2004;183(3):691–8.

65. Kogut MJ, Bastawrous S, Padia S, et al. Hepatobiliary oncologic emergencies: imaging appearances and therapeutic options. Curr Probl Diagn Radiol 2013;42(3):113–26.

66. Lam C, Yuen A, Wai A, et al. Gallbladder cancer presenting with acute cholecystitis: a population-based study. Surg Endosc Other Interv Tech 2005;19(5): 697–701.

67. Gore RM, Yaghmai V, Newmark GM, et al. Imaging benign and malignant disease of the gallbladder. Radiologic Clin 2002;40(6):1307–23.

68. Liang J-L, Chen M-C, Huang H-Y, et al. Gallbladder carcinoma manifesting as acute cholecystitis: clinical and computed tomographic features. Surgery 2009;146(5):861–8.

69. Kim SJ, Lee JM, Lee JY, et al. Analysis of enhancement pattern of flat gallbladder wall thickening on MDCT to differentiate gallbladder cancer from cholecystitis. Am J Roentgenol 2008;191(3):765–71.

70. Venkatanarasimha N, Damodharan K, Gogna A, et al. Diagnosis and management of complications from percutaneous biliary tract interventions. RadioGraphics 2017;37(2):665–80.

71. Oh JG, Choi S-Y, Lee MH, et al. Differentiation of hepatic abscess from metastasis on contrast-enhanced dynamic computed tomography in patients with a history of extrahepatic malignancy: emphasis on dynamic change of arterial rim enhancement. Abdom Radiol 2019;44(2):529–38.

72. Lee C-M, Kang B-K, Kim M. Differentiation of small hepatic abscess from hepatic metastasis with a combination of imaging parameters. J Comput Assist Tomogr 2022;46(4):514–22.

73. Lahoti A. Nephro-urologic emergencies in patients with cancer. In: Todd KH, Thomas JCR, editors. Oncologic emergency medicine: principles and practice. Cham: Springer International Publishing; 2016. p. 273–83.

74. Allen D, Longhorn S, Philp T, et al. Percutaneous urinary drainage and ureteric stenting in malignant disease. Clin Oncol 2010;22(9):733–9.

75. Chlapoutakis K, Theocharopoulos N, Yarmenitis S, et al. Performance of computed tomographic urography in diagnosis of upper urinary tract urothelial carcinoma, in patients presenting with hematuria: systematic review and meta-analysis. Eur J Radiol 2010;73(2):334–8.

76. Sudah M, Masarwah A, Kainulainen S, et al. Comprehensive MR urography protocol: equally good diagnostic performance and enhanced visibility of the upper urinary tract compared to triple-phase CT urography. PLoS One 2016;11(7): e0158673.

77. Misra S, Coker C, Richenberg J. Percutaneous nephrostomy for ureteric obstruction due to advanced pelvic malignancy: have we got the balance right? Int Urol Nephrol 2013;45(3):627–32.

78. Eitan R, Galoyan N, Zuckerman B, et al. The risk of malignancy in post-menopausal women presenting with adnexal torsion. Gynecol Oncol 2007;106(1): 211–4.

79. Oltmann SC, Fischer A, Barber R, et al. Pediatric ovarian malignancy presenting as ovarian torsion: incidence and relevance. J Pediatr Surg 2010; 45(1):135–9.

80. Park SB, Kim JK, Kim K-R, et al. Imaging findings of complications and unusual manifestations of ovarian teratomas. Radiographics 2008;28(4):969–83.

81. Zorzi D, Laurent A, Pawlik T, et al. Chemotherapy-associated hepatotoxicity and surgery for colorectal liver metastases. J Br Surg 2007;94(3):274–86.

82. Weijl NI, Rutten MF, Zwinderman AH, et al. Thromboembolic events during chemotherapy for germ cell cancer: a cohort study and review of the literature. J Clin Oncol 2000;18(10):2169–78.

83. Reginelli A, Sangiovanni A, Vacca G, et al. Chemotherapy-induced bowel ischemia: diagnostic imaging overview. Abdom Radiol 2022;47:1556–64.

84. Deshaies I, Malka D, Soria JC, et al. Antiangiogenic agents and late anastomotic complications. J Surg Oncol 2010;101(2):180–3.

85. Benveniste MF, Gomez D, Carter BW, et al. Recognizing radiation therapy–related complications in the chest. RadioGraphics 2019;39(2):344–66.

86. Stacey R, Green JT. Radiation-induced small bowel disease: latest developments and clinical guidance. Ther Adv Chronic Dis 2014;5(1):15–29.

Starting an Emergency Radiology Division

Scheduling and Staffing, Compensation, and Equity and Parity

Marc A. Camacho, MD, MS, FACR[a], Jeffrey W. Dunkle, MD, FACR[b],
Rawan Abu Mughli, MD[c], Jamlik-Omari Johnson, MD, FASER[d],
M. Stephen Ledbetter, MD, MPH, FASER[e], Savvas Nicolaou, MD, FASER[f],
Aaron D. Sodickson, MD, PhD[e], Suzanne T. Chong, MD, MS, FASER[b],
Ferco H. Berger, MD, EDER, FASER, FESER[c,*]

KEYWORDS

- Emergency radiology division • Management • Scheduling • Staffing • Compensation • Equity
- Parity

KEY POINTS

- Emergent imaging volumes and complexity for acutely ill and injured patients and demands for rapid final report turnaround times continue to increase.
- Many practices have established emergency radiology divisions to cope with these needs, and many other departments are considering doing so.
- Establishing a new division of emergency radiology in a practice with long standing traditional operations practices poses both challenges and opportunities.
- A panel of experts share their experiences with establishing, growing and managing an emergency radiology division in a question and answer format.

INTRODUCTION

Emergency radiology divisions provide subspecialty care tailored to the unique imaging needs of acutely ill and injured patients. Emergency radiology mainly involves coverage of emergency departments, trauma centers, and urgent care centers,[1] supporting referring services such as emergency medicine, trauma surgery, acute care surgery and critical care services. The evolution has included a transformative change, one in which radiology faculty are routinely available 24/7/365, paralleling the approach taken by other specialties like emergency medicine and trauma surgery.[2]

Expert Panel questions and answers.
Authors in order of authorship, Ferco H. Berger is the corresponding author.
[a] Departments of Radiology, University of South Florida Morsani College of Medicine and Florida State University College of Medicine, and Radiology Partners/Radiology Associates of Florida, 2700 University Square Drive, Tampa, FL 33612, USA; [b] Department of Radiology & Imaging Sciences, Indiana University School of Medicine and Indiana University Health, IUH University Hospital, 550 N. University Boulevard, Suite UH 0663, Indianapolis, IN 46202, USA; [c] Department of Medical Imaging, Sunnybrook Health Sciences Centre, University of Toronto, 2075 Bayview Avenue, Room AG-58c, Toronto, Ontario M4N 3M5, Canada; [d] Department of Radiology and Imaging Sciences, Emory University School of Medicine, 500 Peachtree RD NE, Atlanta, GA 30308, USA; [e] Department of Radiology, Brigham and Women's Hospital, Mass General Brigham, Harvard Medical School. Brigham and Women's Hospital, 75 Francis Street, Boston, MA 02115, USA; [f] Department of Radiology, Vancouver General Hospital, University of British Columbia, 899 West 12th Avenue, Vancouver, British Columbia V5Z 1M9, Canada
* Corresponding author.
E-mail address: ferco.berger@sunnybrook.ca

Radiol Clin N Am 61 (2023) 111–118
https://doi.org/10.1016/j.rcl.2022.07.005
0033-8389/23/© 2022 Elsevier Inc. All rights reserved.

In academic models, emergent cases were historically covered during daytime hours by radiology divisions organized by organ system or modality, such as neuroradiology or thoracic imaging, and after-hours by in-house trainees. In that model, it was acceptable for the final report to be available the following morning after attending radiologist review.[3] Increases seen in emergent imaging volume and case complexity,[4–6] along with the increased demand for shorter turnaround times of final reports, has brought an emphasis to adapting this model to include after-hours attending radiologist coverage.[7] In the authors' experience, such a model contributes to successfully meeting these increasing demands, with resultant marked decrease of final report turnaround times[8] as well as a 90% decrease in the emergency department patient recall rate, thus indicating improved quality of service provision.[9]

In private practices, after-hours coverage was historically handled by radiologists performing call shifts. These radiologists typically held variable levels of subspecialization. Although private practice radiologists historically have interpreted a wider breadth of imaging examinations compared with academic radiologists, the trend in radiology is toward ever greater subspecialization and the subsequent increased proportion of time during daytime hours spent in narrower scopes of practice. This trend, when combined with the widening breadth and scope of after-hours imaging studies, has created a situation that may challenge comfort zones and competencies in the call model scheme.

In addition to these options, practices (academic or private) may opt to outsource some or all of their after-hours work to a teleradiology company. These companies may be based wholly within the United States, wholly outside the United States, or some combination thereof. They may provide preliminary or final reports, or a combination. They may charge the local practice fees per case interpreted or bill patients directly. In either case, the cost to the local practice is an important consideration. Another consideration is that remote teleradiology coverage may promote decreased interaction between the emergency radiologist and referring physicians, which can diminish one of the core benefits of on-site emergency radiology faculty.[3] Further discussion of teleradiology services is beyond the scope of this article.

This article assumes that a decision has been made to form an emergency radiology division. Some authors feel this is the most consistent manner to address emergency radiology coverage.[10] Regardless of practice setting type, the development of an emergency radiology division involves consideration of many different factors, focusing heavily on personnel and operational concerns.

Implementing 24/7 coverage is expensive and is typically only feasible in larger practices.[3] If the hospital or health system is mandating the creation or expansion of the clinical service, there may be an opportunity to negotiate an institutional financial commitment to offset the cost. If a decision to add after-hours staffing is being made by the radiology department or practice itself, efforts could be made to secure additional contracts to offset the cost, for example, by covering regional facilities and in effect operating as a regional teleradiology service. This latter approach may require additional investment in information technology and support if the remote facilities are not already within the radiology group's practice sphere. The demand for after-hours work uniformly outstrips the available supply of radiologists willing to work at night and market forces generally require compensation packages that reflect this reality for practices to recruit and retain with success.

After ensuring that a practice can afford to start an ER division, scheduling and staffing are two of the greatest challenges facing a new division. The practice scope and times of clinical service provision need to be determined. Essential scheduling and staffing questions to consider include: Is the service 24/7/365? Will the division cover daytime and evening hours only, evening and overnight only, or overnight only? Will staff be onsite, remote, or a combination? Will imaging be reported only for patients in the emergency department, with or without the inclusion of trauma and stroke patients, or also include inpatients and/or intensive care units?

Granular staffing considerations include determining the total number of shifts at various times of day needed to achieve parity within the rest of the radiology group, allowing for adequate recovery so that night work is sustainable and enables radiologist retention, and calibrating a good mix of onsite and remote reading capabilities to afford greater flexibility. Right-sizing staffing to imaging volume and expected report turnaround times typically requires a detailed understanding of the volumes and their variability, including volumes stratified by hour of day; this should include current data but also build in reasonable growth projections.

Although many early overnight staffing models followed the pattern of 7 consecutive shifts on followed by 7 consecutive shifts off (7 on/7 off), this model has fallen out of favor owing to concerns over sustainability and burnout, with 7 on/14 off now predominating in the market. With the ever-increasing literature regarding the deleterious health effects of overnight shift work and informed by the lived experiences of emergency radiologists in the last 20 or more years of experiences, some sites more recently have been rolling out 7 on/21 off overnight models. Many practices have shifted to shorter blocks of shifts worked more frequently. Alternatively, in the interest of long-term sustainability, some practices use a hybrid model in which radiologists work a mix of shifts throughout the 24/7 cycle, which decreases the overall burden of night work for each radiologist. The length of shifts can vary depending on need, but generally last 8 to 12 hours, with 8 to 10 hours predominating. Shift lengths of more than 9 hours and higher imaging volumes have been shown to significantly increase major interpretative discrepancies as well as degraded job satisfaction.[11] The effect of night shifts on cognitive function is in line with other professions, such as emergency medicine and nursing.[12,13]

Hiring enough radiologists to maintain coverage can be one of the biggest challenges when establishing a new emergency radiology division. Given the relatively early phase of emergency radiology as a subspecialty, even despite growth in number of fellowship programs,[14] the supply of emergency radiology fellowship trained providers is woefully inadequate to meet demand.[1,10]

Staffing emergency radiology divisions can be accomplished entirely with permanent positions or be supplemented by temporary or rotating positions via call coverage by daytime staff, independent contractors, and/or moonlighting radiologists.[1,10] The resulting division may consist of a composite of radiologists with emergency radiology focus and those with other areas of primary expertise. As mentioned elsewhere in this article, rotating radiologists from other subspecialties may not be comfortable covering the multisystem imaging performed in the emergency department.[1,10] Quality may also be an issue; a prior study has demonstrated considerable discordance between interpretations from subspecialized emergency radiologists and nonsubspecialized radiologists.[15]

When recruiting emergency radiologists, it is important to keep in mind that certain personality and sleep physiology traits can help some radiologists to thrive better than others.[5,11] Indeed, as most emergency radiology models include a substantial proportion of after-hours work, it is often beneficial to recruit self-designated "night owls" who tend to be more alert later at night. Emergency radiologists often thrive in the fast pace and adrenaline of the emergency department setting, and should generally be able to maintain calm demeanor in the face of a high-acuity and high-volume workload, and not be easily agitated or distracted.

Compensation methodologies for after-hours work are highly variable and include both monetary and nonmonetary components. These components may include regular salary and bonuses, as well as benefits such as insurance coverage, retirement, and business expense accounts. In the case of private practices and venture capital-backed practices, there may be a third element in the form of ownership through shares.[16] To account for the time needed to recover from the overnight work, after-hours radiologists should work fewer night shifts per year for similar or higher compensation than the number of day shifts other radiologists work. They also work disproportionately more weekends and holidays. The physiologic hardship of working after-hours on a regular basis, especially when past midnight and overnight to the morning, cannot be overstated. Even for night owls, staying up past 2 or 3 AM is physiologically unnatural. It is critical for the radiology practice to recognize that not all hours, nor all days, are created equal. The relevant stakeholders together should establish an acceptable conversion factor[17] that reflects the inherent differences in shifts to best achieve equity and parity in the group.

Finally, a successful emergency radiology division requires validation and endorsement from the department or group and from the institution. The emergency radiologists should feel just as valued as other radiologists in the practice. Creating an environment of equity and mutual respect is key in this regard. Otherwise, the practice may experience poor retention and the challenges of constant recruitment. Inconsistent service delivery may, in turn, lead to a poor relationship with referring services and the health care system. Emergency radiology divisions may themselves help to garner support from their own referring base. This support may manifest by showcasing the value of subspecialized emergency radiology expertise in the form of education, such as delivering grand rounds or lectures to emergency medicine residents, or via hospital committee service, such as trauma surgery and/or emergency department quality assurance committees.

To summarize, starting a new emergency radiology division requires the vision, time, money, and cooperation with other colleagues in radiology and referring services.[10] In the remainder of this article, a panel of experts shares their experiences and opinions on how to create sustainable and successful emergency radiology divisions. Items were discussed by the panel in a questions and answers format in multiple sessions of varying panel constitution. The report of these discussions below will focus on the challenges faced by existing departments in North America, with paragraphs that address a few key questions on topics of how to start an emergency radiology division, staffing and scheduling, compensation, as well as equity and parity with colleagues in their practices.

EXPERT PANEL QUESTIONS AND ANSWERS

Here, panelists share their experience gained over the past 3 decades by establishing, growing, and managing emergency radiology divisions at multiple institutions of varying type and size in North America and Europe. Paragraphs on specific topics detail questions that were discussed in multiple sessions with varying compositions of panelists. The questions are stated at the outset, followed by a synopsis and common themes in the ensuing discussions.

STARTING AN EMERGENCY RADIOLOGY DIVISION
What Is the Single Biggest Piece of Advice you Would Give to Someone Who Is Asking You How to Start an Emergency Radiology Division?

It is important to understand the driving forces necessitating after-hours coverage to ensure that those needs are being met. A hospital may have different needs (which are often focused around emergency department and STAT examination coverage) than the radiology practice (which may desire a clean worklist when the day shift arrives). Recruited members of an emergency radiology division may have an even different set of priorities. So, it is important to strategically consider and balance these differing needs. Many panelists cautioned against trusting that your excellent service delivery will, by itself, be sufficient for garnering sufficient institutional support to succeed. Aligning your plans with the priorities of the hospital system and practice will increase your likelihood of success.

It is also important to consider that future needs may change. For example, many emergency radiology divisions start out covering just nights, but eventually grow to cover 24/7/365. It is worthwhile to take this into account and to include this expansion as part of your planning. The panel agrees that it is important to set out a vision that can form the basis for a negotiated timeline for specific milestones, including the required number of people to staff that envisioned long-term model. It is important to use data analytics to support reasoning for these needs, and it is important to have a physician champion for the emergency radiology division who can lead these efforts.

Support from the other divisions in the radiology department is essential for success. The breadth of after-hours imaging can sometime exceed the skillset of emergency radiologists. It is in the best interest of the patients and the department to have systems in place by which emergency radiologists can consult their other subspecialty colleagues. Depending on the local setup, it may help to have emergency radiologists reciprocate and help cross-cover other divisions. This can broaden understanding and connections across the department, and cross-trained faculty can be ambassadors for the emergency room division in other areas.

Finally, it is important to not spend too much effort in trying to compare an after-hours position with a normal daytime job. It is best to consider it a different position entirely, with its own requirements, pros, cons, and so on.

What Would You Do Differently If You Had To Do It Over?

If staffing levels permit, it would be best to deploy a 24/7/365 model, allowing flexibility in scheduling day, evening, and night shifts, including some sort of shift count and/or compensation differential that values night shifts more than evening, and evening more than day time.

The panel uniformly described regret from those who initially deployed 7 on/7 off staffing models. These have all transitioned over time to other models, with 7 on/14 off predominating. This transition has not always been straightforward to implement, so it is best to avoid 7 on/7 off models for night coverage altogether.

In the negotiation to set up an emergency radiology division, be wary not to concede too much when it comes to matters of equity, parity, or recognition as a valuable and equal division in your practice. You may think that you will eventually be able to prove your value and regain what was lost. However, resources tend to be sparse in health care. So, you may instead find yourself permanently disadvantaged and without the tools and resources you need to create a stable group. Be sure to advocate for yourself and your division. Participate in practice governance and be sure to share your successes with departmental and health care system leadership.

What Are the Biggest Misconceptions or Hurdles to Getting a New Emergency Radiology Division Established?

One of the biggest misconceptions is the idea that emergency radiologists are simply general radiologists who work at night. However, this idea ignores the very specific expertise necessary to become an expert in trauma and emergency imaging, as well as the experience and skills necessary to be successful in an environment typified by high volume and high acuity. Additionally, emergency radiology benefits certain patient groups and their referring acute care teams, like trauma surgery, stroke teams, or emergency physicians. Emergency radiologists provide a dedicated counterpart to those services that fully understand their work environment and priorities.

Another misconception is that it is difficult to retain emergency radiologists for more than 1 or 2 years, especially when they have to work overnights. If practice leadership designs an emergency radiology division well, is responsive to the concerns of the radiologists, and is focused on delivering high-quality service, these divisions can thrive and turnover can be avoided. This notion is substantiated by the success of many divisions and the growth of the subspecialty. The common skepticism is similar to what emergency medicine went through as a specialty, though today it is among the most successful and popular specialties in medicine.

Do You Think It Is Useful to Mobilize the Referring Specialties and Were You Able To?

If your referring services, such as emergency medicine and acute care surgery, have not had any experience elsewhere with what emergency radiologists can offer, getting their support may be difficult. Once you have established the service and proven the added value as a dedicated counterpart, it becomes easier to find support from these services, especially when it comes to expansion plans. At that point, they become powerful allies, especially in advocating to hospital or institutional leadership. That said, it is uncommon for those other services to financially support emergency radiology divisions, even when they benefit most from the clinical service.

SCHEDULING AND STAFFING

What are Your Main Concerns for Scheduling and Staffing of Your Emergency Radiology Division?

Faculty member preferences vary with regard to which type of shifts they prefer to work, as well

as shift frequency. These preferences may change over time. It is important to be able to provide flexibility so that faculty wellness and retention can be maximized. This flexibility comes at the expense of schedule complexity, which can occupy a significant portion of a division chief's administrative time. It is important to be transparent as to how scheduling decisions are made and to be mindful of the importance of treating division members consistently and fairly.

The approach to scheduling days, evenings, and nights should be different. Dedicated night shift work requires more recovery time and associated longer off periods. The panel generally agrees that a model of 7-on/7-off (1-in-2) staffed by 2 dedicated overnight radiologists is unsustainable. In the last decade, the model of 7-on/14-off (1-in-3) staffed by 3 dedicated overnight radiologists has predominated for night shift work. Even that is now under reevaluation; some sites have begun offering longer recovery periods.

If insufficient attention is provided for recovery time and the well-being of night shift workers, it can prompt burnout and turnover. Practices deploying smaller cohorts of night shift workers may be at operational risk from this turnover. For example, an emergency room group of 3 faculty working 1-in-3, upon departure of 1 member, would immediately need to switch to 1-in-2. This situation could accelerate burnout in the remaining faculty, possibly leading to more departures and compromised care of patients.

Strict adherence to a 7-on/14-off model may also be suboptimal, because some faculty prefer shorter blocks of overnight shifts, whereas others prefer longer runs. In larger groups that incorporate evening shift and day shift responsibilities into the rotation with night shifts, decreasing the total number of nights per faculty member may improve sustainability.

A clear-eyed understanding of the job market and labor shortages should be a focus of emergency radiology leaders. Few if any of the panel members have ever experienced an extended period of being fully staffed. If economic conditions allow, it is worthwhile to pursue a model that is somewhat overstaffed to volume, realizing that this may never be fully achieved. This approach may have an added benefit of reducing the pressure on new or junior staff, allowing a longer grace period to increase their reading speed. Staffing to a level of 80% to 90% of what would be needed for peak volume has worked well for most panel members.

Do You Have Any Advice Around Recruitment and Retention, and Keeping Your Team Engaged and Happy?

To a large extent, the schedule considerations as detailed elsewhere in this article influence success in recruiting and retaining division members. With the subspecialty growing and the knowledge around the negative physiologic impacts of overnight work expanding, it is important to staff your division to such a level that burnout is prevented and flexibility is provided.

It is important to know what is happening in the job seekers' market so as to not be blindsided by changes you did not anticipate and are not prepared to counter. The impact of the coronavirus disease 2019 pandemic on radiology operations has even further emphasized how highly mobile radiology service provision has become. This is especially important to consider if you manage a smaller division, where the loss of 1 or 2 people owing to correctable factors in your model could compromise your division's survivability.

Good communication between leadership and division members is important, especially when it comes to assessing workload and how that impacts burnout. Using analytics to drive decision making can ensure that load balancing different shifts is successful and that groups do not become overburdened during certain coverage hours.

Emergency radiology divisions at institutions with training programs can leverage access to learners to develop a pipeline for recruitment. Ensuring that trainees have positive experiences on emergency radiology rotations can facilitate this. It is also helpful to advertise your good works. A social media presence and updated on-line content can be a draw to candidate pools.

Is There a Remote Work Component and How Do You Balance that with On-site Work?

Working remotely is a hot topic and the situation is in evolution nationwide. Many practices have deployed remote reading models to be able to cope with expanding volumes and a mobile workforce. Offering the ability to work from home (or from a different state) can assist with recruitment by broadening the pool of potential candidates. It can also assist with radiologist retention.

Before the coronavirus disease 2019 pandemic, remote work was uncommon in academic practices. Things have changed dramatically, with numerous radiologists now able to read from home, including emergency radiologists. The number of on-site radiologists is diminishing. Although initially there was more emphasis on taxing people who did not have to commute by asking to report

slightly higher case volumes, thinking has now changed to incentivizing the people that do work on site. This is reflective of additional on-site expectations for in-person staffing, including increased consultations and often training expectations.

There is a risk with moving too many readers off site. This practice may diminish the perception of buyin and availability, especially to referring services. Radiology technologists, as well as trainees, may feel insufficiently supported if their radiologists are not on site with them. Also, division culture is more difficult to maintain if people rarely work side by side with each other or get to interact in-person. Remote teleradiology has proven to be valuable tool and better video consultation tools likely have a place. That being said, there is unease in the panel about the increased numbers of remote-only radiologists in emergency radiology.

COMPENSATION
What are Your Thoughts on Compensation for After-hours Work?

Many practices that cover shifts during the day, evening, and/or night, have developed so-called conversion, or weighing factors for each shift, that recognize the sleep and other life impacts of working nonstandard hours. This process may allow flexibility to division members as to what they prioritize. If the weighing factor is expressed by differences in monetary compensation, people could, for example, work more days and fewer overnights for the same income. People working more nights do not have to work as many shifts to earn the same income, or could work more shifts overall to earn extra income. Alternatively, if the goal is to justify a lower number of total shifts per annum to earn a standard salary consistent with individuals with more traditional schedules, the conversion factor can help illustrate the equivalency of earning the same salary while working a lower number of shifts.

For purposes of equity, it is important to anchor the value of the daytime shifts to that of radiologists in other divisions (ie, the local market). Overnight shifts are valued more highly, and is largely dictated by the external market, insofar as value is determined by the number of radiologists required to cover a certain shift.

It can be difficult to get people who do not work nights to understand that time off after working nights is not vacation or typically productive nonclinical time. It is recovery time, and the need for such time is well-documented in the literature. This point has particular importance in discussions with leadership who, if not aware of these issues, may feel justified in offering compensation that is not appropriate. When trying to help leadership or other radiologists understand the need for adequate differential shift counts or compensation, many panelists have at some point implied: "If it is so easy to work overnights, please come and join our team."

One issue unique to private practices forming and maintaining after-hours emergency radiology sections is the question of partnership. In keeping with the themes presented elsewhere in this article, it is optimal for practices offering partnership to traditional schedule radiologists to also do so for those hired for after-hours emergency radiology coverage. Excluding those that provide this valuable service to the practice simply because they are working a sustainable and reasonable schedule reflects a lack of value for such work and could promote high turnover and a lack of sectional continuity.

To create acceptance of differing compensation models in emergency radiology, it may be helpful to create awareness that, although this practice may be perceived as unusual for radiology, it is quite normal in other disciplines, like emergency medicine and hospitalists services. Aligning staffing models and what defines full time effort with what is normal in these other shift work or nocturnal professions can be very helpful.

EQUITY AND PARITY
What Do You Believe Is the Biggest Challenge of Members of Your Team Being Treated Fair and Comparable to Other Radiologists in Your Group or Institution?

There are deficiencies in benchmarking in emergency radiology insofar as metrics do not differentiate between day and nighttime work, which can have very different relative value unit production. The fact that many emergency radiology divisions are also understaffed leads to an artificial overestimate of average relative value units and full-time equivalent production.

The panel is of the opinion that the services from emergency radiology divisions and their radiologists in general are undervalued in many practices, not necessarily from a monetary point of view, but in terms of respect and consideration of their value as a subspecialty. Additionally, the lack of understanding about the need for recovery time for night shift workers is an ongoing challenge.

Are Chances for Research, Promotion, Management, and a Reasonable Work–Life Balance Equal to Other Radiologists in Your Group or Institution?

Especially in divisions where there is a major component of nighttime work, it is very difficult to fulfill academic roles in research, education and management. This hampers promotion of academic ranks. However, it is important to assign tasks to division members to lead components of the division as directors (eg, education, research, quality, fellowship), provided you have been able to hire the right candidates for those positions.

DISCLOSURE

The authors do have no disclosures relevant to the content of this article.

REFERENCES

1. Robinson JD, Gross JA, Cohen WA, et al. Operational considerations in emergency radiology. Semin Roentgenol 2020;55(2):83–94.
2. Scheinfeld MH, Dym RJ. Update on establishing and managing an overnight emergency radiology division. Emerg Radiol 2021;28(5):993–1001.
3. Dunkle J, Jackson VP. Special Focus—outsourcing after hours radiology: a third point of view—twenty-four-hour attending radiology coverage: physical, financial, and educational issues. J Am Coll Radiol 2007;4(10):678–9.
4. Chaudhry S, Dhalla I, Lebovic G, et al. Increase in utilization of afterhours medical imaging: a study of three Canadian academic centers. Can Assoc Radiol J 2015;66(4):302–9.
5. Rohatgi S, Hanna TN, Sliker CW, et al. After-hours radiology: challenges and strategies for the radiologist. Am J Roentgenol 2015;205(5):956–61.
6. Bruls RJM, Kwee RM. Workload for radiologists during on-call hours: dramatic increase in the past 15 years. Insights Imaging 2020;11(1):121.
7. Chong ST, Robinson JD, Davis MA, et al. Emergency radiology: current challenges and preparing for continued growth. J Am Coll Radiol 2019;16(10):1447–55.
8. Mughli RA, Durrant E, Medeiros DTB, et al. Overnight attending radiologist coverage decreases imaging-related emergency department recalls by at least 90. Emerg Radiol 2021;28(3):549–55.
9. Medeiros DTB, Durrant E, Carter M, et al. The impact of overnight in-house attending radiologist coverage on emergency imaging turnaround times during night and next morning. Presented at American Society of Emergency Radiology Annual Meeting and Postgraduate Course, September 11-14, 2019, Scottsdale, AZ.
10. Mueller CF, Yu JS. The concept of a dedicated emergency radiology section: justification and blueprint. Am J Roentgenol 2002;179(5):1129–31.
11. Hanna TN, Lamoureux C, Krupinski EA, et al. Effect of shift, schedule, and volume on interpretive

accuracy: a retrospective analysis of 2.9 million radiologic examinations. Radiology 2017;287(1):205–12.

12. Dula DJ, Dula NL, Hamrick C, et al. The effect of working serial night shifts on the cognitive functioning of emergency physicians. Ann Emerg Med 2001;38(2):152–5.

13. Niu SF, Chu H, Chen CH, et al. A comparison of the effects of fixed- and rotating-shift schedules on nursing staff attention levels. Biol Res Nurs 2013;15(4):443–50.

14. Kennedy P, Vijayasarathi A, Hamid S, et al. Canadian and American emergency radiology fellowship websites: an evaluation of content. Curr Probl Diagn Radiol 2021;50(5):576–9.

15. Robinson JD, Linnau KF, Hippe DS, et al. Accuracy of outside radiologists' reports of computed tomography exams of emergently transferred patients. Emerg Radiol 2018;25(2):169–73.

16. Abbott R., Running a busy private practice emergency radiology service. RC208 Hot Topics in Emergency Radiology Practice. Presented at: 106th Scientific Assembly and Annual Meeting of the Radiological Society of North America, November 29. 2020, Chicago, IL (Virtual).

17. Knaub J. Partner compensation — changing radiology practice may call for changing income division strategy.pdf. Radiol Today 2013;14(9):16. Available at: https://www.radiologytoday.net/archive/rt0913p16.shtml. Accessed June 12, 2022.

Understanding Ballistic Injuries

Noah Ditkofsky, MD, FRCPC*, Jaykumar Raghavan Nair, MD, Yigal Frank, MD,
Shobhit Mathur, MD, Bipin Nanda, MD, Robert Moreland, MD, FRCPC, Jessica A. Rotman, MD

KEYWORDS

• Gunshot wound • RIP • GSW • Bullet • Lead arthropathy • Plumbism • MRI

INTRODUCTION

Ballistic injuries do not discriminate. They are observed in all age groups (including the unborn[1]) and all practice environments.[2,3] In 2016, ballistic trauma resulted in an estimated 276,000 deaths[3] worldwide, and it is impossible to estimate the number of injuries, as many may go unreported. It is consequently reasonable to assume that most radiologists will encounter ballistic trauma at some point in their career.

Ballistic Projectile Types

Ballistic projectiles can be broken down into two broad categories: those discharged from rifles and handguns and those discharged from shotguns. Shotguns fire "pellets," which are effectively small ball bearings (**Fig. 1**) that are most commonly composed of lead or steel.[4] Rifle and handgun rounds are commonly composed of one or a combination of lead, copper, and steel and have a variety of designs.[5–9] The most encountered bullet designs in clinical practice are as follows (**Fig. 2**):

- Lead bullets (LBs): Composed entirely of lead, these bullets deform and fragment as they pass through tissues.
- Full metal jacket (FMJ): A lead core clad in a copper or steel jacket. These bullets are designed to remain intact and penetrate through targets with little if any deformation.
- Semijacketed (SJ): A lead core partially clad with copper, having an exposed lead tip. These bullets are designed to spread and flatten or "mushroom" at the front, resulting in a deformed bullet with an increased surface area and less penetration. These bullets, in practice, often shed pieces as they pass through tissues and can be recognized on radiographs by their debris trail composed of high-density lead and lower-density copper.
- Controlled deformation (CD): Composed of copper, or lead and copper, sometimes with a polymer tip. These bullets are designed to deform and fragment in a controlled manner, leading to characteristic radiographic appearances. At present, the most commonly encountered CD bullet is the radically invasive projectile (RIP) bullet (G2 research) that is composed entirely of copper and breaks into components consisting of a base and several trocars that spiral away from the bullet base.

Mechanism of Wounding

Trauma is generally categorized as blunt or penetrating, with a gunshot wound (GSW) usually included in the latter. However, GSWs are a unique form of injury that has features of both blunt and penetrating trauma and should be separately characterized as "missile injury". When a bullet passes through tissue, it converts its kinetic energy into injury as it crushes and emulsifies the tissues that it directly contacts creating what is known as the permanent cavity.[10] The shape of the permanent cavity is dictated by the orientation and flight stability of the bullet at the point of contact. When bullets are fired, their initial orientation is such that their long axis is nearly perfectly aligned to the direction of flight. However, owing to imperfections in the bullet, over time that bullet will begin to yaw about its direction of flight and eventually it

Division of Emergency, Trauma & Acute Care Radiology, St. Michael's Hospital, 36 Queen Street East, Toronto, Ontario M5B 1W, Canada
* Corresponding author.
E-mail address: ditkofsky@gmail.com

Radiol Clin N Am 61 (2023) 119–128
https://doi.org/10.1016/j.rcl.2022.08.005
0033-8389/23/© 2022 Elsevier Inc. All rights reserved.

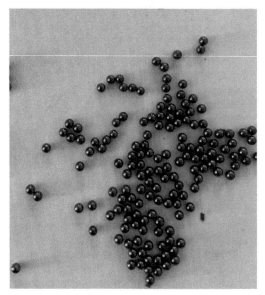

Fig. 1. Shot pellets.

are exceeded, injuries occur. Consequently, highly elastic tissues such as the bowel and the lung are more resistant to temporary cavity-related injury in contrast to relatively inelastic tissues such as the liver.[13]

Bullet construction also contributes to the mechanism of wounding. FMJ bullets are designed to stay intact, causing less of a secondary cavity than SJ bullets or CD bullets. SJ bullets are designed to increase their surface area on contact, which maximizes the diameter of the primary cavity, resulting in greater tissue destruction than would have resulted had the bullet not deformed.[12] This expansion also results in the deposition of a larger volume of energy for a given depth of penetration and a larger temporary cavity.

Imaging Gunshot Wounds

There are two roles for radiology in the management of acute GSW. The first is identifying and characterizing ballistic injuries. The second is vascular intervention to control bleeding and rarely to retrieve an intravascular bullet or shotgun pellet.[14–17] In this article, the authors will focus on the former.

Radiographs are usually the first imaging modality deployed in the evaluation of GSW. Although two orthogonal views will provide the most information, it is more common to acquire only a single view projection using portable techniques. In patients who are hemodynamically unstable, radiographs may be the only preoperative imaging that is performed.

will begin to tumble.[6,10,11] This tumble will be exaggerated by contact with tissues. The consequence of this is permanent cavities that are shaped somewhere between a cylinder and an ellipse.[12]

However, the permanent cavity is only half the story. As the bullet expands its kinetic energy, a "shock wave" known as the secondary or temporary cavity occurs around the permanent cavity. This temporary cavity is the result of tissues stretching before snapping back to their normal configuration. When the elastic limits of tissue

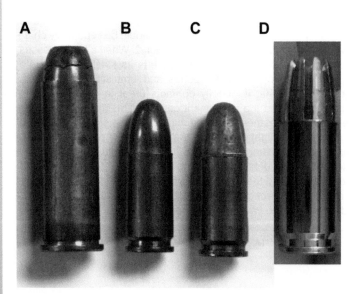

Fig. 2. Commonly encountered bullet constructions include semi-jacketed (*A*), full metal jacketed (*B*) lead (*C*). Less commonly encountered are controlled deformation bullets such as the RIP bullet (*D*).

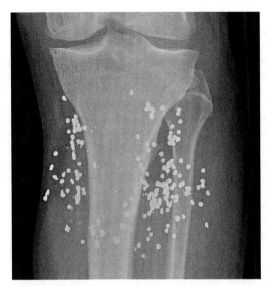

Fig. 3. Multiple shotgun pellets in the soft tissue of the upper calf. Note that many of these are no longer round but are broken or deformed. This is characteristic of a bullet shot composed of lead.

The first step in the analysis of ballistic injuries is identifying the number and location of entry/exit wounds and the number of retained bullets. This requires close coordination with the trauma team and is best achieved by marking each entry/exit site with a BB, a nipple marker, surgical gauze containing a radiopaque marker or an unfolded paperclip on the skin surface. Our institutional preference is an unfolded paperclip, as marking entry/exit sites with BBs or nipple markers can cause confusion in cases of patients who have been shot with shotgun pellets. In addition, in a patient imaged with overlying support apparatus, it is easy to overlook or have support apparatus obscure, a small BB or the marker in surgical gauze. Once each entry/exit wound has been marked, the second step is to apply the "even number rule."[18] Simply stated, the number of entry wounds, exit wounds, and retained bullets/debris fields should be an even number. An odd number implies that there is an unaccounted-for entry/exit wound or a bullet has traveled beyond the imaged region and additional radiographs encompassing a larger field of view should be acquired.[19] Rarely, two bullets entering/exiting at the same location or a vascular bullet embolism (with the bullet lying outside the imaged region) may also result in an odd number. Our experience has been that as simple as the even number rule sounds, it can be devilishly difficult to apply in cases where multiple fragmenting bullets are partially retained within the patient. In these cases, analysis of the scout computerized tomographic

(CT) image and the large field of view it provides may provide a better overview than the limited field of view afforded by trauma bay radiographs. It is important at this juncture to define a "through and through" wound as those in which ballistic material passes through the patient instead of being wholly retained.

Analysis of the plain films and scout CT images is also useful in assessing the type of bullet or pellets with which the patient has been injured . Shotgun pellets can be readily differentiated from bullets as they appear quite different. Shotgun pellets are usually multiple and appear as small rounded metallic densities (**Fig. 3**). The important thing to note on the radiograph is whether the individual pellets have deformed. Deformed pellets imply that they are composed of lead and are consequently nonferromagnetic. Undeformed shotgun pellets imply that they are composed of steel and are likely magnetic.[20] Bullets that remain intact and undeformed are typically FMJ construction (**Fig. 4**). Although many FMJ bullets are composed of copper-clad lead, some are constructed of steel-clad lead, and differentiating between the two requires using CT techniques, which are at the time of writing, still experimental.[21–27] SJ bullets have a variety of designs but are all composed of a lead core with partial copper cladding. The exposed lead tip expands or mushrooms on contact and the bullet increases its surface area. On imaging these bullets can be identified by the "three Ds": deformation, disintegration, and debris (**Fig. 5**). When these bullets disintegrate, it is often possible to differentiate the lower-density copper jacket, from the higher-density lead core. CD bullets are designed to deform and fragment in predictable ways and can consequently be recognized by characteristic deformation patterns. At present, the most commonly encountered CD bullet in our experience is the "RIP bullet" and consequently the authors will focus our discussion on this bullet. RIP bullets are composed entirely of copper and are constructed with a base and trocars. The trocars are designed to separate and spiral out from the bullet base resulting in multiple primary cavities.[7,28] These bullets can be readily identified by the characteristic appearance of the separated trocars (**Fig. 6**).

CT is the gold standard in imaging ballistic injuries. Its high spatial and anatomic resolution allows for the analysis of ballistic trajectories as well as the identification of end-organ injuries. All patients with GSW undergoing CT should be imaged using a metal artifact reduction algorithm if possible. These algorithms decrease the corrupt projection data resulting from metal bullets

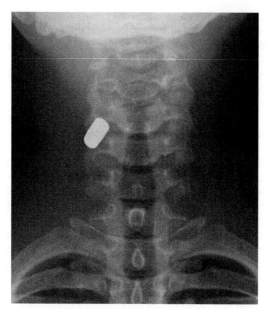

Fig. 4. A full metal jacket bullet within the soft tissues of the neck. Note that the bullet is not deformed or accompanied by any debris.

attenuating photons, consequently reducing artifacts.[29,30] GSW to the head and neck region should be imaged with a noncontrast head CT followed by CT angiography (CTA) of the head and neck.[31]

There is no consensus on the best imaging protocol for imaging the thorax, abdomen, and pelvis, with some advocating for the use of a combination of enteric and intravenous contrast,[32–34] and others questioning the utility of enteric contrast material.[35,36] What is uniformly accepted is the utility of intravenous contrast. At our institution, we have adopted a split bolus IV contrast only technique, with contrast timed to opacify the aorta and pulmonary arteries as well as the portal venous system. The scan is monitored during the acquisition by the radiologist on duty (or a radiology trainee) to determine the need for delayed phase imaging or a CT cystogram. The authors administer enteric contrast on a case-by-case basis as a problem-solving tool.

MR imaging is infrequently used in patients suffering from acute GSW as a result of the length of time needed to perform the MR imaging as well as safety concerns surrounding the support apparatus and the imaging compatibility of retained ballistic debris of unknown composition (RBUC).

Trajectory Analysis and Wound Patterns

Understanding the trajectory of each bullet is the key to ensuring that all injuries are identified and appropriately managed.[37–41] CT tractography has been proposed as a method of evaluating bullet

trajectory[42] that has automated analysis[43,44]; however, these techniques are infrequently applied in routine clinical practice. Instead, it is best to rely on routine CT techniques and an understanding of the wounding mechanism of bullets. Bullets travel in straight lines. However, they can deflect, when moving at lower velocities or when encountering dense bone (**Fig. 7**). When assessing a bullet's trajectory, it is important to look for evidence of deflection anytime a bullet encounters bone. It is also important to understand that patients are usually imaged in a position different than the position in which they were shot. This can result in bullet paths that are bent or curved. The respiratory cycle should also be considered when seeking to understand the course of a bullet through a patient.

Earlier, the authors discussed the importance of marking surface wounds to ensure that the "even number rule" is satisfied and these marked surface wounds are the starting point in the analysis of bullet trajectory. Starting with the marked surface wounds, examine the orientation of stranding in the subcutaneous fat and look for a low-density linear tract through the deeper muscle. This can then be used to infer the initial bullet trajectory. In the context of a single GSW with a retained bullet, the course of the bullet can then be easily extrapolated. In patients injured with SJ or LBs, it is not uncommon to see shed debris along the bullet tract which provides an additional clue to the course taken by the bullet. In patients who have sustained

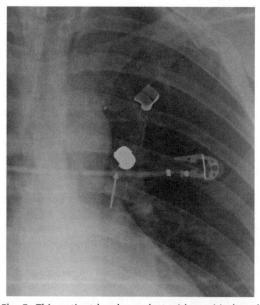

Fig. 5. This patient has been shot with semi-jacketed bullet as evidenced by the bullet disintegration, deformation, and debris. Note how the high-density lead (*green arrow*) can be differentiated from the low-density copper (*red arrow*).

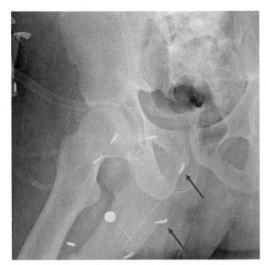

Fig. 6. This patient has been shot by a RIP bullet. Note the characteristic appearance of the trocars (*red arrows*) that have separated from the bullet base (*green arrow*). (*Courtesy of* Hillel S. Maresky, MD, Philadelphia, PA.)

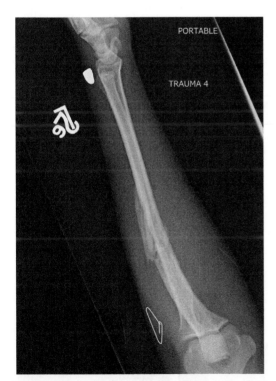

Fig. 7. In this patient with a single GSW to the forearm, the entry wound (marked by an unfolded paperclip) is proximal to the fractured ulna. The ulnar fracture is in turn proximal to the retained bullet. This appearance could only occur if the bullet deflected off of the ulna.

multiple GSW, it is important to repeat this process for each ballistic tract scrutinizing not only the crushed tissues along the permeant tract, but surrounding structures for evidence of injury related to the temporary cavity (Fig. 8). In patients who have had bullets pass cleanly through them, a "through and through GSW," the authors advocate describing surface wounds as "entry/exit" wounds as opposed to specifying which is which.

Bullets passing through bone provide an additional clue to determine bullet trajectory. As bullets pass through bone, they tend to pull pieces into the permanent cavity in the direction of bullet travel.[20] In addition, when bullets pass through flat bones, such as the calvarium, scapula, and iliac wings, they frequently create a beveled wounding pattern with the site of penetration into the bone having a narrower aperture than the site of exit from the bone[20,45,46] (Fig. 9)—this permits assessment of bullet's direction of travel and a clue to the bullet's paths. When patients have been injured with FMJ bullets and have through and through injuries, there is unlikely to be a debris trail (as these bullets stay intact). Consequently, knowing the site of entry/exit wounds is critical to ensure accurate image interpretation.

When bullets pass in close proximity to the gas-containing structures of the respiratory or gastrointestinal tract, the presence of extraluminal gas often results in much consternation. In our experience, it is not unusual for a small volume of gas to be pulled into the patient by the bullet; however, large volumes of gas in the peritoneal cavity or increasing gas on follow-up imaging typically indicate a perforated hollow viscus. GSWs to the neck are a particular challenge as soft tissue swelling can impede detection of injuries[46] to the trachea or aerodigestive tract. The authors strongly suggest that any GSW to the head and neck region be evaluated with both precontrast imaging and a CTA with a metal artifact reduction technique. This will allow for the most accurate determination of trajectory and permit optimal evaluation for vascular injuries despite streak artifacts from metal. Any structure in the direct path of the bullet should be considered as injured[47] and a low threshold for endoscopically evaluating injuries to the esophagus should be maintained.

Long-Term Complication of Retained Ballistic Material

Although acute GSW has been colloquially referred to as "acute lead poisoning", lead poisoning or plumbism is a true long-term complication of GSW. Symptoms are variable and include reproductive difficulties, anemia,

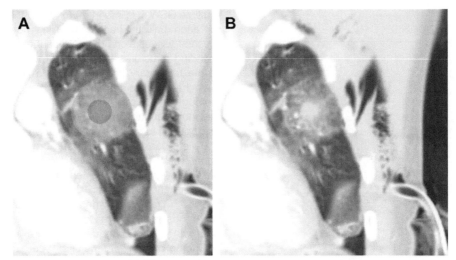

Fig. 8. Annotated (A) and nonannotated images (B) demonstrate a single transthoracic GSW. The permanent cavity of crushed tissue (red circle, A) is surrounded by pulmonary contusion resulting from the temporary cavity (green circle, A).

abdominal pain, nephropathy, encephalopathy, and neuropathy.[48,49] These symptoms may be intermittent, manifesting at times of metabolic stress[50,51] leading to repeated workups with the root cause being overlooked. Bullets that have been extensively fragmented, sit near or within joint spaces, or have lodged in bones put patients at increased risk of elevated serum lead levels.[52–54] Consequently, correlation with serum lead levels should be considered in patients with retained ballistic debris and nonspecific symptoms that could be attributed to lead poisoning.

Bullets within joint spaces are not inert and should be removed when encountered to mitigate lead arthropathy, a chronic complication associated with a retained lead within a joint space.[55] LBs bathed in the synovial fluid will dissolve over time, resulting in a cascade of foreign body

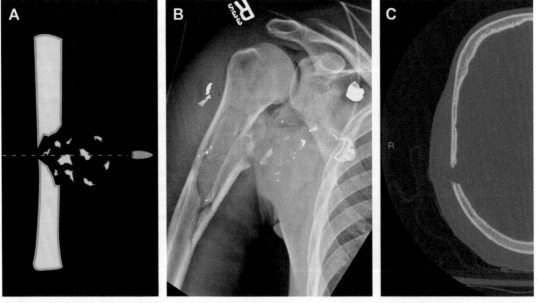

Fig. 9. (A) Illustration of the radiographic features commonly encountered when a bullet passes through bone. Note the beveled appearance of the injury with the narrower aperture at the site of entry and the bone fragments moving in the direction of bullet travel. (B) Radiographic example of this pattern. (C) Classic beveled appearance associated with ballistic injuries to flat bones.

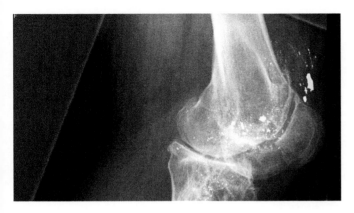

Fig. 10. Patient with a remote gunshot wound to the knee showing the classic findings of lead arthropathy. The bullet has eroded and fragmented and there is synovial staining by dissolved lead. Note the preserved bone mineral density. (*Courtesy of* M. Christakis, MD FRCP(c), Toronto, ON.)

reactions, articular cartilage damage, proliferative synovitis, and finally destructive arthritis.[55–57] As the bullet dissolves, it breaks into smaller fragments increasing the surface area of lead exposure and resulting in the characteristic diffused staining of the synovium and the characteristic radiographic appearance of the "lead arthrogram"[48,55,56,58–60] (Fig. 10). Although not typically a diagnostic dilemma, due to the presence of a high density of metal and history of GSW, the radiographic features of lead arthropathy include preserved bone mineral density in the presence of joint space narrowing, subchondral sclerosis, and cyst/erosion formation. Early in the disease process, the articular cartilage may increase in density similar to the appearances seen in chondrocalcinosis.[60] The CT and MR imaging findings of lead arthropathy are less well described, but mimic those seen on radiographs. Cross-sectional imaging will better delineate joint effusions, synovial inflammation, and some of the more subtle degenerative changes.[55] When CT is performed, metal artifact reduction algorithms should be used to optimize image reconstruction.

MR Imaging in Post-Gunshot Wound Patients

Retained ballistic debris of unknown composition (RBUC) should no longer be considered an absolute contraindication to MR imaging. Instead, any patient with retained ballistic debris should be considered as MR imaging conditional. MR imaging should only be performed in these patients when there is a clear indication, and the results of the MR imaging are likely to influence the patient's management. At our institution, we counsel the patient on the risks of potential RBUC migration and heating and require informed consent before imaging. Shotgun pellets that have lost their normal rounded contour on radiographs are likely

to be made of soft lead and are MR imaging compatible, whereas shotgun pellets made of steel or tungsten do not deform or fragment and are MR imaging incompatible. Bullets that have not fragmented but have maintained their characteristic shape should be considered FMJ bullets. FMJ bullets are typically composed of lead and copper and are MR imaging compatible[61]; however, a subset of these bullets have jacketing material that contains cheaper steel.[62] These bullets have been described as MR imaging incompatible[63] but may still be imaged in some circumstances with extreme caution.[8,62] Bullets that have irregularly disintegrated or disintegrated into two densities of metal on radiographs are likely to be composed of a combination of lead and copper and are consequently MR imaging compatible.[5] However, the presence of debris alone should not confer a false sense of security. Bullets passing through vehicles or jewelry can result in debris that is not MR imaging compatible mixed with bullet fragments[9] (Fig. 11) and a discussion with the patient surrounding the circumstances of their injury, as well as evaluation of the radiographs, should be part of the MR imaging screening process. As an additional precaution, the authors advise restricting these patients to scanning at 1.5 T.

Recent research into material decomposition and dual-energy CT techniques has shown great promise as a means of discriminating between ferromagnetic and nonferromagnetic materials; however, at present these studies have all been performed in vitro.[24–26,64] In the future, these techniques, possibly aided by machine learning, are likely to make the jump from the laboratory to the clinical environment and will likely increase radiologist comfort and influence institutional policy pertaining to the MR imaging of patients suffering from GSWs.

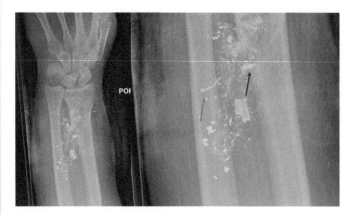

Fig. 11. Patient who has sustained a GSW to the wrist. At first glance, the disintegration of the bullet would suggest that the patient is MR imaging compatible. However, in discussion with this patient's care team, the additional history of the patient having been shot through their wristwatch was obtained. Close inspection of the image demonstrated ferromagnetic watch parts such as the watch hand (*green arrow* on magnified view) and the pusher (*red arrow* on magnified view) that made the patient ineligible for wrist MR imaging.

SUMMARY

Accurate imaging evaluation of GSWs requires a thorough knowledge of the pathophysiology of this disease as well as a mechanism-based approach to uncovering injuries. Close integration with the trauma team will help to ensure that all surface wounds are marked and that appropriate imaging protocols using metal artifact reduction are used. It is important to remember that patients suffering from GSW in the acute phase can also have long-term complications such as plumbism and lead arthropathy. Consequently, the role of the radiologist should be expanded to not only identifying the acute injuries but also identifying injuries that might lead to future degenerative joint disease and systemic illness. Finally, radiologists act as gatekeepers to MR imaging, and recent research has shown that patients with retained ballistic debris can be safely imaged if appropriate precautions are taken.

CLINICS CARE POINTS

- Ballistic wounding can be broadly characterized as injuries related to the permanent cavity and the secondary cavity related to tissue stretching that surrounds the permanent cavity.
- The even number rule states that each bullet entering the patient must either exit the patient or be retained within the patient. Consequently, a tally of the number of surface wounds and retained bullets/debris fields should result in an even number.
- Radiographs should be the initial imaging modality used in the assessment of patients with gunshot wound, with two orthogonal views acquired if possible.

- Computerized tomographic scans should be acquired using intravenous contrast material with metal artifact reduction techniques if available.
- Retained bullets can result in plumbism and lead arthropathy.
- Retained ballistic debris is no longer considered an absolute contraindication to MR imaging. These patients can usually be safely imaged if appropriate precautions are taken.

ACKNOWLEDGMENTS

The authors would like to thank Dr Hillel Maresky (Temple University) and Dr Monique Christakis (University of Toronto) for contributing images to this study.

DISCLOSURE

None of the authors has any commercial or financial conflicts of interest.

REFERENCES

1. Molina GA, Aguayo WG, Cevallos JM, et al. Prenatal gunshot wound, a rare cause of maternal and fetus trauma, a case report. Int J Surg Case Rep 2019; 59:201–4.
2. Kaufman EJ, Wiebe DJ, Xiong RA, et al. Epidemiologic Trends in Fatal and Nonfatal Firearm Injuries in the US, 2009-2017. JAMA Intern Med 2021; 181(2):237–44.
3. Global Burden of Disease Injury C, Naghavi M, Marczak LB, et al. Global Mortality From Firearms, 1990-2016. JAMA 2018;320(8):792–814.
4. Mann M, Espinoza EO, Ralston RM, et al. Shot pellets: an overview. Assoc Firearm Tool Mark Examiners J 1994;26(3).

5. Fountain AJ, Corey A, Malko JA, et al. Imaging Appearance of Ballistic Wounds Predicts Bullet Composition: Implications for MRI Safety. AJR Am J Roentgenol 2021;216(2):542–51.

6. Ditkofsky NG, Maresky H, Mathur S. Imaging Ballistic Injuries. Can Assoc Radiol J 2020;71(3):335–43.

7. Ditkofsky N, Maresky HS, Steenburg S. Radically Invasive Projectiles-first reports and imaging features of this new and dangerous bullet. Emerg Radiol 2020;27(4):393–7.

8. Ditkofsky N, Colak E, Kirpalani A, et al. MR imaging in the presence of ballistic debris of unknown composition: a review of the literature and practical approach. Emerg Radiol 2020;27(5):527–32.

9. Ditkofsky N, Gross JA, Dodge JP. Ballistic Debris of Unknown Composition Should Be Considered MRI Conditional. AJR Am J Roentgenol 2021; 217(2):W6.

10. Fackler ML. Wound ballistics. A review of common misconceptions. JAMA 1988;259(18):2730–6.

11. Ditkofsky N, Elbanna KY, Robins J, et al. Ballistic Injury Imaging: The Basics. Curr Radiol Rep 2018;6(12):45.

12. Hollerman JJ, Fackler ML, Coldwell DM, et al. Gunshot wounds: 1. Bullets, ballistics, and mechanisms of injury. AJR Am J Roentgenol 1990;155(4):685–90.

13. Fackler ML, Surinchak JS, Malinowski JA, et al. Wounding potential of the Russian AK-74 assault rifle. J Trauma 1984;24(3):263–6.

14. Treto K, Bhullar IS, Lube MW. Iliac Artery Bullet Embolus after Isolated Thoracic Ballistic Injury. Am Surg 2017;83(7):253–4.

15. Beatty JS, Mitchell JW, Bates WB, et al. Left profunda femoris artery bullet embolus resulting from a 0.22 caliber gunshot wound to the back. Am Surg 2013;79(9):e310–1.

16. Frenkel A, Shaked G, Shelef I, et al. Missile Embolism to the Pulmonary Artery. Am Surg 2017;83(2):54–6.

17. de Oliveira RM, Drumond DAF. Considerations about ballistic embolism: experience at the João XXIII Hospital. Rev Med Minas Gerais 2014;24(4):527–34.

18. Folio L, McHugh C, Hoffman MJ. The even-number guide and imaging ballistic injuries. Radiol Technol 2007;78(3):197–203.

19. Hynes AM. Finding the missing bullet: A case report of an unusual trajectory from the left scapula into the left orbit. Trauma Case Rep 2021;35:100530.

20. Wilson AJ. Gunshot injuries: what does a radiologist need to know? Radiographics 1999;19(5):1358–68.

21. Patino M, Prochowski A, Agrawal MD, et al. Material Separation Using Dual-Energy CT: Current and Emerging Applications. Radiographics 2016;36(4): 1087–105.

22. Ognard J, Dissaux B, Diallo I, et al. Manual and Fully Automated Segmentation to Determine the Ferromagnetic Status of Bullets Using Computed Tomography Dual-Energy Index: A Phantom Study. J Comput Assist Tomogr 2019;43(5):799–804.

23. McCollough CH, Leng S, Yu L, et al. Dual- and Multi-Energy CT: Principles, Technical Approaches, and Clinical Applications. Radiology 2015;276(3):637–53.

24. Winklhofer S, Stolzmann P, Meier A, et al. Added value of dual-energy computed tomography versus single-energy computed tomography in assessing ferromagnetic properties of ballistic projectiles: implications for magnetic resonance imaging of gunshot victims. Invest Radiol 2014;49(6):431–7.

25. Gascho D, Zoelch N, Richter H, et al. Identification of Bullets Based on Their Metallic Components and X-Ray Attenuation Characteristics at Different Energy Levels on CT. AJR Am J Roentgenol 2019; 213(3):W105–13.

26. Gascho D, Zoelch N, Richter H, et al. Heavy metal in radiology: how to reliably differentiate between lodged copper and lead bullets using CT numbers. Eur Radiol Exp 2020;4(1):43.

27. Gascho D. Lodged bullets on computed tomography: Three classification procedures for the virtual investigation of bullets or their fragments that cannot be recovered from the living patient. Med Sci Law 2020;60(4):245–8.

28. Zhang X, Cain MD, Williams CD, et al. G2 Research Radically Invasive Projectile: The Importance of Recognizing Its Imaging and Autopsy Patterns. Am J Forensic Med Pathol 2021;42(3):248–51.

29. Gjesteby L, De Man B, Jin Y, et al. Metal artifact reduction in CT: where are we after four decades? Ieee Access 2016;4:5826–49.

30. Berger F, Niemann T, Kubik-Huch RA, et al. Retained bullets in the head on computed tomography - Get the most out of iterative metal artifact reduction. Eur J Radiol 2018;103:124–30.

31. Offiah C, Hall E. Imaging assessment of penetrating injury of the neck and face. Insights Imaging 2012; 3(5):419–31.

32. Munera F, Morales C, Soto JA, et al. Gunshot wounds of abdomen: evaluation of stable patients with triple-contrast helical CT. Radiology 2004; 231(2):399–405.

33. Saksobhavivat N, Shanmuganathan K, Boscak AR, et al. Diagnostic accuracy of triple-contrast multi-detector computed tomography for detection of penetrating gastrointestinal injury: a prospective study. Eur Radiol 2016;26(11):4107–20.

34. Shanmuganathan K, Mirvis SE, Chiu WC, et al. Penetrating torso trauma: triple-contrast helical CT in peritoneal violation and organ injury–a prospective study in 200 patients. Radiology 2004;231(3): 775–84.

35. Jawad H, Raptis C, Mintz A, et al. Single-Contrast CT for Detecting Bowel Injuries in Penetrating Abdominopelvic Trauma. AJR Am J Roentgenol 2018; 210(4):761–5.

36. Ramirez RM, Cureton EL, Ereso AQ, et al. Single-contrast computed tomography for the triage of

patients with penetrating torso trauma. J Trauma 2009;67(3):583–8.

37. Chittiboina P, Banerjee AD, Zhang S, et al. How bullet trajectory affects outcomes of civilian gunshot injury to the spine. J Clin Neurosci 2011;18(12):1630–3.

38. Grandinetti H, Zanetti G, Marchiori E. Tubular Opacity in the Lung Along a Bullet Trajectory. Arch Bronconeumol (Engl Ed 2021;57(4):305.

39. Khan MS, Khan BM, Naz S, et al. Is estimated bullet trajectory a reliable predictor of severe injury? Case report of a thoraco-abdominal gunshot with a protracted trajectory managed nonoperatively. BMC Res Notes 2013;6:63.

40. Hirshberg A, Wall MJ Jr, Mattox KL. Bullet trajectory predicts the need for damage control: an artificial neural network model. J Trauma 2002;52(5):852–8.

41. Duz B, Cansever T, Secer HI, et al. Evaluation of spinal missile injuries with respect to bullet trajectory, surgical indications and timing of surgical intervention: a new guideline. Spine (Phila Pa 1976) 2008;33(20):E746–53.

42. Bruckner BA, Norman M, Scott BG. CT Tractogram: technique for demonstrating tangential bullet trajectories. J Trauma 2006;60(6):1362–3.

43. Folio L, Solomon J, Biassou N, et al. Semi-automated trajectory analysis of deep ballistic penetrating brain injury. Mil Med 2013;178(3):338–45.

44. Folio LR, Fischer TV, Shogan PJ, et al. CT-based ballistic wound path identification and trajectory analysis in anatomic ballistic phantoms. Radiology 2011;258(3):923–9.

45. Pinto A, Russo A, Reginelli A, et al. Gunshot Wounds: Ballistics and Imaging Findings. Semin Ultrasound CT MR 2019;40(1):25–35.

46. Reginelli A, Russo A, Maresca D, et al. Imaging assessment of gunshot wounds. Semin Ultrasound CT MR 2015;36(1):57–67.

47. Steenburg SD, Sliker CW, Shanmuganathan K, et al. Imaging evaluation of penetrating neck injuries. Radiographics 2010;30(4):869–86.

48. Linden MA, Manton WI, Stewart RM, et al. Lead poisoning from retained bullets. Pathogenesis, diagnosis, and management. Ann Surg 1982;195(3):305–13.

49. Weiss D, Tomasallo CD, Meiman JG, et al. Elevated Blood Lead Levels Associated with Retained Bullet Fragments - United States, 2003-2012. MMWR Morb Mortal Wkly Rep 2017;66(5):130–3.

50. Dillman RO, Crumb CK, Lidsky MJ. Lead poisoning from a gunshot wound. Report of a case and review of the literature. Am J Med 1979;66(3):509–14.

51. Cagin CR, Diloy-Puray M, Westerman MP. Bullets, lead poisoning and thyrotoxicosis. Ann Intern Med 1978;89(4):509–11.

52. Apte A, Bradford K, Dente C, et al. Lead toxicity from retained bullet fragments: A systematic review and meta-analysis. J Trauma Acute Care Surg 2019;87(3):707–16.

53. Yen JS, Yen TH. Lead poisoning induced by gunshot injury with retained bullet fragments. QJM 2022;114(12):873–4.

54. McQuirter JL, Rothenberg SJ, Dinkins GA, et al. Change in blood lead concentration up to 1 year after a gunshot wound with a retained bullet. Am J Epidemiol 2004;159(7):683–92.

55. Fernandes JL, Rocha AA, Soares MV, et al. Lead arthropathy: radiographic, CT and MRI findings. Skeletal Radiol 2007;36(7):647–57.

56. DeMartini J, Wilson A, Powell JS, et al. Lead arthropathy and systemic lead poisoning from an intraarticular bullet. AJR Am J Roentgenol 2001;176(5):1144.

57. Leonard MH. The solution of lead by synovial fluid. Clin Orthop Relat Res 1969;64:255–61.

58. Ramji Z, Laflamme M. Ankle Lead Arthropathy and Systemic Lead Toxicity Secondary to a Gunshot Wound After 49 Years: A Case Report. J Foot Ankle Surg 2017;56(3):648–52.

59. McAninch SA, Adkison J, Meyers R, et al. Bullet fragment-induced lead arthropathy with subsequent fracture and elevated blood lead levels. Proc (Bayl Univ Med Cent) 2017;30(1):88–91.

60. Sclafani SJ, Vuletin JC, Twersky J. Lead arthropathy: arthritis caused by retained intra-articular bullets. Radiology 1985;156(2):299–302.

61. Dedini RD, Karacozoff AM, Shellock FG, et al. MRI issues for ballistic objects: information obtained at 1.5-, 3- and 7-Tesla. Spine J 2013;13(7):815–22.

62. Karacozoff AM, Pekmezci M, Shellock FG. Armor-piercing bullet: 3-T MRI findings and identification by a ferromagnetic detection system. Mil Med 2013;178(3):e380–5.

63. Eggert S, Kubik-Huch RA, Klarhofer M, et al. Fairly direct hit! Advances in imaging of shotgun projectiles in MRI. Eur Radiol 2015;25(9):2745–53.

64. Gascho D, Zoelch N, Deininger-Czermak E, et al. Visualization and material-based differentiation of lodged projectiles by extended CT scale and the dual-energy index. J Forensic Leg Med 2020;70:101919.

Imaging of Trauma in Pregnancy

Devang Odedra, MD, MASc, FRCPC[a,*], Vincent M. Mellnick, MD, FSAR[b],
Michael N. Patlas, MD, FRCPC, FASER, FCAR, FSAR[c]

KEYWORDS

- Pregnancy • Trauma • Diagnostic imaging • Ultrasound • Multidetector computed tomography
- Magnetic resonance imaging

KEY POINTS

- A pregnant trauma patient is essentially 2 patients—the mother and the fetus. The mother should be the primary patient in the initial assessment and management.
- The fear of radiation should not preclude an appropriate assessment of the mother.
- Radiologists should be familiar with multimodality findings of placental injuries.
- Once the mother is stabilized, fetal well-being should be assessed with physical examination, external fetal monitoring, and a dedicated fetal ultrasound examination.

INTRODUCTION

Trauma and unintentional injury are leading causes of death in women of reproductive age in the United States and affect up to 7% of all pregnancies.[1–4] In a large series based in the United States, women of reproductive age comprised 9.8% of all trauma patients and, within this cohort, 5.3% patients were pregnant.[1] At the same time, in comparison with all of the trauma patients encountered by clinicians and radiologists, pregnant trauma patients comprise a very small percentage (0.5%).[1] This infrequency can translate into less experience and preparedness when a pregnant trauma patient is brought through the emergency department doors. The most common mechanisms of trauma in pregnancy include motor vehicle accidents, falls, and domestic violence.[1,4–6] Blunt trauma is much more common, comprising up to 90% to 96% of cases, compared with penetrating trauma.[1,4] Pregnancy causes several unique physiologic and structural changes that increase the risk of certain traumatic injuries and pose certain challenges in the

management.[1,4,7] There are 2 patients in this scenario, the mother, and the fetus, and each warrant a thorough clinical and, potentially, imaging workup.[8–10]

This review outlines the special considerations when it comes to imaging a pregnant trauma patient. The role of radiography, ultrasound, computed tomography (CT) scan, and MRI in the imaging of pregnant trauma patients will be discussed. A special focus will be given to obstetric injuries such as placental abruption, uterine rupture, and direct fetal injuries. Other pregnancy-related topics such as ectopic pregnancy in trauma are also covered briefly.

CLINICAL MANAGEMENT OF THE PREGNANT TRAUMA PATIENT

The primary focus of the initial management of a pregnant trauma patient is on the mother. The primary assessment includes ensuring the mother's airway, breathing, and circulation. The patient is placed in a left oblique decubitus position to decrease compression of the inferior vena cava

a Department of Medical Imaging, North York General Hospital, 4001 Leslie Street, North York, Ontario M2K
1E1, Canada; b Abdominal Imaging Division, Mallinckrodt Institute of Radiology, Washington University
School of Medicine, 510 S. Kingshighway Boulevard, Campus Box 8131, St. Louis, MO 63110, USA; c Division
of Emergency/Trauma Radiology, Department of Radiology, McMaster University, Hamilton General Hospital,
237 Barton Street East, Hamilton, Ontario L8L 2X2, Canada
* Corresponding author.
E-mail address: devang.odedra@medportal.ca

Radiol Clin N Am 61 (2023) 129–139
https://doi.org/10.1016/j.rcl.2022.07.006

by the fetus.[11] A careful physical examination of the abdomen is then performed to check for any signs of seat-belt injury or bruising.

During the secondary survey, a detailed obstetric history is taken along with the performance of a detailed head-to-toe physical examination. Signs of uterine injuries such as vaginal bleeding, ruptured membranes, or a bulging perineum are assessed. Fetal heartbeat auscultation is performed, and fetal monitoring is initiated.

Appropriate management of a pregnant trauma patient requires a multidisciplinary approach. Members from the obstetric team are routinely involved in the primary assessment of the trauma patient. Certain sites also involve the neonatal intensive care unit in the event of an emergency Caesarean delivery.[3,4,12] Radiology and anesthesiology are also crucial in the imaging assessment and hemodynamic management of the patient. In addition to providing acute care, physicians should engage social and psychological support services in ensuring patient's safety and preventative strategies.[7]

IMAGING OF THE PREGNANT TRAUMA PATIENT
General Principles

A main consideration that differentiates the sequence of imaging assessment of a pregnant trauma patient from a nonpregnant trauma patient is the heightened concern for radiation exposure in pregnancy.[13] However, the fear of radiation should not be a barrier to appropriate diagnostic workup of the patient.[14] Care should be taken, when possible, to use as low as reasonably achievable radiation dose to minimize the exposure to the mother, and more importantly, the fetus. Ultrasound examination and radiography certainly have their roles in the imaging of a pregnant trauma patient, although a CT scan remains the ultimate modality of choice for a thorough assessment of potential injuries.[12,15]

The type and severity of adverse effects of radiation on the fetus depends on the gestational age and the amount of radiation dose. During the first 2 weeks of gestation, the main risk is fetal death at thresholds of 50 to 100 mGy of dose. If the fetus survives past this period, there are likely no long-term detrimental effects. During 2 to 20 weeks of gestation, the primary concern from radiation exposure is that of fetal malformations, with a threshold of 50 to 150 mGy. At any point during the pregnancy, there is a risk of fetal carcinogenesis, approximated as an increased lifetime risk

Table 1
Estimated radiation dose to the fetus from common trauma-related radiographical and CT studies

Examination	Estimated Fetal Dose (mGy)
Radiography	
Cervical spine (AP, lateral)	<0.001
Extremities	<0.001
Chest (PA, lateral)	0.002
Thoracic spine (AP, lateral)	0.003
Abdomen (AP)	1–3
Lumbar spine (AP, lateral)	1
CT scan	
Head	0
Chest (routine)	0.2
Chest (pulmonary embolism)	0.2
Abdomen (routine)	4
Abdomen and pelvis (routine)	25
Abdomen and pelvis (renal colic)	10
CT angiography of total aorta	34

(Data from[16,18])

of cancer by 2% with a fetal dose exposure of 50 mGy.[16,17]

Adverse effects of radiation on the fetus were a bigger concern in the past when the doses from earlier generations of CT scanners were generally higher. With the newer generation technology, the radiation dose exposure to the fetus for any single study is generally considerably less than 50 mGy (**Table 1**).[16,18] Hence, when it is clinically indicated, the risk of adverse events from radiation exposure to the fetus is generally outweighed by the benefits of detecting life-threatening injuries, and a thorough radiological workup of the patient should not be avoided.

Ultrasound Examination

The ready availability of ultrasound examinations in the emergency department and its real-time capability renders it the modality of choice in the primary screening of a trauma patient regardless of their pregnancy status. A focused assessment with sonography for trauma provides a good screening assessment of the internal injuries by assessing presence of free fluid in the 4 quadrants of the abdomen.[19] It has a sensitivity of up to 83% in the detection of free fluid in pregnant trauma patients.[20] In pregnant patients, a small amount of physiologic free fluid may be present; however, it is usually low in volume. Therefore, any fluid detected on a focused assessment with sonography for trauma examination should be regarded as potentially pathologic.[4,21]

Ultrasound examinations can also assess the solid organs for any direct signs of injuries such as lacerations or contusions. The sensitivity of an ultrasound examination in detecting intra-abdominal traumatic injuries in pregnant patients range from 61% to 86%, with a specificity ranging from 94% to 100%.[20,22,23] It serves as a good initial screening test and, when positive, can expedite the care of the patient. However, owing to its relatively poor sensitivity, it cannot substitute for a CT assessment of the patient.

Ultrasound examination has the advantage over any other modality in obstetric assessment of the mother and the fetus. It allows the assessment of the gestational age, fetal cardiac rate and rhythm, placental localization and exclusion of placenta previa, assessment of amniotic fluid, cervical length, fetal well-being, vascular flow with Doppler imaging, direct fetal injuries, and fetal demise.[3] Hence, a dedicated obstetric sonographic examination is recommended in all cases of significant maternal trauma. As per the American College of Radiology (ACR) Appropriateness Criteria on major blunt trauma, an ultrasound focused assessment with sonography for trauma examination and ultrasound examination of the pelvis are usually appropriate in the initial evaluation of a pregnant trauma patient.[24]

Radiography and Computed Tomography Scans

Radiography is portable, fast, and low in radiation. Similar to nonpregnant patients, chest and pelvic radiographs are standard in the initial assessment of a pregnant trauma patient. Some institutions also routinely obtain cervical spine radiographs. Additional radiographs can be performed based on the suspected sites of injuries in the extremities.[3,25]

A CT scan is the workhorse of trauma imaging in the emergency department. Although radiography and ultrasound examination have their roles in the initial assessment of the pregnant trauma patient, a CT scan should be the modality of choice for any patient with a major trauma or suspected injuries.

In any woman of childbearing age and particularly in pregnant women, reasonable strategies to minimize radiation dose should be used during a CT scan. Diagnostic images at the lowest possible dose should be obtained by using both hardware and software optimization techniques. When multiple scanners exist in the radiology department, the scanner with the most optimized dose profile should be reserved for imaging of the pregnant trauma patient. The scan parameters, including the tube potential, tube current–time product, pitch, and limiting the z-axis coverage should be tailored to the patient and the area of interest. Iterative reconstruction techniques have been shown to decrease the radiation dose without compromising image quality and should be used when available.[26] The standard trauma protocol varies by institution, but often includes 2 phases (arterial and portal venous) through the abdomen and pelvis with intravenous contrast.[27] Intravenous contrast has not been shown to have any adverse effects on the mother or the fetus and the ACR does not recommend against it.[28,29] Multiple scans through the abdomen and pelvis can potentially be avoided by using a split bolus technique or by obtaining a single, late arterial phase acquisition with selective later scans if needed.[30,31] Dual-energy CT scanning is a promising technique that has the potential to reduce dose by generating virtual unenhanced images based on postcontrast images.[32] Extra caution should be practiced in repeating CT studies because cumulative doses from multiple studies can easily surpass the 50 mGy threshold.

MRI

Given its lack of universal availability, slower image acquisition, and the need to remove the patient from clinical care, MRI is usually not the first-line modality and is reserved as a problem-solving tool. The ACR Appropriateness Criteria also recommend against its use in the initial assessment of pregnant trauma patients.[24] It has a complementary role in the assessment of complex neurologic and musculoskeletal injuries. It can also be used as a troubleshooting tool for abdominal injuries, for example, assessing the integrity of the main duct in the setting of high-grade pancreatic trauma.[33,34] Finally, it can be used as a follow-up imaging tool for the reassessment of injuries in stable patients to avoid further radiation dose.

No definite adverse events associated with MRI on the mother or the fetus have been shown. However, there are theoretic risks of overheating the fetus and potential effects of acoustic noise.[35] The ACR White Paper for safe MR practices recommends MRI at any stage in the pregnancy if the benefits outweigh the risks and if the information cannot be obtained with another modality.[36] The use of intravenous gadolinium-based contrast agents should be avoided unless necessary because adverse outcomes associated with gadolinium-based contrast agents have been shown in animal studies.[36,37]

IMAGING OF PREGNANCY-SPECIFIC INJURIES
Placental Abruption

Placental abruption is the most common cause of fetal death in trauma.[3] It is more common after 16 weeks of gestation, and affects 1% to 5% of minor trauma patients and 30% to 50% of major trauma patients during pregnancy.[16,38] Fetal mortality in cases of traumatic placental abruption is up to 67% to 75%.[14] The term placental abruption refers to complete or partial detachment of the placenta from the underlying myometrium before the expected delivery time.[39] It results from the shear forces between relatively inelastic placental tissue and the elastic myometrium, with a rapidly accumulating intervening hemorrhage.[3] Risk factors other than trauma include advanced maternal age, smoking, alcohol and cocaine use, hypertension, in vitro fertilization, and preeclampsia.[38,39] Typical clinical signs and symptoms include abdominal pain, uterine tenderness, uterine contractions and hypertonicity, vaginal bleeding, preterm labor, or an abnormal external fetal monitoring tracing. However, it can also be clinically occult and a high index of suspicion is warranted.[40] Complications of placental abruption include preterm labor, fetal distress, low birth weight, oligohydramnios, fetal death, and maternal coagulopathy.[38,41] Placental abruption can be classified into 4 types based on the location of the hemorrhage in relation to the placenta: retroplacental, marginal subchorionic, preplacental, and intraplacental.[39] A retroplacental hematoma is located deep to the basal plate of placenta. Its size correlates with fetal outcomes. with a hematoma larger than 50 mL in size or causing more than 50% placental detachment associated with poor outcomes.[42] A marginal subchorionic hematoma elevates the placenta, but also extends behind the chorion. A preplacental hematoma is relatively uncommon. Intraplacental hematoma is noted in the intervillous space of the placenta and carries a worse prognosis than retroplacental hematoma.[43]

Ultrasound examination is the primary modality of choice in assessing obstetric traumatic injuries. However, it suffers from poor sensitivity in the detection of placental abruption, as low as 24%.[39,44] It

does, however, have a high specificity of up to 96%.[17,45] A normal placenta at ultrasound examination appears as an echogenic structure relative to the underlying myometrium with a hypoechoic retroplacental zone.[39,46,47] The ultrasound appearance of a placental hemorrhage depends on the age of the hematoma and can vary from echogenic to isoechoic and eventually hypoechoic over time. In the acute to subacute setting, the hematoma can be similar in echogenicity to the placenta, making its detection challenging. A maneuver has been described as an aid to differentiating between the hematoma and the placenta, whereby gently pushing on the hematoma demonstrates softness, like a Jell-O effect, whereas the normal placenta is relatively firm.[39] Besides the direct visualization of a periplacental hematoma, the radiologist should also look for focal thickening of the placenta, because it may suggest an underlying placental abruption. Potential mimics of periplacental hematoma include myometrial contraction or a tumor such as chorioangioma or leiomyoma; however, the use of Doppler imaging helps in differentiating them; a hematoma should not have vascularity, whereas the other two should.[43]

The reported sensitivities and specificities of a CT scan for placental abruption are much better, ranging from 86% to 100% and 56% to 98%,[15,48–50] respectively. Radiologists should be familiar with the appearances of placental abruption on a CT scan because it is the workhorse of trauma imaging. However, owing to the general infrequency of pregnant trauma patients, radiologists often do not have enough experience for assessing placenta on a CT scan and can overlook these important injuries. Earlier in the pregnancy, a normal placenta on contrast-enhanced CT scan appears as a homogenous ring of tissue surrounding the gestational sac. With time, the placenta becomes increasingly heterogenous and develops placental cotyledons, which are seen as rounded areas of low attenuation with surrounding enhancing placenta (**Fig. 1**).[51] With time, indentations of the placenta form on the fetal side and venous lakes form on the maternal side.[16,39] Placental hemorrhage appears as areas of hypoenhancement, forming acute angles with the myometrium on a CT scan. Like ultrasound examination, a focal thickening of the placenta should also raise suspicion for an underlying hematoma (**Fig. 2**). Occasionally, hyperdense layering hemorrhagic contents may be seen within the amniotic fluid.[39] Placental venous lakes and myometrial contractions may mimic placental hematoma on the CT scan. Venous lakes can be characterized with ultrasound imaging; they have a characteristic appearance of hypoechoic areas with flow.

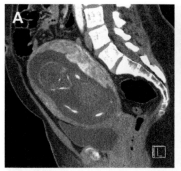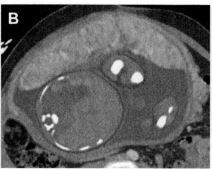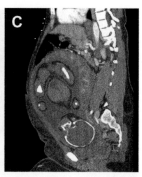

Fig. 1. Examples of normally enhancing placenta on CT from 3 different patients who sustained blunt trauma but whose pregnancies were unaffected. Note that placental enhancement can be heterogeneous, as shown in all 3 examples. Partial thickness areas of placental enhancement greater than (*A*), or less than (*B, C*) skeletal muscle may be normal. Note the absence of full-thickness perfusion defect or hematoma.

Myometrial contractions form obtuse angles with the myometrium without an associated hematoma.[49] Saphier and colleagues[52] has proposed a standardized CT grading system for the evaluation of placenta in trauma, based on the placental surface enhancement. Placental abruption may manifest on a CT scan with full-thickness foci of hypoenhancement in the placenta. Occasionally, it may present with global placental nonenhancement (**Fig. 3**). It may be accompanied by hemorrhage in the myometrium or amniotic sac.

MRI has a good accuracy for placental abruption with specificity and a sensitivity of up to 100%.[53] At MRI, normal placenta is slightly hyperintense to myometrium on T2-weighted imaging and slightly hypointense on T1-weighted images. The placenta is initially quite homogenous and with time becomes heterogenous. The normal myometrium has 3 layers with a middle hyperintense layer on T2-weighted imaging and becomes thinner with progressive gestational age.[39,54] Periplacental hemorrhage signal varies based on the age, but usually appears as hypointense on T2-weighted images and hyperintense on T1-weighted images (**Fig. 4**). Diffusion-weighted and gradient echo imaging can demonstrate restricted diffusion and susceptibility artifact within the hematoma, respectively.[53,55] Uterine contractions can mimic placental hematoma; however, they can also be distinguished by its T2 hypointense signal like the myometrium (see **Fig. 4**).

Uterine Rupture and Penetrating Injury

Uterine rupture is a rare but catastrophic diagnosis, affecting less than 1% of pregnant trauma cases.[2,9] It is associated with nearly 100% fetal and up to 10% maternal mortality.[16] The spectrum of rupture can vary from partial serosal lacerations to complete uterine avulsion. Signs and symptoms include maternal shock, abdominal distension, irregular uterine contour, palpable fetal parts, sudden abnormal fetal heart rate pattern, ascent of fetal presenting part, and peritoneal irritation.[3]

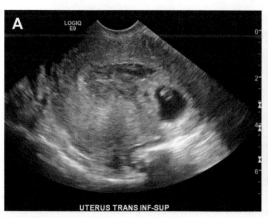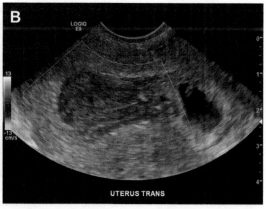

Fig. 2. Subchorionic hemorrhage after trauma in a pregnant patient, 6 weeks estimated gestational age. Ultrasound images show a large, heterogenous echogenicity collection in the uterus subjacent to the gestation sac (*A*) without associated color flow (*B*). This hematoma was observed conservatively.

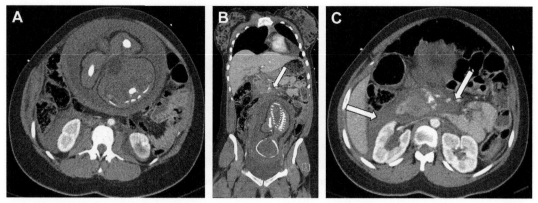

Fig. 3. Placental abruption after motor vehicle collision in a patient 32 weeks pregnant. Contrast-enhanced CT scan shows nonenhancement of the placenta (*A, B*), compatible with abruption. This led to intrauterine fetal demise. The mother also sustained an injury to the root of the small bowel mesentery (*B, C*) with associated mesenteric and retroperitoneal hematomas (*arrows*).

Ultrasound imaging is limited in the assessment of uterine rupture.[16] On a CT scan, the areas of laceration or rupture are noted as focal regions of hypoenhancement. A frank rupture may be seen as a focal defect in the uterus and protrusion of fetal parts outside the uterus (**Fig. 5**). In cases of penetrating injuries, the radiologist should be extra diligent in following the trajectory of the wound and searching for gas or foreign bodies surrounding the uterus, given the high fetal mortality of 71% to 73% for uterine gunshot wounds and 27% to 42% for stabbings.[9,38,56–58]

Fetal Injuries

Direct fetal injuries are overall uncommon because the fetus is cushioned by the maternal body wall,

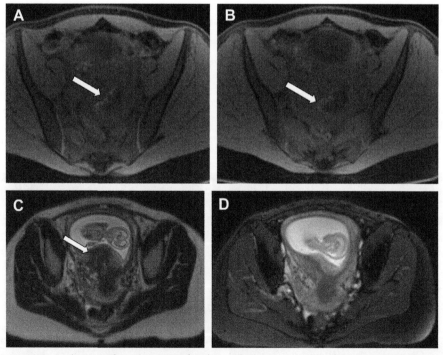

Fig. 4. Two separate patients undergoing MRI after low-velocity trauma. The first patient (*A, B, arrows*) had a small amount of T1 bright subchorionic hemorrhage adjacent to her first trimester gestational sac. This small hematoma was managed conservatively without incident. The second patient has a myometrial contraction (*C, arrow*), characterized by a contour abnormality of the myometrium that is T2 hypointense and which resolves on subsequent sequence performed 10 minutes later (*D*).

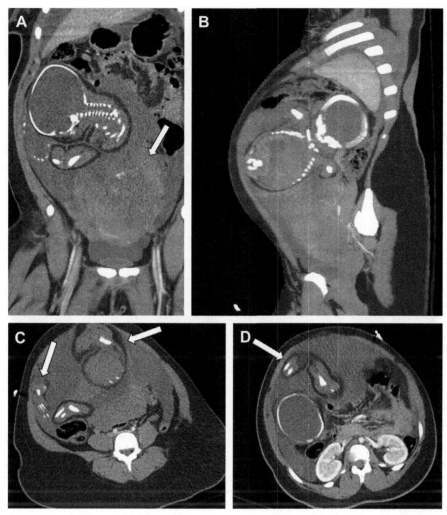

Fig. 5. Uterine rupture. A 17-year-old, 36-week pregnant woman presented to the emergency department after a motor vehicle collision. Contrast-enhanced CT scan demonstrates hemoperitoneum and a fetus external to an ill-defined uterus (*A, arrow*) with fetal parts touching the peritoneal surfaces (*C, D, arrows*). The fetus did not survive this severe trauma with uterine rupture.

uterus, and the amniotic fluid. Later in the pregnancy, the amount of amniotic fluid in relation to the fetus decreases, increasing the risk of direct injury. The most common injury observed is fetal head injury and skull fractures.[16,38] Ultrasound examination can visualize a focal step-off or overlap with a change in the shape of the fetal skull. It can also demonstrate signs of intracranial hemorrhage such as an intracranial mass, hydrocephalus, or an echogenic hematoma. A CT scan can directly visualize the fractures with cortical breach and demonstrate a hyperdense space occupying hemorrhagic collection (**Fig. 6**).[59,60] The normal suture pattern should not be confused with fractures. A fetal MRI allows good detection of intracranial pathology in the fetus and injuries may manifest as hemorrhage, hydrocephalus, or mass effect.[61,62]

Trauma and Ectopic Pregnancy

Ectopic pregnancy has an incidence of 19.7 cases per 1000 pregnancies and may be encountered in an acute trauma setting.[63] Trauma can precipitate the rupture of a preexisting ectopic pregnancy, causing a medical and surgical emergency. The findings at ultrasound examination or on the CT scan of a ruptured ectopic pregnancy include free fluid, which may be complex, the absence of an intrauterine gestation sac, and the presence of an adnexal mass.[64,65]

Imaging of Nonobstetric Injuries

Several physiologic changes take place during pregnancy, which increase the risk for certain traumatic injuries. The cardiac output increases during

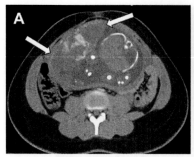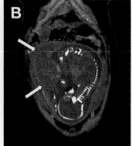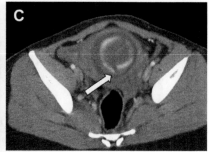

Fig. 6. Fetal injury from blunt abdominal trauma. A 20-year-old pregnant woman involved in motor vehicle collision. Contrast-enhanced CT scan shows full-thickness defects in placental enhancement (*A, B, arrows*) compatible with abruption. There is also a mildly displaced parietal bone fracture involving the fetal skull (*C, arrow*). The fetus did not survive this traumatic injury.

the pregnancy from 4.5 to 6.0 L/min and the uterine flow increases from 1% to 10% of the cardiac output. This results in dilated inferior vena cava and pelvic vasculature, increasing the risk of a retroperitoneal hematoma in blunt or penetrating trauma.[9,38,41,66] The spleen enlarges by up to 50%, which increases the likelihood and severity of the splenic injuries.[67] As the gravid uterus enlarges, it displaces the solid organs upward, closer to the rib cage, making them susceptible to injuries (see **Fig. 3**).[2,3,16,50] The urinary bladder is displaced lower in the pelvis, increasing the risk of bladder injury in the setting of pelvic trauma.[25,68] The uterus also exerts a mass effect on the ureters, causing dilatation of the proximal collecting system, increasing the risk of injury to the kidneys.[69,70]

In contrast, the enlarging uterus provides some protective effect to the maternal body, especially in the setting of penetrating trauma. The incidence of maternal visceral injury with penetrating abdominal trauma is 15% to 40% in pregnant women compared with 80% to 90% in nonpregnant women.[71] Owing to the displacement by the uterus, the risk of serious injury to the solid organs is lower in the setting of penetrating trauma. Additionally, the uterine musculature absorbs the large part of a projectile's momentum and cushions its effect on the maternal structures. This naturally increases the risk of injury to the fetus, with 60% to 70% fetal injuries in penetrating traumas compared with only 20% maternal injuries.[3]

SUMMARY

The pregnant patient with acute trauma is not a common demographic encountered by clinicians or radiologists. However, there are important clinical and imaging considerations for this special population that are vital in ensuring the

maternal and fetal well-being. A multidisciplinary approach with close involvement of obstetrics and psychosocial personnel is key. Although radiography and ultrasound examination are frequently used modalities in the setting of maternal–fetal trauma, the fear of radiation should not preclude one from carrying out a thorough diagnostic workup of the patient with a CT scan. MRI mainly serves as a problem solving and follow-up modality. After stabilizing the mother, fetal well-being should be assessed with external fetal monitoring and a dedicated obstetric ultrasound examination. Radiologists should be familiar with the sonographic and CT findings of catastrophic entities such as placental abruption and uterine rupture.

CLINICS CARE POINTS

- During the first 2 weeks of gestation, the main risk of radiation exposure is fetal death at thresholds of 50 to 100 mGy of dose.
- Placental abruption is the most common cause of fetal death in trauma. Ultrasound has relatively low sensitivity (24%) but a high specificity (96%) for the detection of placental abruption. The sensitivity and specificity of CT is 86-100% and 56-98%, respectively, and of MRI up to 100%.

DISCLOSURE

The authors have nothing to disclose.

REFERENCES

1. Maxwell BG, Greenlaw A, Smith WJ, et al. Pregnant trauma patients may be at increased risk of mortality compared to nonpregnant women of reproductive

age: trends and outcomes over 10 years at a level I trauma center. Womens Health (Lond) 2020;16. 1745506520933021.

2. Brown HL. Trauma in pregnancy. Obstet Gynecol 2009;114(1):147–60.

3. Jain V, Chari R, Maslovitz S, et al. Guidelines for the Management of a Pregnant Trauma Patient. J Obstet Gynaecol Can 2015;37(6):553–74.

4. Lucia A, Dantoni SE. Trauma Management of the Pregnant Patient. Crit Care Clin 2016;32(1): 109–17.

5. El-Kady D, Gilbert WM, Anderson J, et al. Trauma during pregnancy: an analysis of maternal and fetal outcomes in a large population. Am J Obstet Gynecol 2004;190(6):1661–8.

6. Deshpande NA, Kucirka LM, Smith RN, et al. Pregnant trauma victims experience nearly 2-fold higher mortality compared to their nonpregnant counterparts. Am J Obstet Gynecol 2017;217(5):590. e591-590 e599.

7. Smith KA, Bryce S. Trauma in the pregnant patient: an evidence-based approach to management. Emerg Med Pract 2013;15(4):1–18 [quiz: 18-19].

8. Petrone P, Talving P, Browder T, et al. Abdominal injuries in pregnancy: a 155-month study at two level 1 trauma centers. Injury 2011;42(1):47–9.

9. Brown S, Mozurkewich E. Trauma during pregnancy. Obstet Gynecol Clin North Am 2013;40(1): 47–57.

10. Karadas S, Gonullu H, Oncu MR, et al. Pregnancy and trauma: analysis of 139 cases. J Turk Ger Gynecol Assoc 2012;13(2):118–22.

11. Murphy NJ, Quinlan JD. Trauma in pregnancy: assessment, management, and prevention. Am Fam Physician 2014;90(10):717–22.

12. Mirza FG, Devine PC, Gaddipati S. Trauma in pregnancy: a systematic approach. Am J Perinatol 2010; 27(7):579–86.

13. Shakerian R, Thomson BN, Judson R, et al. Radiation fear: impact on compliance with trauma imaging guidelines in the pregnant patient. J Trauma Acute Care Surg 2015;78(1):88–93.

14. Puri A, Khadem P, Ahmed S, et al. Imaging of trauma in a pregnant patient. Semin Ultrasound CT MR 2012;33(1):37–45.

15. Kopelman TR, Bogert JN, Walters JW, et al. Computed tomographic imaging interpretation improves fetal outcomes after maternal trauma. J Trauma Acute Care Surg 2016;81(6):1131–5.

16. Raptis CA, Mellnick VM, Raptis DA, et al. Imaging of trauma in the pregnant patient. Radiographics 2014; 34(3):748–63.

17. Barraco RD, Chiu WC, Clancy TV, et al. Practice management guidelines for the diagnosis and management of injury in the pregnant patient: the EAST Practice Management Guidelines Work Group. J Trauma 2010;69(1):211–4.

18. Kelaranta A, Kaasalainen T, Seuri R, et al. Fetal radiation dose in computed tomography. Radiat Prot Dosimetry 2015;165(1–4):226–30.

19. Richards JR, McGahan JP. Focused Assessment with Sonography in Trauma (FAST) in 2017: what radiologists can learn. Radiology 2017;283(1): 30–48.

20. Goodwin H, Holmes JF, Wisner DH. Abdominal ultrasound examination in pregnant blunt trauma patients. J Trauma 2001;50(4):689–93 [discussion: 694].

21. Hussain ZJ, Figueroa R, Budorick NE. How much free fluid can a pregnant patient have? Assessment of pelvic free fluid in pregnant patients without antecedent trauma. J Trauma 2011;70(6):1420–3.

22. Richards JR, Ormsby EL, Romo MV, et al. Blunt abdominal injury in the pregnant patient: detection with US. Radiology 2004;233(2):463–70.

23. Meisinger QC, Brown MA, Dehqanzada ZA, et al. A 10-year retrospective evaluation of ultrasound in pregnant abdominal trauma patients. Emerg Radiol 2016;23(2):105–9.

24. American College of Radiology. ACR Manual on Contrast Media. American College of Radiology; 2021. Available at: https://www.acr.org/-/media/ ACR/Files/Clinical-Resources/Contrast_Media.

25. Tejwani N, Klifto K, Looze C, et al. Treatment of Pregnant Patients With Orthopaedic Trauma. J Am Acad Orthop Surg 2017;25(5):e90–101.

26. Greffier J, Macri F, Larbi A, et al. Dose reduction with iterative reconstruction: optimization of CT protocols in clinical practice. Diagn Interv Imaging 2015;96(5): 477–86.

27. Vu M, Anderson SW, Shah N, et al. CT of blunt abdominal and pelvic vascular injury. Emerg Radiol 2010;17(1):21–9.

28. American College of Radiology. ACR Manual on Contrast Media. American College of Radiology; 2021.

29. Chen MM, Coakley FV, Kaimal A, et al. Guidelines for computed tomography and magnetic resonance imaging use during pregnancy and lactation. Obstet Gynecol 2008;112(2 Pt 1):333–40.

30. Corwin MT, Seibert JA, Fananapazir G, et al. Journal club: quantification of Fetal Dose Reduction if Abdominal CT Is Limited to the Top of the Iliac Crests in Pregnant Patients With Trauma. AJR Am J Roentgenol 2016;206(4):705–12.

31. Jeavons C, Hacking C, Beenen LF, et al. A review of split-bolus single-pass CT in the assessment of trauma patients. Emerg Radiol 2018;25(4): 367–74.

32. Megibow AJ, Kambadakone A, Ananthakrishnan L. Dual-energy computed tomography: image acquisition, processing, and workflow. Radiol Clin North Am 2018;56(4):507–20.

33. Gupta A, Stuhlfaut JW, Fleming KW, et al. Blunt trauma of the pancreas and biliary tract: a

multimodality imaging approach to diagnosis. Radiographics 2004;24(5):1381–95.

34. Odedra D, Mellnick VM, Patlas MN. Imaging of blunt pancreatic trauma: a systematic review. Can Assoc Radiol J 2020;71(3):344–51.

35. De Wilde JP, Rivers AW, Price DL. A review of the current use of magnetic resonance imaging in pregnancy and safety implications for the fetus. Prog Biophys Mol Biol 2005;87(2–3):335–53.

36. Manlove W, Fowler KJ, Mellnick VM, et al. Role of MRI in Trauma in the Pregnant Patient. In: Masselli G, editor. MRI of fetal and maternal Diseases in pregnancy. Cham: Springer International Publishing; 2016. p. 491–7.

37. Sundgren PC, Leander P. Is administration of gadolinium-based contrast media to pregnant women and small children justified? J Magn Reson Imaging 2011;34(4):750–7.

38. Sadro C, Bernstein MP, Kanal KM. Imaging of trauma: part 2, Abdominal trauma and pregnancy–a radiologist's guide to doing what is best for the mother and baby. AJR Am J Roentgenol 2012; 199(6):1207–19.

39. Fadl SA, Linnau KF, Dighe MK. Placental abruption and hemorrhage-review of imaging appearance. Emerg Radiol 2019;26(1):87–97.

40. Kettel LM, Branch DW, Scott JR. Occult placental abruption after maternal trauma. Obstet Gynecol 1988;71(3 Pt 2):449–53.

41. Pearlman MD, Tintinalli JE, Lorenz RP. Blunt trauma during pregnancy. N Engl J Med 1990;323(23): 1609–13.

42. Podrasky AE, Javitt MC, Glanc P, et al. ACR appropriateness Criteria(R) second and third trimester bleeding. Ultrasound Q 2013;29(4):293–301.

43. Ott J, Pecnik P, Promberger R, et al. Intra- versus retroplacental hematomas: a retrospective case-control study on pregnancy outcomes. BMC Pregnancy Childbirth 2017;17(1):366.

44. Boisrame T, Sananes N, Fritz G, et al. Placental abruption: risk factors, management and maternal-fetal prognosis. Cohort study over 10 years. Eur J Obstet Gynecol Reprod Biol 2014; 179:100–4.

45. Glantz C, Purnell L. Clinical utility of sonography in the diagnosis and treatment of placental abruption. J Ultrasound Med 2002;21(8):837–40.

46. Zaidi SF, Moshiri M, Osman S, et al. Comprehensive Imaging Review of Abnormalities of the Placenta. Ultrasound Q 2016;32(1):25–42.

47. Kanne JP, Lalani TA, Fligner CL. The placenta revisited: radiologic-pathologic correlation. Curr Probl Diagn Radiol 2005;34(6):238–55.

48. Manriquez M, Srinivas G, Bollepalli S, et al. Is computed tomography a reliable diagnostic modality in detecting placental injuries in the setting of

acute trauma? Am J Obstet Gynecol 2010;202(6): 611 e611–615.

49. Wei SH, Helmy M, Cohen AJ. CT evaluation of placental abruption in pregnant trauma patients. Emerg Radiol 2009;16(5):365–73.

50. Jha P, Melendres G, Bijan B, et al. Trauma in pregnant women: assessing detection of post-traumatic placental abruption on contrast-enhanced CT versus ultrasound. Abdom Radiol (Ny) 2017;42(4): 1062–7.

51. Kopelman TR, Berardoni NE, Manriquez M, et al. The ability of computed tomography to diagnose placental abruption in the trauma patient. J Trauma Acute Care Surg 2013;74(1):236–41.

52. Saphier NB, Kopelman TR. Traumatic Abruptio Placenta Scale (TAPS): a proposed grading system of computed tomography evaluation of placental abruption in the trauma patient. Emerg Radiol 2014;21(1):17–22.

53. Masselli G, Brunelli R, Di Tola M, et al. MR imaging in the evaluation of placental abruption: correlation with sonographic findings. Radiology 2011;259(1): 222–30.

54. Allen BC, Leyendecker JR. Placental evaluation with magnetic resonance. Radiol Clin North Am 2013; 51(6):955–66.

55. Masselli G, Brunelli R, Parasassi T, et al. Magnetic resonance imaging of clinically stable late pregnancy bleeding: beyond ultrasound. Eur Radiol 2011;21(9):1841–9.

56. Zhu HB, Jin Y. Uterine rupture following a road traffic accident. Ir J Med Sci 2011;180(3):745–7.

57. Gallo P, Mazza C, Sala F. Intrauterine head stab wound injury resulting in a growing skull fracture: a case report and literature review. Childs Nerv Syst 2010;26(3):377–84.

58. Naeem M, Hoegger MJ, Petraglia FW 3rd, et al. CT of Penetrating Abdominopelvic Trauma. Radiographics 2021;41(4):1064–81.

59. Zeina AR, Kessel B, Mahamid A, et al. Computed tomographic diagnosis of traumatic fetal subdural hematoma. Emerg Radiol 2013;20(2):169–72.

60. Joseph JR, Smith BW, Garton HJ. Blunt prenatal trauma resulting in fetal epidural or subdural hematoma: case report and systematic review of the literature. J Neurosurg Pediatr 2017;19(1): 32–7.

61. Sanapo L, Whitehead MT, Bulas DI, et al. Fetal intracranial hemorrhage: role of fetal MRI. Prenat Diagn 2017;37(8):827–36.

62. Kirkinen P, Partanen K, Ryynanen M, et al. Fetal intracranial hemorrhage. Imaging by ultrasound and magnetic resonance imaging. J Reprod Med 1997;42(8):467–72.

63. Tenore JL. Ectopic pregnancy. Am Fam Physician 2000;61(4):1080–8.

64. Pham H, Lin EC. Adnexal ring of ectopic pregnancy detected by contrast-enhanced CT. Abdom Imaging 2007;32(1):56–8.

65. Lin EP, Bhatt S, Dogra VS. Diagnostic clues to ectopic pregnancy. Radiographics 2008;28(6):1661–71.

66. Ryo E, Unno N, Nagasaka T, et al. Changes in the size of maternal inferior vena cava during pregnancy. J Perinat Med 2004;32(4):327–31.

67. Maymon R, Zimerman AL, Strauss S, et al. Maternal spleen size throughout normal pregnancy. Semin Ultrasound CT MR 2007;28(1):64–6.

68. Leggon RE, Wood GC, Indeck MC. Pelvic fractures in pregnancy: factors influencing maternal and fetal outcomes. J Trauma 2002;53(4):796–804.

69. Kawashima A, Sandler CM, Corl FM, et al. Imaging of renal trauma: a comprehensive review. Radiographics 2001;21(3):557–74.

70. Bailey RR, Rolleston GL. Kidney length and ureteric dilatation in the puerperium. J Obstet Gynaecol Br Commonw 1971;78(1):55–61.

71. Stone IK. Trauma in the obstetric patient. Obstet Gynecol Clin North Am 1999;26(3):459–67, viii.

Computer Tomography Angiography of Peripheral Vascular Injuries

Fabio M. Paes, MD, MBA[a,b,*], Felipe Munera, MD[a,b]

KEYWORDS

- CTA • Trauma • Peripheral vascular injury

KEY POINTS

- CTA is a highly effective tool for the detection and characterization of peripheral vascular injuries.
- Extremity vascular injury is more often associated with penetrating trauma (75% to 80% of cases) than blunt trauma (5%–25% of cases).
- Peripheral vascular injuries account for 40% to 75% of all vascular injuries treated in civilian trauma centers.

INTRODUCTION

Peripheral vascular injuries are defined as injuries to the axillary-brachial trunk and its branches in the upper extremity, and femoral-popliteal trunk and its branches in the lower extremity.[1] Overall, injury to the extremity arteries is a rare finding in the setting of trauma but an important source of morbid and mortality when present. Fast and accurate diagnosis followed by rapid repair of vascular injuries are important for achieving the best clinical outcomes. The advancements in computer tomography (CT) imaging and decades of experience on traumatic vascular imaging have allowed emergency and trauma radiologists to become important contributors for the diagnosis and characterization of peripheral vascular injury. In the next sections, we review the epidemiology and demographics of patients presenting with peripheral vascular injuries, discuss the indications for imaging, factors to optimize CT angiography (CTA) technique, imaging findings, and common challenges for accurate diagnosis and characterization of such injuries. Finally, we briefly present recent advancements in CT imaging of vascular injuries with focus on the increasing role of dual-energy CT (DECT) in the trauma setting.

Epidemiology

The incidence of peripheral vascular injury varies by population (adult vs pediatric; military vs civilian; urban vs rural), upper versus lower extremity location, as well as trauma mechanism (penetrating vs blunt).

A large systematic review of the National Trauma Databank reported a prevalence of 0.5% of patients with at least one extremity vascular injury out of 1,861,799 trauma cases.[2] Although rare, peripheral vascular injuries account for 40% to 75% of all vascular injuries treated in civilian trauma centers.[1] They occur more often in young adult men (mean age of 35 years), with a slightly higher prevalence in the lower extremity than upper extremity.[1–4] Extremity vascular injury is more often associated with penetrating trauma (75% to 80% of cases in urban trauma centers) than blunt trauma (5%–25% of cases), and among the penetrating mechanisms, more often after a gunshot wound than stab wound.[1,5] Among the cases of blunt trauma of the extremity, the prevalence of

[a] Department of Radiology, Jackson Memorial Hospital, University of Miami-Miller School of Medicine, 1611 Northwest 12th Avenue, West Wing 279, Miami, FL 33136, USA; [b] Department of Radiology, Ryder Trauma Center, 1115 Northwest 14th Street, Miami, FL 33136, USA
* Department of Radiology, Jackson Memorial Hospital, University of Miami-Miller School of Medicine, 1611 Northwest 12th Avenue, West Wing 279, Miami, FL 33136
E-mail address: fpaes@med.miami.edu

Radiol Clin N Am 61 (2023) 141–150
https://doi.org/10.1016/j.rcl.2022.08.006
0033-8389/23/© 2022 Elsevier Inc. All rights reserved.

peripheral vascular trauma varies depending on the presence of associated osseous injuries. Arterial damage is encountered in less than 1% of cases of long bone fracture, 9% of cases of severe open tibial fractures, and as high as 16% of cases of knee dislocation.[6,7]

The morbidity and mortality of cases of peripheral vascular trauma are mostly a result of exsanguination, compartment syndrome, ischemia, and amputation. Timely and accurate diagnosis of peripheral vascular injury followed by prompt intervention have proven to reduce complications and improve prognosis. Delays in diagnosis are associated with amputation rate as high as 86% in the lower extremities.[6,8]

Triage of Peripheral Vascular Injury

The appropriate treatment strategy for patients with trauma to the extremities depends on rapid detection, localization, and characterization of a possibly accompanying vascular injury. The decision of whether to pursue CTA in the setting of a suspected peripheral vascular injury largely depends on the patient's presentation and physical examination findings. On arrival to the trauma center, the patient is triaged through the primary and secondary advance trauma life support (ATLS) surveys and immediate interventions are performed on clinically unstable and/or actively bleeding patients. On clinically stable patients, most trauma teams rely on physical examination to determine the presence of "hard" or "soft" signs of peripheral vascular injury and decide whether imaging is necessary (Table 1). The "hard" or overt signs of extremity arterial injury include active pulsatile bleeding; rapidly expanding hematoma; palpable thrill/audible bruit; or classic signs of severe acute limb ischemia (a.k.a. 5 "P": pulselessness, pallor, paresthesia, pain, and paralysis).

The presence of these hard signs correlates with high probability of vascular injury and need of invasive management.[1] In cases where hard signs are present and intervention is indicated, exact localization and characterization of the vascular injury is necessary (ie, multiple extremity fractures or shotgun wound), and the trauma team may pursue CTA imaging if the clinical condition permits and the study can be obtained in a timely fashion.

The "soft" signs of extremity arterial injury include history of arterial bleeding at the scene of trauma or in transit; proximity of a penetrating wound or blunt injury to an artery; small nonpulsatile hematoma over an artery; and neurologic deficit originating in a nerve adjacent to a named artery. The incidence of arterial injuries in such trauma patients ranges from 3% to 25%, depending on which individual soft sign or combination of signs is present. In patients presenting with soft signs and ankle brachial index (ABI) or arterial pressure index (API) less than 0.9, further imaging (CTA or duplex ultrasound) is usually indicated. Imaging is also recommended when the ABI/API or pulses are unclear and/or the extremity remains cool. The presented algorithm follows the expert recommendations from the Western Trauma Association/Critical Decisions in Trauma[1] (Fig. 1)

In cases of polytrauma where the decision for whole body CTA has already been made, the trauma team may decide to include injured extremities in the imaging protocol, regardless of the degree of suspicion for vascular injury, to save time, benefit from the administered contrast injection, obtain better characterization of the underlying soft tissues and osseous injuries, and, furthermore, ultimately affect patient disposition.[3]

Value of Computer Tomography Angiography for Extremity Vascular Injury

Historically, digital subtraction angiography (DSA) was the diagnostic modality of choice for the evaluation of suspected arterial injury in trauma patients. During the past 2 decades with the universal availability of CT scanners in emergency rooms and continuous advancement of CT technology, DSA has largely been replaced by CTA for investigation of upper and lower extremity vascular injuries. Among the advantages of CTA, the ability to simultaneously visualize soft tissues and bone structures and seamless integration of extremity CTA with torso imaging in trauma patients make it preferable for use, particularly for the holistic evaluation of polytrauma patients. In comparison to DSA, CTA is also less expensive, faster to perform and is not associated with potential iatrogenic complications of catheter

Table 1 Physical signs of peripheral arterial injury	
Hard Signs	**Soft Signs**
Active pulsatile bleeding	Stable hematoma
Expanding hematoma	Nonpulsatile bleeding
Palpable thrill	Cool or pale limb
Audible bruit	Neurologic deficit
5 "P" of ischemic limb: Pulselessness, pallor, paresthesia, pain, and paralysis	Diminished distal pulses

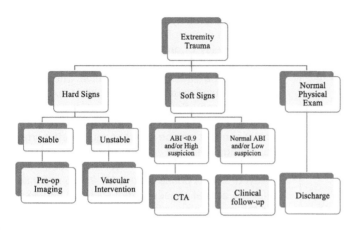

Fig. 1. Triage algorithm for peripheral vascular injury.

angiography, such as dissection, pseudoaneurysm, thrombotic occlusion, access hematoma, and peripheral embolization.[3] The continuous advances of CT technology have improved image quality, permitted faster acquisition and imaging reconstruction times, and allowed incorporation of postprocessing techniques to routine readings with the use of curved multiplanar reformats, maximum intensity projection (MIP), bone subtraction, trajectography, and three dimensional (3D) volume-rendering.[3,9–11] The inability to perform concurrent percutaneous intervention at the time of diagnosis constitutes the main disadvantage of CTA in comparison to conventional angiography. In the minority of cases where subsequent embolization and/or stenting is required, performing CTA first increases the overall radiation and contrast exposure.

Current CTA technology and protocols have proven to be highly sensitive, specific, and accurate for the detection of peripheral vascular injuries. Multiple studies of trauma patients who underwent extremity CTA for vascular injury evaluation showed outstanding sensitivities in the range of 95% to 100%, specificities of 87% to 100%, and accuracy around 93%. They also showed low nondiagnostic imaging yield of less than 5% and good interobserver agreement between different readers.[12–14] Although some small injuries can be missed by CTA, none of the missed injuries were deemed clinically significant in the landmark studies.[13,15,16]

Computer Tomography Angiography Imaging Technique and Protocol

Angiographic imaging of the extremity arteries should be acquired on newer 64-slice or above CT scanners, even though most multidetector CT scanners with at least 16 slices can render adequate diagnostic images when the protocols are optimized.[3,14] In order to provide the

necessary steady and homogenous flow of contrast required for opacification of the smaller branches of the peripheral arteries, patients should have adequate large gauge peripheral intravenous (IV) access, typically 18-gauge or 20-gauge for average-sized adults, and power injector with sufficient iodine concentration contrast (at least 300 mg/mL) must be used. The exact CTA protocols for extremity imaging will vary among institutions and scanners, although the principles for imaging optimization are the same. The parameters used in our institution are listed in **Box 1**.

Patient preparation is key to obtain optimal diagnostic images of the peripheral vessels. The contrast should be injected through a peripheral line placed on the contralateral side of the injured extremity to prevent dense venous contrast from obscuring the adjacent arterial findings. Adequate position and lack of motion are important to avoid the formation of imaging artifacts. Ideally, for imaging evaluation of the upper extremities, the arms should be raised above the head, palm facing upward with fingers extended in order to limit streak artifacts arising from the denser body. When this position is not possible due to injuries, the scan can be performed with arms down positioned along the torso and palms facing up. For lower extremity evaluation, the patient is usually positioned supine with both legs together. Concomitant imaging acquisition of both lower extremities is recommended, even if only one leg has sustained injury, mostly to allow intrastudy control of contrast opacification of the distal arteries. The extremity in question can be immobilized if the patient is unable to remain still for the examination.

In most large trauma centers, the exact protocol of CTA of the extremities will depend on the need of concomitant images of the torso as part of a whole-body scan. For most trauma patients, we can acquire adequate CTA images of the upper and/or lower extremity concomitantly with our

> **Box 1**
> **Optimized CTA protocol for peripheral arterial trauma**
>
> Scanning Parameters (multi detector computer tomography (MDCT) 64 and 128 slices)
>
> Voltage: 120 kVp
>
> Current: 250 mAs
>
> Tube Current Modulation
>
> Pitch: 0.7
>
> Revolution Time: 0.5 sec
>
> Collimation: 0.6 mm
>
> Contrast Administration
>
> 18–20-gauge IV line
>
> 100–120 mL of iodine contrast (Ioversol 350 mg/mL, Mallinckrodt)
>
> Contrast rate of 4.0 mL/s for 15 s, decreased to 3.0 mL/s, followed by 30 mL of saline at 4.0 mL/s
>
> Injection on the contralateral extremity of the side of interest
>
> Contrast Trigger:
>
> Whole-body scanning: Fixed delay of 25 s for arterial phase. Usually adequate for upper extremity. Sequential scanning for lower extremities. Immediate rescanning of the lower extremities when outrun contrast bolus.
>
> Isolated extremity: Fixed delay as above or bolus trigger in the aortic arch/subclavian for upper extremity and distal abdominal aorta/common iliac for lower extremity.
>
> Delay imaging of the extremity may be acquired on request of the radiologist
>
> Reconstruction Parameters
>
> 1.5 mm and 3.0 mm axial images
>
> 1.5 mm coronal and sagittal multiplanar reformat (MPRs)
>
> Routine 3 planes MIPs
>
> 3 D and curved reformats by request

routine whole-body trauma scan by adjusting the contrast injection rate and timing of acquisition. In our institution, we use fixed scan timing of 25-second delay for optimal mid-to-late arterial phase imaging for most of our whole-body trauma cases. Time is often critical in the emergent polytrauma setting and a preset delay is most expedient and supported by available literature.[14,16] This can be adjusted depending on the additional extremity being imaged. In cases of injuries to the upper extremity, the delay can be the same or shorter, whereas in cases of distal lower extremity injury a longer delay of around 40 to 45 seconds may be necessary. Bolus tracking or test bolus can be used as a satisfactory alternative when clinically possible, particularly on isolated extremity trauma cases. Sequential dedicated extremity scanning with or without a separate second injection of contrast may be used to acquire better arterial images if the initial scan is deemed nondiagnostic.[14,17] Dual phase acquisition with delayed venous phase images (ie, 25–35 seconds after the arterial phase) are not routinely acquired for the extremities, although they may be useful and can be requested by the emergent radiologist in selected cases.[14]

At our institution, the submillimeter isotropic voxel data set is routinely reconstructed at 1.5 and 3.0 mm in the conventional axial plane and submitted for evaluation. Multiplanar reconstructions on sagittal and coronal planes along the axis of the extremity as well as MIP images are also obtained by technologists at the scanner. 3D volume rendering images and curved planar reformats, including trajectography, can be requested or constructed using postprocessing software available on the workstations.

Imaging Findings

There are 5 recognized types of acute vascular injuries with corresponding imaging findings (**Figs 2–8**).: (1) intimal tears (intimal flaps, surface disruptions, or subintimal/intramural hematomas), (2) full thickness vessel wall defects with pseudoaneurysms or hemorrhage, (3) complete transections with active hemorrhage and/or occlusion, (4) arteriovenous fistulas (AVF), and (5) spasm. Low-grade intimal injuries and/or intramural hematomas are more often associated with blunt trauma and can lead to secondary occlusion. Full thick wall defects, complete transections, and AVF usually occur with penetrating trauma. Spasm is a temporary finding more common in young patients, which can occur after blunt or penetrating trauma. On imaging and clinically, spasm may be confused with intimal injury or intramural hematoma causing significant stenosis and reversible decreased peripheral flow. A traumatic true peripheral artery aneurysm is a rare and late finding that occurs when intimal or intimal-media injury leads to dilation of an artery with no extraluminal extravasation of contrast. Full-thickness defect in the arterial wall with extraluminal extravasation and pooling of contrast corresponds to active arterial bleed and is responsible for an acute pulsatile hematoma immediately after injury. A traumatic

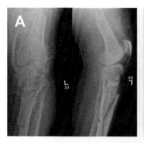 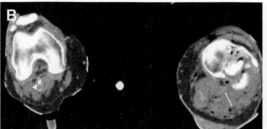 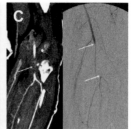

Fig. 2. A 43-year-old man hit by a car. (*A*) antero-posterior (AP) and lateral radiographs of the left knee showing comminuted fractures of the left tibial plateau, proximal fibula diaphysis, and distal femoral diaphysis. Comminuted fractures of the tibia have an elevated risk of concomitant arterial injury. (*B*) Axial CTA image at the level of the popliteal fossa shows lack of opacification of the left popliteal artery (*arrow*). Note the patent opacified right popliteal artery on the contralateral extremity (*arrowhead*). (*C*) Coronal MPR and corresponding DSA images show the segmental traumatic occlusion of the left popliteal artery (*arrows*). Traumatic occlusions can occur due to intimal injury or transection followed by thrombosis.

pseudoaneurysm corresponds to a similar traumatic arterial injury but the extraluminal blood is encapsulated and contained by the surrounding tissues. Arterial transections occur when the circumference of the vessel is disrupted and usually leads to active contrast extravasation from the proximal segment and/or thrombotic occlusion of the disconnected distal artery. As for traumatic venous injuries in the extremity, wall defects in many peripheral veins seem to heal when local tissue pressure is applied which prevents significant extravasation of blood in most traumatic cases.

Adequate characterization of vascular injuries relies on optimal opacification of the arteries on CTA and sometimes multiphasic acquisition. Intimal injuries seem as contour irregularity and/or intraluminal linear defects with or without segmental narrowing of the traumatized arterial segment and may be differentiated from external

soft tissue compression and spasm, which usually involves a longer segment and present as smooth or concentric narrowing. The term "traumatic dissection" to describe an arterial flap in the setting of trauma is controversial among emergency radiologists and surgeons, and furthermore should not be used. Instead, intimal injury with a flap is preferred to describe the traumatic imaging finding.

The presence of complete lack of opacification of an arterial segment at the injured extremity is usually due to thrombotic occlusion from intimal injury, focal wall defect, or transection, or due to embolism from a proximal injury. Posttraumatic thrombotic occlusions should be differentiated from suboptimal opacification of the vessels in cases where the scanner outruns the contrast bolus, severe hypotension, severe spasm and/or proximal bleeding, which decreases the flow to

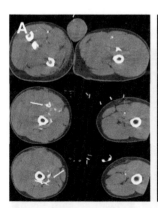 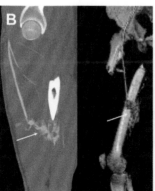 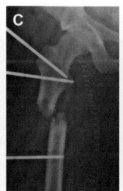 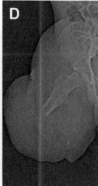

Fig. 3. A 35-year-old man after a motor vehicle accident presenting with an enlarging right thigh hematoma. (*A*) Sequential axial CTA images show abrupt cut-off of the right superficial femoral artery (SFA) and active contrast extravasation (*arrows*) at the level of the femoral fracture. (*B*) Sagittal MIP and 3D-volume rendering images demonstrate the SFA transection and the active arterial extravasation (*arrows*). Distal lower extremity arteries are not opacified. (*C*) Patient underwent initially open revascularization and external fixation of the right femur. (*D*) Unfortunately, the patient did not progress well and an above the knee amputation was performed.

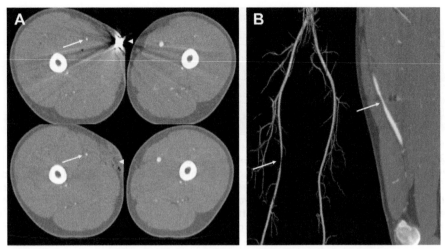

Fig. 4. A 21-year-old man status after gunshot wound to the right thigh. Diminished distal pulses. (*A*) Sequential axial CTA images shows smooth reduced caliber of the right SFA (*arrows*) when compared with the contralateral side. Note the superficial track and retained bullet in the medial soft tissues of the right thigh (*arrowheads*). (*B*) 3D-volume rendering and sagittal MPR again show the segmental smooth narrowing of the right SFA compatible with spasm. The patient was treated conservatively and the distal pulses improved.

the suspected arterial bed. Additional delayed imaging, comparison to the contralateral side and/or duplex sonography can be used as adjunctive in some cases and help differentiate.

Pseudoaneurysms present as round foci of pooled contrast material in the injured region, following the density of the adjacent normal artery and retaining a constant shape in all phases. In contrast, active arterial extravasation changes in morphology, increases in size/spreads and shows higher attenuation than the adjacent artery on delayed phase images. Traumatic AVF present as early opacification of venous structures during the arterial phase of imaging, implying direct communication between injured artery and vein at the site of trauma. Although always present, the direct arteriovenous channel may be small and not seen on the CT images. AVF is differentiated from asymmetric hyperemia and early venous return on the injured extremity by having the contrast density in the opacified venous segment of the fistula approaching of the adjacent artery. In cases where multiphasic images are acquired, newer or more conspicuous areas of irregular high attenuation in delayed images, not corresponding to arterial contrast enhancement foci on earlier phase, usually represent hemorrhage of venous origin or from osseous fractures.[18,19]

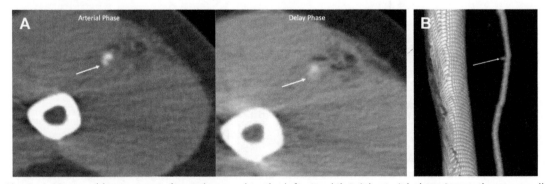

Fig. 5. A 28-year-old man status after stab wound to the left arm. (*A*) Axial arterial phase image shows a small focal outpouching of contrast arising from the brachial artery at the site of the stab wound (*arrow*). No notable change in morphology or blooming of the contrast outpouching on the delay image (*arrow*) confirming the presence of a small pseudoaneurysm of the brachial artery. (*B*) 3D-volume rendering image again depicts the small pseudoaneurysm (*arrow*). It was treated successfully with external pressure only.

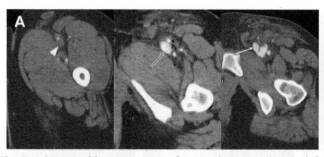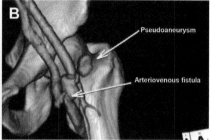

Fig. 6. A 26-year-old woman status after gunshot wound to the left upper thigh and buttock. (*A*) Sequential axial CTA images demonstrate the soft tissue wound in the left groin, irregular morphology and outpouching of the proximal SFA (*solid arrow*), and early opacification of the adjacent femoral vein (*open arrow*). Note the nonopacified femoral vein below the level of the injury (*arrowhead*). The findings depict an AVF between the SFA and femoral vein with a presence of a pseudoaneurysm. (*B*) 3D-volume rendering image shows the AVF connection, the SFA pseudoaneurysm, and the antegrade early opacification of the common femoral and external iliac veins.

The following cases illustrate the different imaging findings of peripheral vascular injuries and exemplify key concepts for accurate diagnosis.

Imaging Analysis Challenges and Pitfalls

The approach to reviewing the hundreds to thousands of CTA images generated from a single trauma patient varies among radiologists but good imaging quality and systematic and comprehensive imaging review methodology are necessary to provide an efficient and accurate report of the vascular injuries to the trauma teams. Despite vigilant attention to protocol and adequate technique, extremity CTAs are more prone to poor diagnostic quality and artifacts in the setting of trauma due to the inherited time limit constraints and critical condition of the patients. Lack of and/ or incomplete contrast opacification of the arteries related to mismatched between the timing of the image acquisition and arrival of the contrast bolus is one of the most common reasons for suboptimal

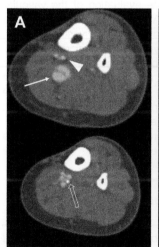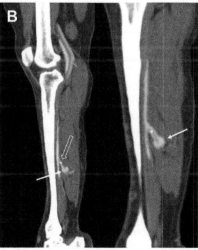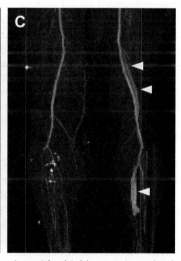

Fig. 7. A 36-year-old man status after gunshot wound to the right calf presenting with a highly comminuted right tibia fracture (not showed). Left leg was deemed intact on initial examination. Bilateral lower extremity CTA was performed to evaluate for vascular injury on the right lower leg. Axial (*A*) and sagittal (*B*) CTA images of the left leg showed unexpected early opacification of the posterior tibial vein (PTV; *arrowhead*), outpouching from the posterior tibial artery (PTA; *solid arrow*) and a small communication between the PTA and PTV, corresponding to a traumatic left PTA-PTV AVF and a PTA pseudoaneurysm. A tiny metallic bullet fragment was seen in the vicinity of the vascular injury (*open arrow*). On reexamination of the left lower leg, a small pinhole defect was identified on the left calf corresponding to the penetrating injury. (*C*) Subtraction MIP image of the lower extremities showed the left leg AVF and corresponding early opacification of the left leg deep venous system proximal to the injury (*arrowhead*).

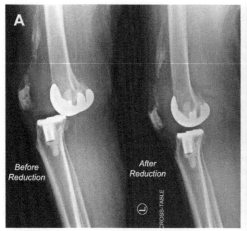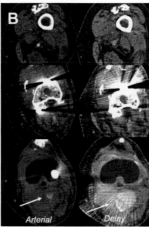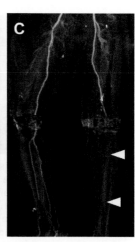

Fig. 8. A 65-year-old woman status after motor vehicle accident presenting with left knee arthroplasty disloca-tion. (A) Radiographs of the left knee before and after reduction. Given the elevated risk for vascular injury, CTA was obtained. (B) Sequential axial arterial and delay images of the left knee are shown. The presence of ar-throplasty creates significant streak artifact obscuring the popliteal artery. However, focal change in caliber of the visualized popliteal segment with blooming of the contrast pooling on the delay phase below the level of the arthroplasty permit the diagnosis of popliteal transection. (C) Subtraction MIP image of the lower extremities shows the abrupt cut-off at the left popliteal artery with no opacification of the distal tibial-peroneal trunk (arrowhead).

CTA evaluation. Incorrect scan trigger time of imag-ing acquisition after injection of contrast is a com-mon cause. This can occur due to variable hemodynamic state of the patients, such as in the presence of congestive heart failure or significant atherosclerosis. Fast CT acquisitions along the z-axis, commonly on new scanners, can "outrun" the contrast bolus leading to incomplete vessel filling in the distal lower extremities, particularly when extremity imaging is combined with whole body CTA acquisition. An immediate delayed CT imaging of the lower extremities using the already given contrast bolus can sometimes solve the issue. Alternatively, a repeat injection with bolus triggering at the distal aorta may be necessary and can provide adequate lower extremity im-ages.[4] The decision to repeat the CTA should be made in agreement with the clinical team.

Motion is a common challenge for adequate im-aging in the trauma setting. Trauma patients are more prone to move during imaging due to altered mental status, pain, and/or inability to follow com-mands. Adherence to adequate patient posi-tioning and immobilization of the extremity in question are necessary in order to obtain diag-nostic CTA images of the extremities in chal-lenging patients. Sometimes, sedation may be required to allow adequate imaging.

Metallic projectiles retained in soft tissues, bone fragments, and orthopedic hardware can result in significant artifacts, commonly limiting the evalua-tion of adjacent vessels, and obscuring or creating "false" vascular injury imaging findings. Often, adequate contrast opacification of the vessels and the use of multiplanar reformats still allow evaluation of large vessels and the diagnosis of major traumatic injuries. In cases where the streak artifact precludes the evaluation of the vascular bed in question, DSA may be indicated to evaluate and exclude the presence of vascular injury. Recent imaging advancements using metal arti-fact reduction algorithms and/or DECT have shown to decrease metal and/or bone fragment artifacts, improving visualization of the of the soft-tissues and bones details, and as such can be useful to evaluate vascular injuries.[20] Unfortu-nately, limited research exists on the use of those techniques for the evaluation of peripheral vascular trauma.

Dual-Energy Computer Tomography in Vascular Trauma

DECT is a process for creating CT images using 2 photon spectra at different kVp during acquisition. Currently, the techniques and hardware used to obtain the different photon spectra vary accord-ingly to the CT vendors, including multiple X-ray tubes and beam split filter by Siemens, fast kV-switching of tube voltage by GE, and dual-layer detector by Philips.[20] The benefit of DECT for vascular imaging revolves around the ability to in-crease the conspicuity of iodine contrast using low–keV monoenergetic iodine mapping and z-effective color mapping reconstruction techniques and also the ability to isolate and suppress certain materials such as iodine, metal, and calcium densities.[21] The theoretic benefits of DECT imaging in trauma for some clinical scenarios, including better visualization of solid-organ, mesenteric, bowel, and vascular injuries, have been demonstrated, although with limited data.[21,22]

For vascular trauma, the presence of active arterial extravasation of iodine contrast remains the most clinically significant finding on imaging, usually correlating with morbidity and associated with the need of intervention. The imaging diagnosis of active extravasation depends on the identification of extraluminal iodine contrast. In routine single-phase CTA, extraluminal foci of high density may represent active arterial bleeding, pseudoaneurysm, or hyperattenuating materials such as bone fragments, enteric material, or foreign bodies. In the presence of bone fractures or penetrating projectiles, the extravasated contrast can be obscure making those trauma scenarios more challenging. Studies have shown that low–keV monoenergetic images from DECT angiography improve general arterial image quality and vascular contrast-to-noise ratios, although those were not performed in trauma setting. Moreover, calcium subtraction techniques have been shown to improve visualization of arterial lumen in patients with severe atherosclerotic disease and as such have a theoretic role in the peripheral artery injury evaluation. Finally, virtual noncontrast images and iodine overlay maps can help with the visualization of active contrast extravasation, by differentiating iodine contrast from noniodine hyperattenuating materials, including bone fragments in the presence of fractures.[22] Unfortunately, limited data evaluating the role and benefits of DECT in peripheral vascular trauma exist. To our knowledge, a recent article by Joshi and colleagues was the first and only study examining the diagnostic quality of DECT imaging compared with conventional CT in the setting of vascular injury secondary to lower extremity trauma.[21] Although with limitations, the authors showed increased contrast density in all evaluated lower extremity vascular segments, reduction in nondiagnostic vascular segments, and subjective improvement in imaging quality for some vascular segments when using DECT compared with conventional CT. No differences in vascular injury detection rates between the 2 CT techniques were encountered in this study.[21]

A more detail discussion of DECT technique, in particular how it generates the imaging maps in the different spectra and its utility in trauma are beyond the scope of this article. For more information on the increased role of DECT in emergency imaging, please refer to 2 excellent articles also part of this Radiology Clinics issue.

SUMMARY

In summary, vascular injuries of the extremities are an important source of morbidity and mortality for trauma patients. CTA plays a fundamental role in the workup and characterization of those injuries. Knowledge of the imaging findings of the diverse types of peripheral arterial injuries is a requirement for radiologists participating in the care of trauma patients. Adequate imaging protocols minimize pitfalls and allow radiologists to provide rapid and accurate diagnosis, which are necessary to expedite patient disposition.

CLINICS CARE POINTS

- Peripheral vascular injuries account for 40% to 75% of all vascular injuries treated in civilian trauma centers.

- Extremity vascular injury is more often associated with penetrating trauma (75% to 80% of cases in urban trauma centers) than blunt trauma (5%–25% of cases), and among the penetrating mechanisms, more often after a gunshot wound than a stab wound.

- CTA is a highly effective tool for the detection and characterization of peripheral vascular injuries with proven outstanding sensitivities in the range of 95% to 100%, specificities of 87% to 100%, and accuracy around 93%.

- Patient preparation is key to obtain optimal diagnostic images of the peripheral vessels. Adequate IV access, iodine contrast flow, patient position, and lack of motion are all important to avoid the formation of imaging artifacts and allow adequate imaging evaluation.

- AVF is differentiated from asymmetric hyperemia and early venous return on the injured extremity by having the contrast density in the opacified venous segment of the fistula approaching the adjacent artery.

DISCLOSURE

All authors certify that they have no competing interests to declare that are relevant to the content of this article.

REFERENCES

1. Feliciano DV, Moore FA, Moore EE, et al. Evaluation and management of peripheral vascular injury. Part 1. Western Trauma Association/critical decisions in trauma. J Trauma 2011;70(6):1551–6.
2. Barmparas G, Inaba K, Talving P, et al. Pediatric vs adult vascular trauma: a National Trauma Databank review. J Pediatr Surg 2010;45(7):1404–12.
3. Walkoff L, Nagpal P, Khandelwal A. Imaging primer for CT angiography in peripheral vascular trauma. Emerg Radiol 2021;28(1):143–52.
4. Pieroni S, Foster BR, Anderson SW, et al. Use of 64-row multidetector CT angiography in blunt and penetrating trauma of the upper and lower extremities. Radiographics 2009;29(3):863–76.
5. Callan AK, Bauer JM, Mir HR. Over-utilization of computed tomography angiography in extremity trauma. OTA Int 2019;2(4):e030.
6. Halvorson JJ, Anz A, Langfitt M, et al. Vascular injury associated with extremity trauma: initial diagnosis and management. J Am Acad Orthop Surg 2011; 19(8):495–504.
7. Allen MJ, Nash JR, Ioannidies TT, et al. Major vascular injuries associated with orthopaedic injuries to the lower limb. Ann R Coll Surg Engl 1984;66(2):101–4.
8. Green NE, Allen BL. Vascular injuries associated with dislocation of the knee. J Bone Joint Surg Am 1977;59(2):236–9.
9. Weger K, Hammer P, McKinley T, et al. Incidence and clinical impact of lower extremity vascular injuries in the setting of whole body computed tomography for trauma. Emerg Radiol 2021;28(2):265–72.
10. Fritz J, Efron DT, Fishman EK. Multidetector CT and three-dimensional CT angiography of upper extremity arterial injury. Emerg Radiol 2015;22(3):269–82.
11. Dreizin D, Munera F. Multidetector CT for Penetrating Torso Trauma: State of the Art. Radiology 2015; 277(2):338–55.
12. Patterson BO, Holt PJ, Cleanthis M, et al. Imaging vascular trauma. Br J Surg 2012;99(4):494–505.
13. Jens S, Kerstens MK, Legemate DA, et al. Diagnostic performance of computed tomography angiography in peripheral arterial injury due to trauma: a systematic review and meta-analysis. Eur J Vasc Endovasc Surg 2013;46(3):329–37.
14. Fishman EK, Horton KM, Johnson PT. Multidetector CT and three-dimensional CT angiography for suspected vascular trauma of the extremities. Radiographics 2008;28(3):653–65. ; discussion 665-656.
15. Colip CG, Gorantla V, LeBedis CA, et al. Extremity CTA for penetrating trauma: 10-year experience using a 64-detector row CT scanner. Emerg Radiol 2017;24(3):223–32.
16. Soto JA, Munera F, Morales C, et al. Focal arterial injuries of the proximal extremities: helical CT arteriography as the initial method of diagnosis. Radiology 2001;218(1):188–94.
17. Bozlar U, Ogur T, Norton PT, et al. CT angiography of the upper extremity arterial system: Part 1-Anatomy, technique, and use in trauma patients. AJR Am J Roentgenol 2013;201(4):745–52.
18. Dreizin D, Munera F. Blunt polytrauma: evaluation with 64-section whole-body CT angiography. Radiographics 2012;32(3):609–31.
19. Gakhal MS, Sartip KA. CT angiography signs of lower extremity vascular trauma. AJR Am J Roentgenol 2009;193(1):W49–57.
20. Wellenberg RHH, Hakvoort ET, Slump CH, et al. Metal artifact reduction techniques in musculoskeletal CT-imaging. Eur J Radiol 2018;107:60–9.
21. Joshi R, LeBedis C, Dao K, et al. Dual energy CT angiography for lower extremity trauma: comparison with conventional CT. Emerg Radiol 2022;29(3): 471–7.
22. Wortman JR, Uyeda JW, Fulwadhva UP, et al. Dual-Energy CT for Abdominal and Pelvic Trauma. Radiographics 2018;38(2):586–602.

Imaging of Soft Tissue Infections

Ninad Salastekar, MBBS, MPH*, Andres Su, MD, Jean Sebastien Rowe, MD,
Aravind Somasundaram, MD, Phillip K. Wong, MD, Tarek N. Hanna, MD

KEYWORDS

• Soft tissue infections • Necrotizing fasciitis • Myositis • Abscess • Tenosynovitis • Bursitis

KEY POINTS

- In the setting of soft tissue infections, physical examination lacks sensitivity and specificity, and imaging is often required to evaluate the depth of involvement and identify complications.
- It is important to identify necrotizing soft tissue infections with a key imaging finding of soft tissue gas along with fluid along fascial planes, as these infections have a more rapid and morbid course.
- Imaging modality should be carefully selected based on the region of infection, and the clinician should be aware that multiple imaging modalities may ultimately be necessary

INTRODUCTION

Soft tissue infections encompass a diverse group of diseases with a broad spectrum of morbidity and mortality, ranging from uncomplicated cellulitis to necrotizing fasciitis (NF).[1] There are many predisposing conditions that make individuals prone to soft tissue infections but the more common risk factors include advanced age, immunosuppression, illicit drug use, peripheral vascular disease, obesity, and malnutrition.[2] Most infections gain access to the body because of skin breakdown from trauma, surgery, or ulceration.[2,3] Much less commonly, infections can seed the soft tissues through hematogenous spread.[2,3]

Although superficial infections can often be diagnosed and managed clinically, physical examination and laboratory findings may lack sensitivity and specificity.[4] As such, imaging is often required to evaluate the extent, depth, and character of soft tissue infection, demonstrating which soft tissue structures are involved and if there are complications. Soft tissue infection may seem to be superficial but in the absence of imaging, clinicians fail to differentiate cellulitis from soft tissue abscess in 22% of cases, which can lead to delayed or incorrect treatment.[5]

In this article, we review the various types of soft tissue infections and provide an overview of both expected imaging findings and complications that may alter clinical management. We provide an overview of the utility of different imaging modalities and review systematically the spectrum of soft tissue infections, from superficial to deep, with multimodality case examples.

IMAGING MODALITIES

Based on physical examination, patient risk factors, and laboratory parameters, the Emergency Department provider must decide if imaging is necessary.

Radiography

Radiographs are not required for the evaluation of soft tissue infection but they are included in the diagnostic pathway and may be the only imaging obtained in cases of mild infection not requiring hospitalization.[6] Plain radiographic findings in the setting of soft tissue infection include nonspecific findings such as swelling, effacement of fat planes, and potentially skin discontinuity in the setting of deep ulcers.[4] The radiologist relies on the provided

Department of Radiology and Imaging Sciences, Emory University School of Medicine, 1364 Clifton Road Northeast, Atlanta, GA 30322, USA
* Corresponding author. Emergency and Trauma Imaging, Department of Radiology and Imaging Sciences, Emory University School of Medicine, Atlanta, GA 30322.
E-mail address: nsalast@emory.edu

Radiol Clin N Am 61 (2023) 151–166
https://doi.org/10.1016/j.rcl.2022.08.003
0033-8389/23/© 2022 Elsevier Inc. All rights reserved.

patient history in these settings, as identical imaging findings can be seen in trauma and venous insufficiency.[4] Radiography can provide 2 valuable pieces of information by identifying radiopaque foreign bodies (which may be a nidus for infection) or soft tissue gas (suggesting necrotizing infection).[2,4,7] Radiographs also provide a high-resolution overview of the osseous structures, help exclude other causes of soft tissue swelling such as fracture, and are the first-line imaging study to evaluate for osteomyelitis.

Sonography

After initial radiographs, ultrasound(US) is often the second modality used to evaluate patients with soft tissue infections. Its advantages include low cost, availability, portability, and utility for real-time guidance of fluid aspiration.[7] Point-of-care ultrasound (POCUS) is widely adopted by emergency or clinic providers at the bedside to garner information in lieu of or before a dedicated US within the radiology department.[8] POCUS allows clinicians to rapidly evaluate for abscess, reduces inappropriate attempts at incision and drainage in the absence of abscess by 20% compared with physical examination alone, and enables screening for superficial foreign bodies.[8]

Computed Tomography

The benefits of computed tomography (CT) include wide availability (both geographic and temporal), short acquisition times, broad anatomic coverage, high spatial resolution, and the capacity for multiplanar reformats. These qualities make CT a mainstay for evaluating potentially complicated soft tissue infections in the emergent setting. The administration of intravenous (IV) contrast improves anatomic delineation and facilitates the diagnosis of abscess. CT has significantly higher sensitivity than radiography for diagnosing necrotizing soft tissue infections.[9] Indeed, a negative contrast-enhanced CT can reliably rule out the need for surgical intervention when there is clinical concern for necrotizing infection.[10]

MR Imaging

MR imaging is the gold standard imaging modality in the evaluation and characterization of soft tissue infections, providing high spatial and contrast resolution for all types of soft tissues, with abundant anatomic detail.[4] The optimal MR imaging protocol depends on the anatomic area of interest and the specific clinical question but at minimum should include T1-weighted images (T1WI) for anatomic evaluation and T2-weighted images (T2WI) or short T inversion-recovery (STIR) sequences to evaluate for edema. Contrast-enhanced MR imaging offers significant advantages when evaluating for fluid collections, fascial enhancement, and pyomyositis or myonecrosis.

Nuclear Medicine

Diagnostic nuclear medicine examinations including Ga-67 and labeled leukocyte Single Photon Emission Computed Tomography (SPECT)/CT, 18F-fluorodeoxyglucose (18F-FDG) PET/CT, and more recently Ga-68 tracers have applications in the assessment of infectious and inflammatory soft tissue disorders.[11] Although these techniques are useful in problem-solving situations, they are not routinely deployed in clinical practice and are outside the scope of this article.

SKIN AND SUBCUTANEOUS INFECTIONS
Cellulitis and Abscess

Cellulitis is a nonnecrotizing infection limited to the skin and subcutaneous fat without the involvement of the underlying fascia or muscles.[4,12] It presents most commonly in the lower extremities as an area of skin demonstrating erythema, swelling, and warmth.[13] The largest insurance claims-based study reports an incidence rate for cellulitis of 24.6/1000 person-years, with a higher incidence in men and adults aged older than 45 years.[13] In immunocompetent adults, the most common causative organisms include *Streptococcus pyogenes* (Group A Streptococci) and *Staphylococcus aureus*. In immunocompromised adults, atypical pathogens such as gram-negative bacilli, anaerobes, and mycobacteria are often encountered.[14] Common risk factors for cellulitis include vascular insufficiency/venous stasis, diabetes, chronic liver disease, IV drug use, and retained foreign body following trauma[1,4,12] (**Fig. 1**). Although the diagnosis of cellulitis is primarily clinical, imaging studies can help to determine the extent and depth of infection, and to evaluate for the presence of retained foreign bodies or complications such as abscess or necrotizing infection.

The US appearance of cellulitis ranges from swelling of the skin and subcutaneous fat to increased echogenicity. The subcutaneous soft tissues may demonstrate a cobblestone appearance arising from the reticular pattern of hypoechoic, edematous connective tissue interspersed between echogenic lobules of subcutaneous fat.[12,15,16] Although nonspecific, hyperemia on color Doppler US favors an underlying infectious cause over noninfectious causes of skin and subcutaneous edema such as venous insufficiency/thrombophlebitis, cardiac failure, or anasarca.[12,16]

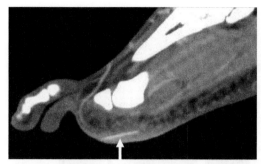

Fig. 1. A sagittal contrast-enhanced CT of the forefoot shows a linear radiopaque density along the plantar surface of the forefoot soft tissues in keeping with a retained foreign body, in this case a wood splinter (*arrow*). There is surrounding inflammatory stranding and skin thickening, however, no organized fluid collection. Imaging may be key to identify retained foreign bodies, which can be a nidus for infection.

Thickening of the skin and superficial fascia, and subcutaneous fat stranding are the most common findings of cellulitis on CT.[16] MR imaging is typically reserved for more serious infections or when complications are suspected. However, typical features of cellulitis on MR imaging include hypointense signal on T1WI and corresponding hyperintensity on T2WI within the affected skin and subcutaneous tissues[17] (**Fig. 2**).

An abscess represents a walled-off collection of inflammatory cells, tissue debris, and causative organisms.[17] Superficial abscesses most commonly result from direct inoculation following penetrating trauma, although deep abscesses are usually sequelae of hematogenous spread of infection.[17] *Staphylococcus* is the most common causative organism identified in abscesses.[14]

An abscess may seem as mass-like soft tissue swelling or a gas–fluid level within soft tissues on radiographs.[17] On US, an abscess's echogenicity varies from anechoic to hyperechoic depending on the contents, although the most common appearance is an anechoic or hypoechoic collection.[15] The presence of gas within a collection (characterized by echogenicity with posterior shadowing) is highly suggestive of abscess in the appropriate clinical setting.[15] Other US features of an abscess include an echogenic rim with increased peripheral vascularity, internal septations, and mobile echogenic debris.[15] The central fluid component of an abscess seems hypoattenuating on CT and T1-hypointense and T2-hyperintense on MR imaging. Both CT and MR imaging typically demonstrate an irregular, thick enhancing wall on postcontrast images and may contain internal gas depending on the organism in question[2,16] (**Figs. 3–6**). US-guided or CT-

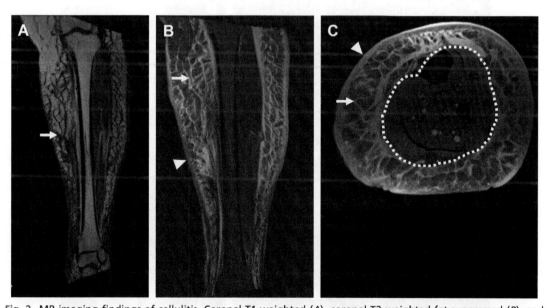

Fig. 2. MR imaging findings of cellulitis. Coronal T1-weighted (*A*), coronal T2-weighted fat suppressed (*B*), and axial T2-weighted fat suppressed sequences demonstrate circumferential skin thickening (*arrowheads*) and infiltrative subcutaneous fat edema (*arrows*) without a focal fluid collection. The subcutaneous edema presents as T1W hypointense and T2W hyperintense lines against a backdrop of fatty lobules. Notice the absence of edema signal deep to the fascia within the intermuscular compartment demonstrating this is a superficial skin and soft tissue infection (*C-dashed lines* demarcate the muscular compartment). Similar imaging findings can also be seen with third spacing (volume overload), chronic lymphedema, and chronic venous stasis.

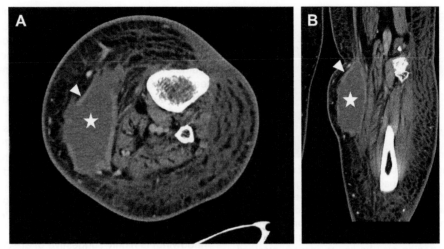

Fig. 3. Lower extremity subcutaneous abscess. Contrast-enhanced axial (*A*) and coronal (*B*) CT shows skin thickening, subcutaneous stranding, and a rim-enhancing (*arrow-head*) subcutaneous abscess (*star*) located in the subcutaneous fat.

guided percutaneous drainage is usually the treatment of choice for larger soft tissue abscesses. Note that there are mimickers for soft tissue infection by imaging, including infiltrative neoplasm, and supportive clinical features are important in making this imaging diagnosis (**Fig. 7**).

Fascial Infections

NF is a soft tissue infection characterized by necrosis of superficial and deep fascia with a fulminant clinical course and high mortality. The pathophysiology of NF involves rapid

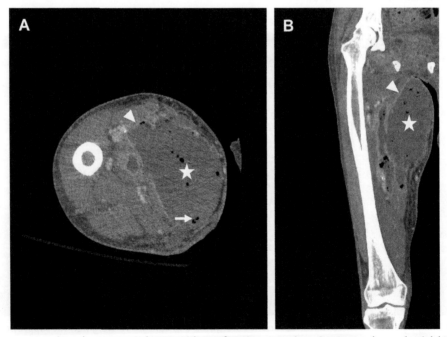

Fig. 4. Lower extremity subcutaneous abscess with gas-forming organism. Contrast-enhanced axial (*A*) and coronal (*B*) CT images of the thigh show a large rim-enhancing (*arrowhead*) fluid collection (*star*) containing foci of gas (*arrow*), compatible with an abscess with subcutaneous fat and intramuscular involvement. Foci of gas in this case are compatible with a gas-forming organism, and foci of gas suspended within the center of the collection (not floating to the top) imply thick viscous material within the abscess cavity compatible in this case with necrotic tissue and thick pus.

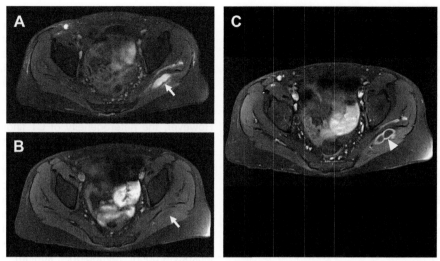

Fig. 5. Left gluteus maximus abscess in an IV drug user with fever and left buttocks pain and swelling. Axial proton-density fat saturated (PDFS) (A), axial T1 fat-saturated precontrast (B), and axial T1 fat-saturated postcontrast (C) demonstrating lobulated PDFS hyperintense and precontrast T1 hypointense (arrows) fluid collection in the left gluteus maximus. This collection demonstrates robust peripheral enhancement (C, arrowhead) in keeping with abscess.

dissemination of infection catalyzed by toxin-mediated activation of cytokines leading to microthrombosis and ischemia, typically following post-traumatic or postsurgical inoculation.[18] Infection is usually polymicrobial (Type 1) or, when monobacterial, commonly caused by Group A β-hemolytic streptococci (Type 2).[19,20] The initial clinical presentation of NF may mimic that of cellulitis or abscess but the disease progresses rapidly (within hours) to systemic toxicity and shock.[20] Reported mortality ranges widely from 9% to 76%, with an average of 25% to 35%.[20] Prompt diagnosis and treatment, and specifically early surgical debridement, are crucial for decreasing mortality. NF is a clinical diagnosis, and prompt surgical treatment should not be delayed by imaging in patients with characteristic clinical signs and symptoms. In equivocal cases, however, imaging is key to the diagnosis of NF and more sensitive than physical examination or clinical scores in diagnosing necrotizing soft tissue infections.[21]

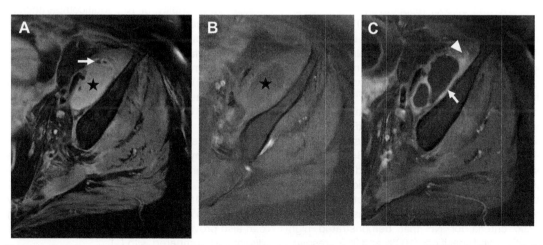

Fig. 6. Left psoas abscess with gas-forming bacteria. Axial PDFS (A) demonstrates an ovoid hyperintense fluid collection (black star) with tiny antidependent foci of hypointensity compatible with gas bubbles (arrow). Axial T1 fat-saturated precontrast (B) and axial T1 fat-saturated post-contrast (C) show this collection to have intrinsic T1 hypointensity (B, black star) with postcontrast peripheral enhancement (arrow) compatible with an abscess in the left psoas. Notice the hazy enhancement in the adjacent psoas muscle compatible with background myositis (C, arrowhead).

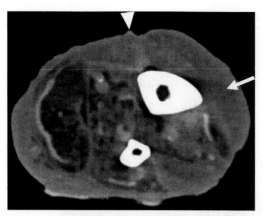

Fig. 7. Mimic of soft tissue infection—Kaposi's sarcoma in an HIV patient. CT extremity showing skin thickening and nodularity (*arrowhead*), with intermediate density haziness of the subcutaneous fat (*arrow*). This appearance is like cellulitis and is included to demonstrate how other conditions, including malignancy, can mimic soft tissue infection. This issue is complicated by the fact that malignant soft tissue involvement can be complicated by infection, and in such cases, comparison of imaging over time and clinical correlation is essential.

The presence of gas in the subcutaneous tissues or along the fascial planes is a highly specific sign of NF. However, soft tissue gas is absent in about half of NF cases,[22] especially in the early stages of disease.[23] Radiography has a limited role and poor sensitivity for the detection of soft tissue gas.[21] CT is the most sensitive modality for the detection of soft tissue gas, with a recent meta-analysis reporting sensitivity and specificity of 88.5% and 93.3%, respectively.[2,9,21,23] Other characteristic findings of NF on CT include the thickening of the superficial and deep fascia, inflammation and fluid along fascial planes extending to the intermuscular septa and muscles, and nonenhancement of fascia (which, when present, differentiates NF from non-NF).[2,10,23,24] The presence of fluid along the deep fascia on CT was the only finding that could reliably differentiate between NF and nonnecrotizing soft tissue infections (N-NSTI) according to a study by Bruls and colleagues[25] (**Fig. 8**). Martinez and colleagues included soft tissue gas, multiple fluid collections, absence or heterogeneity of enhancement, and inflammatory changes deep to the fascia as diagnostic criteria for NF that demonstrated high sensitivity and specificity (100% and 98%, respectively).[10] McGillicuddy and colleagues proposed the NSTI CT Scoring System that assigned points to findings of fascial air,[5] muscle/fascial edema,[4] fluid along fascial planes,[3] lymphadenopathy,[2] and subcutaneous edema.[1] A composite score

of greater than 6 had a sensitivity and specificity of 86.3% and 91.5%, respectively, with area under the curve of 0.928 (95% confidence interval [CI] 0.893–0.964).[26] A subsequent meta-analysis found that including multiple imaging findings in addition to fascial gas marginally improves the sensitivity of CT for the diagnosis of necrotizing soft tissue infections, at the cost of specificity.[21] However, the heterogeneity of CT findings used as criteria to diagnose NF in previous studies limits the accuracy of these sensitivity/specificity metrics.[21] CT was also found to be superior when differentiating NF from N-NSTI when compared with the Laboratory Risk Indicator for Necrotizing Fasciitis score, a retrospectively developed, externally validated, diagnostic and prognostic scoring system incorporating values of C-reactive protein, leukocyte count, hemoglobin, sodium, creatinine, and glucose.[25,27] CT is also useful to evaluate the extent of the disease, which helps surgical planning and treatment.

US is not commonly used to diagnose NF, and there is limited data evaluating the sensitivity/specificity of US in the diagnosis of NF. Common findings of NF on US include fluid along fascia and soft tissue gas that may appear as hyperechoic foci with "dirty" posterior shadowing, and muscle edema/early necrosis.[12,28,29]

Although MR imaging offers superior soft tissue contrast and potentially higher sensitivity for the detection of soft tissue infections such as NF, CT is often the preferred cross-sectional imaging modality because of its easy availability, faster image acquisition, and lower cost,[24] especially as delayed diagnosis and treatment significantly increase the mortality of NF. Multicompartmental (>2) involvement of the deep fascia, with 3 mm or greater of fascial thickening, low-signal intensity of the deep fascia on fat-suppressed T2WI, and nonenhancement of the affected fascia on post-contrast T1WI help distinguish NF from N-NSTI.[30] Gas along the fascial planes, when present, can be detected as areas of signal void or susceptibility on gradient echo sequences.[2] According to a systematic review by Kwee and colleagues, T2 hyperintensity of deep fascia was the most commonly used diagnostic MR imaging criterion for NF, with a pooled sensitivity of 86.4% (95% CI 76.1%–92.7%) and a pooled specificity of 65.2% (95% CI 35.4%–86.6%).[31] MR imaging can also provide superior evaluation for extent of disease as compared with CT.[30]

Fournier's Gangrene

Fournier's gangrene (FG) is a NF of the external genitalia and perineum that constitutes an urologic

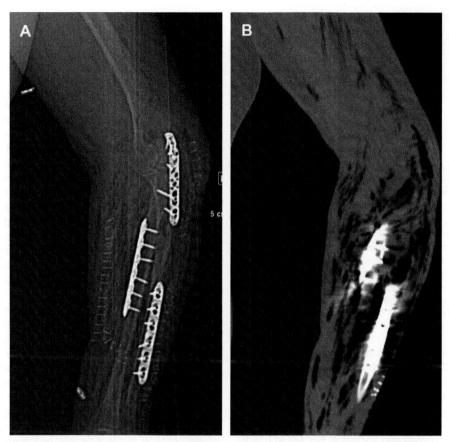

Fig. 8. NF of the left arm after surgery to repair forearm fractures. The patient had increasing pain, swelling, and rapid development of crepitus following surgery. Scout (*A*) and coronal noncontrast CT (*B*) show extensive gas throughout the deep soft tissues of the forearm, the upper arm, and extending up into the axilla. Notice how the gas is distributed throughout multiple compartments, along both fascial planes and within the muscular fibers. Patient required amputation of the arm.

emergency, with rapid progression (over hours) and mortality ranging from 20% to 40%.[32] FG is uncommon with an incidence of 1.6 per 100,000 and accounts for only 0.02% of hospital admissions in the United States.[32] The disease has a male predominance (men to women ratio 10:1–42:1), notwithstanding the underreporting of female cases.[28,32,33] A minority of studies do report a higher proportion of female patients (up to 55%).[34] Diabetes is the most associated comorbid condition in patients with FG.[32,35] Other comorbid conditions include obesity, cardiac and renal disease, alcoholism, peripheral vascular disease and immunosuppression.[28,32,35,36]

Sources of infection typically include perianal, ischiorectal or periurethral sites.[28,33,37] Infection is often polymicrobial (54%), followed by *Escherichia coli* (47%) and *Streptococcus* (37%).[38] Although specific inciting factors cannot be determined in some cases, urogenital and perineal trauma or interventions, indwelling catheters,

prolonged hospitalization, and pressure sores increase risk of FG.[28,33,36,39,40] Previous case series have reported high mortality rates of up to (88%) but the largest population-based study in the United States reported a case fatality rate of 7.5%.[32] Diabetes, cardiac and renal disease, renal failure, and sepsis are associated with increased mortality.[35,41]

Diagnosis of FG is primarily clinical. Patients may present with scrotal/perineal pain and tenderness with a poorly demarcated area of swelling and erythema.[36] Sepsis; multiorgan failure; skin blisters, bullae, and necrosis; and putrid discharge may be present in advanced disease.[36,42] Pain out of proportion with physical findings should raise the suspicion for FG.[36] Crepitus is present in up to 36% of cases[43] and highly specific for anaerobic infections.[36] Treatment consists of early surgical debridement and broad-spectrum antibiotics.

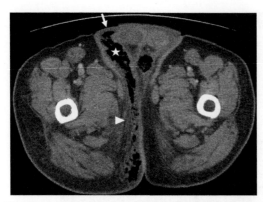

Fig. 9. FG in a male with diabetes presenting to the emergency department with perineal pain, redness, swelling, and crepitus. Skin thickening (*arrow*) and regions of hazy subcutaneous fat stranding (*arrowhead*) are present, with extensive gas throughout the perineum, worse on the right (*star*). This patient required extensive surgical debridement, and it can be helpful for the surgeons to clearly demarcate the extend of infection by imaging.

CT is the imaging modality of choice to evaluate the extent of disease and to help establish the diagnosis in equivocal cases. Findings of FG on CT include subcutaneous and fascial thickening/edema, fluid collection/abscess, and soft tissue gas[22,28,34] (**Fig. 9**). Although soft tissue gas in the scrotum is a common finding in FG, up to 5% to 20% of cases may not demonstrate this finding.[22,37] Ballard and colleagues validated the NSTI CT score (developed by McGillicuddy and colleagues) in 38 patients with FG and demonstrated high interobserver variability for the detection of most of the CT findings/components of the score.[26,34] CT is also useful to identify the source of infection and to evaluate extent of disease by detecting subcutaneous or fascial air tracking along the anterior abdominal wall and inguinal canals.[28] Retroperitoneal spread has been reported in a small number (8%) of patients.[34] Spread to the thighs, chest wall, and axilla has also been reported.[33]

Other modalities such as radiography, US, and MR imaging have limited utility in the diagnosis of FG, especially when CT is readily available, and demonstrate findings of NF in the scrotum and perineum as described above. US can help distinguish FG from a bowel-containing inguinoscrotal hernia and other causes of testicular/scrotal pain such as testicular torsion and epididymo-orchitis.[28,37] However, US is limited by a smaller field of view, operator dependence, and potential intolerance by patients due to exacerbation of scrotal/perineal pain.[37,44,45] MR imaging of the scrotum and perineum in cases of FG requires

longer acquisition times and rarely provides additional information compared with CT[45] (**Fig. 10**).

MUSCULAR INFECTIONS
Infectious Myositis and Pyomyositis

Infectious myositis is an infection of skeletal muscle[46] caused by a range of pathogens and introduced by various mechanisms. Pyomyositis specifically refers to an acute bacterial infection of skeletal muscle (most commonly S aureus) that often arises from hematogenous seeding.[47]

Normal skeletal muscle tends to resist infection but becomes vulnerable when its architecture is disrupted by an external insult. Antecedent blunt trauma is implicated in many cases of pyomyositis,[48,49] followed by a presumed transient bacteremia. Systemic factors can also predispose to muscle infection. In a study of hospitalized patients in the United States from 2002 to 2014, the risk factors most associated with pyomyositis were human immunodeficiency virus (HIV), hematologic malignancy, diabetes mellitus (types I and II), organ transplantation, and malnutrition.[47] Cases occur in both children and adults but in multiple settings, peaks have been observed in pediatric populations under the age of 10.[47,50]

Pyomyositis evolves in 3 stages following the initial episode of bacterial seeding. Stage 1, the invasive stage, is characterized by low-grade fever and dull pain in the affected muscle(s), persisting for up to 3 weeks. The absence of skin changes at this stage can make clinical diagnosis difficult but if pyomyositis is suspected, conservative treatment with antibiotics may suffice. In Stage 2, the purulent or suppurative stage, local pain and tenderness worsen along with fevers and chills, coinciding with the development of an intramuscular abscess. This feature differentiates bacterial pyomyositis from viral myositis, which does not progress to abscess formation. Patients frequently present for imaging at this stage, and surgical or image-guided drainage becomes critical. By Stage 3, the late stage, local erythema and fluctuance usually manifest, and disseminated infection can lead to sepsis and other systemic complications requiring intensive care.[50,51]

The lower extremities are the most common site of infection, with the quadriceps muscles predominating, followed by the gluteal and iliopsoas muscles. In children, this clinical picture may prompt evaluation according to the limping child algorithm, including with initial radiography to assess for fracture.[52] Although historically iliopsoas infection was associated with spinal tuberculosis, most iliopsoas infections today originate in the gastrointestinal and urinary tracts. Pyomyositis most often

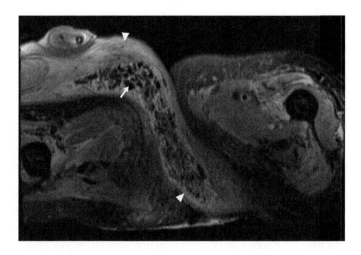

Fig. 10. FG on MR imaging. A single axial PDFS sequence shows diffuse PDFS hypo-intense foci throughout the soft tissue of the perineum (*arrow*) compatible with foci of gas. Throughout the perineum and surrounding these foci of gas, there is PDFS hyperintensity compatible with edema and fluid (*arrowhead*).

involves a single muscle but up to 40% may be multifocal.[4]

Radiography is of limited utility for diagnosing pyomyositis but can detect other, especially osseous, pathologic conditions. US can be used to visualize soft tissue fluid collections but is limited by depth of penetration. As such, abscesses in the deep muscles or extending into the pelvis may not be adequately visualized, necessitating cross-sectional imaging. Sonographic findings that suggest infected fluid include peripheral hyperemia, internal debris and septations, and internal gas. The absence of these findings, however, does not exclude infection.[53]

CT is often obtained initially in the emergency department demonstrating enlargement and hypoattenuation of the affected muscle, and effacement of adjacent fat planes. An intramuscular abscess is usually present, with peripheral rim enhancement and central nonenhancement following administration of IV-iodinated contrast[4] (Fig. 11).

On MR imaging, muscle edema is evident as high signal on T2-weighted or fat-suppressed long-TR sequences and may be the sole or principal imaging finding in Stage 1 pyomyositis. Edema in adjacent subcutaneous soft tissues suggests associated cellulitis but may not be present in patients with HIV. Abscesses demonstrate rim enhancement with administration of gadolinium-based contrast. Microvascular hemorrhage accounts for features such as T1-hyperintense foci within the muscle, or a T1-hyperintense and T2-hypointense rim around the abscess.[54]

Differential Diagnosis for Pyomyositis

Several noninfectious diseases have imaging features overlapping with pyomyositis. Differentiation is facilitated by clinical factors including history and laboratory findings but imaging can provide clues.

Hematoma is in the differential diagnosis for an intramuscular fluid collection and may be difficult to distinguish from abscess on imaging. Correlation with infectious symptoms and laboratory values is often key, and follow-up to resolution should be considered. A spontaneous hematoma in the absence of anticoagulation raises concern for an underlying tumor, which should be excluded with follow-up imaging. Internal enhancement, especially mass-like or nodular enhancement, suggests neoplasm over hematoma or abscess. Various patterns of internal enhancement can also be seen in myositis ossificans and myonecrosis, both discussed below. Subcutaneous edema is usually not associated with intramuscular tumors but

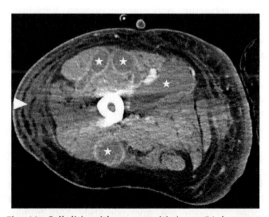

Fig. 11. Cellulitis with pyomyositis in an IV drug user with MRSA bacteremia. Contrast-enhanced axial CT demonstrates subcutaneous fat stranding (*arrowhead*) with multiple rim-enhancing fluid collections within the anterior, adductor, and posterior thigh muscle compartments (*stars*).

tumor-related T2-hyperintense signal within muscle may be difficult to distinguish from edema.[4]

Traumatic or sports-related injuries, such as muscle strain or tears, can produce high T2 signal within the muscle on MR imaging. A detailed history, however, generally suggests acute muscle injury over infection. Characteristic locations of muscle injury, for example, at the myotendinous junction, and US maneuvers to visualize muscle tears can assist.[54]

The following noninfectious muscle pathologic conditions should also be considered in the differential diagnosis for pyomyositis.

Inflammatory Myopathy

Among the noninfectious, immune-mediated myopathies, the 3 most common are polymyositis, dermatomyositis, and inclusion body myositis. Patients classically present with proximal muscle weakness in the extremities. Dermatomyositis occurs in both children and adults, whereas polymyositis occurs in adults and inclusion body myositis in predominantly adults aged older than 50 years. In acute disease, MR imaging is sensitive for detecting muscle edema. In the chronic phase, affected muscles may undergo fatty infiltration and atrophy. Concurrent edema in the subcutaneous soft tissues and fascial lining characterizes dermatomyositis but not polymyositis. Linear or reticular soft tissue calcification suggests juvenile dermatomyositis over polymyositis, is apparent on radiography, and may be subtly visible on MR imaging as low T1 and T2 signal. Muscle involvement in the inflammatory myopathies is characteristically bilateral and can be symmetric or asymmetric. Pyomyositis, however, is more often unilateral and focal.[54]

Myositis Ossificans

Blunt trauma may precede the development of pyomyositis but can also precipitate myositis ossificans. Defined by gradual mineralization and heterotypic bone formation within injured skeletal muscle, myositis ossificans also develops in the setting of severe burn injuries or paralysis. In the acute or pseudo-inflammatory phase, patients present with rapid-onset pain and swelling.[54] Early imaging findings can resemble those of infection and/or neoplasm, with intramuscular edema and/or a T2-hyperintense mass-like intramuscular lesion.[4] Gadolinium enhancement can be peripheral or diffuse.[55] In the subacute and chronic phases, the classic peripheral rim of calcification develops, evident on radiographs. Internal T1-hyperintense and T2-hyperintense areas of fatty marrow develop in the chronic phase. As imaging findings are nonspecific early in the course, short-interval follow-up with repeat imaging is useful.[54]

Diabetic Muscle Infarction, Myonecrosis

Muscle infarction occurs most commonly in patients with uncontrolled diabetes mellitus types I or II and is termed diabetic myonecrosis in these cases. It is rare compared with other diabetic complications, and nephropathy, retinopathy, and/or neuropathy are often already present. Myonecrosis presents with acute onset of severe pain and swelling usually in the lower extremities, persisting for several weeks.[56] Fever and leukocytosis tend to be absent.[4] On MR imaging, T2 hyperintensity is seen in the affected muscle with associated perifascial or subcutaneous edema. Signal characteristics may resemble those of pyomyositis but involvement of multiple noncontiguous muscles is more common in myonecrosis.[54] Moreover, the enhancement pattern of myonecrosis varies from diffuse enhancement to intense rim enhancement with linear internal enhancing streaks.[4] On US, linear echogenic structures traversing the lesion have been described, and internal mobile or swirling fluid is usually absent. Differentiation from pyomyositis is important because myonecrosis resolves with conservative treatment, including glycemic control. Muscle biopsy is not recommended because of the risk of complications and prolongation of symptoms.[56]

Denervation

Denervation of a muscle group can result in pain and/or weakness, sometimes with accompanying sensory deficits depending on the nerve affected. MR imaging abnormalities can be seen in the acute, subacute, and chronic phases. Intramuscular edema with T2 hyperintensity develops within 1 to 2 days. Affected muscles can become paradoxically enlarged in the following 2 to 4 weeks, reflecting hypertrophy/pseudohypertrophy.[4] If untreated, denervation results in muscle atrophy over months. Subcutaneous edema is notably absent in denervation, helping to differentiate it from infection.[54]

BURSAL INFECTIONS

Bursae are closed, extra-articular, fluid-filled sacs that reduce the friction between soft tissues and bones.[57] There are approximately 150 bursae located throughout the body. Bursitis is the inflammatory process incited by overuse, trauma, or prolonged pressure, characterized by overproduction of fluid from the synovial cells that line the bursae. The most common sites include the olecranon,

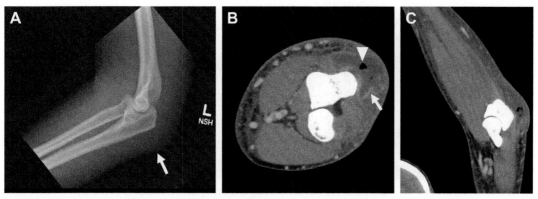

Fig. 12. Septic olecranon bursitis. Lateral elbow radiograph (A) with diffuse swelling posteriorly with more rounded soft tissue density within the region of the olecranon bursa (*arrow*). Contrast-enhanced axial (B) and sagittal (C) CT demonstrating peripherally enhancing (*B, arrow*), gas-containing fluid collection (*B, arrowhead*) within the olecranon bursa with surrounding skin thickening and subcutaneous fat stranding.

prepatellar and trochanteric bursae, given their superficial location and susceptibility to trauma.[58] Septic bursitis occurs when the bursae become infected, with *S aureus* and the *Streptococcus* species being the most common causative organisms.[59] Superficial bursitis occurs most often when there is direct inoculation through trauma or micropuncture of the skin. Deep bursitis occurs when there is hematogenous contamination or contiguous spread from bone or soft tissue infections.[60] It is estimated that approximately one-third of cases of olecranon and prepatellar bursitis are septic, resulting in an estimated annual incidence of 0.1/1000 in the population.[61] Epidemiologically, bursitis is more common in men in the age range of 40 to 80 years. This can be attributed to the fact that most cases are caused by repetitive trauma, commonly seen in occupational labor

such as plumbing and roofing. Imaging plays a critical role in the evaluation of septic bursitis.[62]

Anteroposterior and lateral radiographs are used in the initial diagnostic imaging workup for septic bursitis, primarily to rule out the presence of a foreign body or acute pathologic fracture because the clinical presentation is nonspecific.[61] Radiography can also detect enthesophytes, or abnormal bony projections at the attachment site of a tendon or ligament, often associated with bursitis. In cases where septic bursitis is caused by a gas-producing organism, gas bubbles may be visualized.

Sonography may reveal a distended bursa, edema around the bursa, and bursal wall thickening, although these findings are nonspecific.[2] Of note, a distended bursa is not pathognomonic for bursitis and may indicate an adjacent

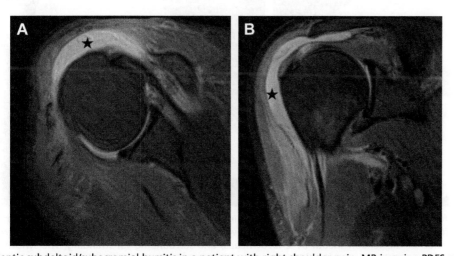

Fig. 13. Septic subdeltoid/subacromial bursitis in a patient with right shoulder pain. MR imaging PDFS sequences in axial (A) and coronal (B) planes of the right shoulder demonstrate marked fluid-filled distention of the subacromial/subdeltoid bursa (*black star*), compatible with bursitis.

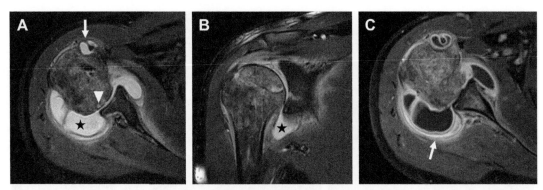

Fig. 14. Septic arthritis of the right shoulder, demonstrating the utility of MR imaging in cases where soft tissue infection has clinical overlap with joint involvement. MR imaging PDFS sequences in axial (*A*) and coronal (*B*) planes of the right shoulder show massive PDFS-hyperintense fluid distending the joint capsule (*black star*). The biceps tendon sheath is also filled with fluid and distended (*A, arrow*). Postcontrast fat-suppressed axial images (*C*) show brisk enhancement of the thickened joint capsule and synovium (*C, arrow*). Tiny foci of PDFS hyperintensity in the humeral head and bony glenoid are compatible with small erosions (*A, arrowhead*).

pathologic condition. Findings more specific for bursitis include mixed-echogenicity material within the bursa or hyperemia of the bursal wall on color Doppler imaging.[2] No sonographic finding reliably differentiates septic bursitis from reactive bursitis, with the exception of rice bodies, which can be seen in the setting of rheumatoid arthritis and tuberculosis.[63] US may also be used for image-guided needle aspiration of the bursal sac.[64]

CT can reveal a fluid distention of the bursa, bursal wall thickening, and surrounding soft tissue changes (**Fig. 12**). CT is most sensitive for detecting small amounts of gas, as in the setting of a gas-forming infection, which is most easily identified on lung windows. In addition, CT can clearly delineate

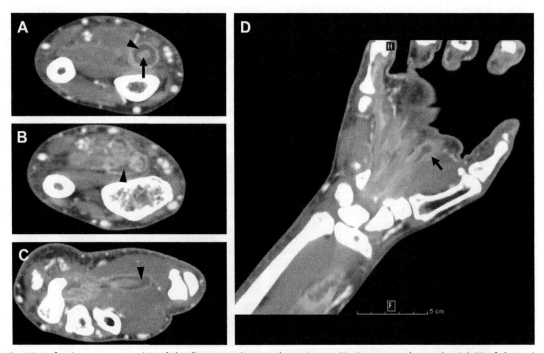

Fig. 15. Infectious tenosynovitis of the flexor tendons in the wrist on CT. Contrast-enhanced axial CT of the wrist and hand from proximal to distal (*A–C*) and coronal view (*D*). There is enlargement of the tendons (*A, arrow*) with fluid distention of the tendon sheath (*A–C arrowheads*) and surrounding fat-stranding. The synovium of the tendon sheaths are thickening and mildly enhancing (*D, arrow*), a feature which is often better appreciated on MR imaging. Note that these findings track proximal and distal to the carpal tunnel—and delineation of extent of infection is important for surgical management.

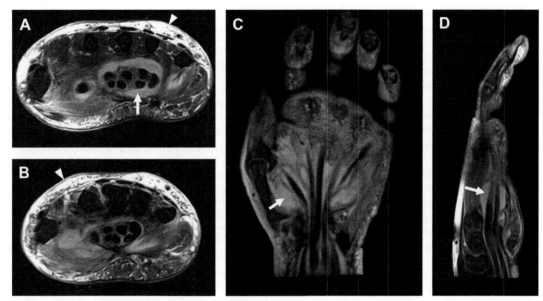

Fig. 16. Infectious tenosynovitis of the flexor tendons in the wrist on MR imaging. Axial (*A*, *B*), coronal (*C*), and sagittal (*D*) MR imaging PDFS sequences demonstrate fluid throughout the flexor tendon sheaths of the hand and wrist (*arrows A, C, D*). The hand and wrist are diffusely swollen with subcutaneous PDFS hyperintensity compatible with edema (*A, B, arrowheads*). Note that this patient did not receive contrast, and the diagnosis is still evident.

skin thickening overlying the affected bursae and reveal sinus tracts or ulcerations.[17]

MR imaging is sensitive for the detection of bursal fluid in the setting of septic bursitis (**Fig. 13**). This fluid demonstrates low signal intensity on T1WI and high signal intensity on T2WI. Following the administration of gadolinium-based contrast, the wall of the bursa and adjacent soft tissues will enhance.[2] Gas, if present, manifests as signal voids in the affected region. In cases of deep bursitis, MR imaging can help detect the development of an abscess or extension of infection into adjacent bone or joints[65] (**Fig. 14**).

TENDON AND TENDON SHEATH INFECTIONS

Infectious tenosynovitis is most often caused by direct inoculation of the tendon sheath with skin flora following penetrating injuries, such as puncture wounds or human/animal bites. In keeping with this mechanism, these infections commonly affect the tendon sheaths of the hand, mostly the flexor tendon sheaths.[66–68] In addition to *S aureus*, which represents 75% of positive cultures, other commonly isolated bacteria include methicillin-resistant *S aureus* (29% of cultures), *Staphylococcus epidermidis*, beta-hemolytic *Streptococcus* species, and *Pseudomonas aeruginosa*. Polymicrobial infections are common, especially in immunocompromised patients, which

underscores the importance of empiric treatment with broad-spectrum antibiotics, before culture and sensitivity results enable targeted antibiotic therapy.[67–69]

The diagnostic criteria for acute bacterial tenosynovitis are primarily clinical and based on the 4 Kanavel signs, described by surgeon Allen B Kanavel in the early 1900s. These include fusiform swelling of the digit, severe tenderness along the course of the tendon sheath, fixed semiflexed posture of the finger, and exquisite pain with attempted passive extension.[68,70,71]

US may assist in diagnosis and is also used for image-guided aspiration. Fluid analysis is required to confirm the diagnosis because infectious and noninfectious tenosynovitis (inflammatory, traumatic, HIV-related/AIDS-related, or sarcoidal tenosynovitis) share the same sonographic imaging findings. On grayscale US images, there is accumulation of fluid/pus in the tendon sheath, enlargement of the tendon relative to the contralateral one, and hyperemia on color Doppler images.[71,72] US can also detect and provide image guidance for the removal of retained foreign bodies, which can compromise treatment if left in place. US guidance can also prove useful in cases of chronic infection, where the scarcity of fluid may necessitate lavage, or where biopsy of the synovial membrane may be needed for diagnosis and targeted antibiotic treatment.[68,70–72]

Plain radiographs are useful in the emergent setting as a rapid, cost-effective method of identifying retained foreign bodies or associated acute osseous injuries. Soft tissue swelling and fixed semiflexion, although nonspecific, may also be evident on plain radiographs to support the diagnosis of acute bacterial tenosynovitis. In chronic or late-presenting cases, osseous erosions can also be detected on plain radiographs, raising suspicion for complications such as septic arthritis or osteomyelitis.[66]

CT and MR imaging provide helpful information when the diagnosis is unclear, or for preoperative planning in severe cases of deep infections violating multiple tissue compartments. CT images show enlargement of the tendons with fluid distention of the synovium and surrounding fat-stranding (**Fig. 15**). MR imaging demonstrates thickening, T2/STIR hyperintensity and contrast enhancement of the affected tendon sheaths (**Fig. 16**). In the hand, infections can spread via anatomic communications between, for example, the flexor pollicis longus and fifth finger flexor tendon sheaths (which represent the radial and ulnar bursae of the carpus, respectively), and CT or MR may best delineate the full extent of infection.[66]

SUMMARY

Soft tissue infections encompass a diverse set of diseases, many of which have nonspecific clinical and laboratory findings that challenge the acute care provider. These entities may be simple, uncomplicated, and self-limited but can also present with or progress to deeper infections, which may have high levels of morbidity and mortality. When deployed appropriately, imaging with radiography, US, CT, or MR imaging can improve diagnostic confidence and accuracy, assist in identifying complications, and guide interventions. The emergency radiologist should be well versed in the imaging of these conditions and serve as a resource to the acute care clinician.

CLINICS CARE POINTS

- Although superficial infections can often be diagnosed and managed clinically, physical examination may lack sensitivity and specificity, and imaging is often required to evaluate the depth of involvement and identify complications. Depending on the area of involvement, radiography, US, CT, MR imaging, or a combination of imaging modalities may be required.

- Soft tissue infections can be nonnecrotizing or necrotizing, with the latter having a morbid and rapid course. Necrotizing soft-tissue infection imaging findings include fascial gas, muscle/fascial edema, fluid along fascial planes, lymphadenopathy, and subcutaneous edema.

- Infectious myositis and pyomyositis occur most frequently in the lower extremities. CT is often obtained initially in the emergency department demonstrating enlargement and hypoattenuation of the affected muscle, and effacement of adjacent fat planes. An intramuscular abscess suggests pyomyositis and is best delineated with postcontrast imaging.

- Bursal and tendon-sheath infections are also important soft tissue infections that require specific clinical management. Bursal infections are characterized by fluid-distention of bursa, which have thick walls, and can be evaluated by US for superficial bursa or CT/MR imaging for deeper bursa. Infectious tenosynovitis most commonly affects the flexor tendon sheaths of the hand, characterized by thickened and enhancing synovium with fluid-filled tendon sheaths.

DISCLOSURE

The authors have no conflicts of interest to disclose.

REFERENCES

1. Bystritsky R, Chambers H. Cellulitis and soft tissue infections. Ann Intern Med 2018;168(3):ITC17–32.
2. Turecki MB, Taljanovic MS, Stubbs AY, et al. Imaging of musculoskeletal soft tissue infections. Skeletal Radiol 2009;39(10):957–71.
3. Hill MK, Sanders CV. Skin and soft tissue infections in critical care. Crit Care Clin 1998;14(2):251–62.
4. Hayeri MR, Ziai P, Shehata ML, et al. Mimics: From Cellulitis to Necrotizing Fasciitis. Radiographics 2016;36(6):1888–910.
5. Sivitz AB, Lam SHF, Ramirez-Schrempp D, et al. Effect of bedside ultrasound on management of pediatric soft-tissue infection. J Emerg Med 2010;39(5):637–43.
6. Vartanians VM, Karchmer AW, Giurini JM, et al. Is there a role for imaging in the management of patients with diabetic foot? Skeletal Radiol 2009;38(7):633–6.

7. Altmayer S, Verma N, Dicks EA, et al. Imaging musculoskeletal soft tissue infections. Semin Ultrasound CT MR 2020;41(1):85–98.

8. Arnold MJ, Jonas CE, Carter RE. Point-of-Care Ultrasonography. Am Fam Physician 2020;101(5): 275–85.

9. Leichtle SW, Tung L, Khan M, et al. The role of radiologic evaluation in necrotizing soft tissue infections. J Trauma Acute Care Surg 2016;81(5):921–4.

10. Martinez M, Peponis T, Hage A, et al. The Role of Computed Tomography in the Diagnosis of Necrotizing Soft Tissue Infections. World J Surg 2018; 42(1):82–7.

11. Arnon-Sheleg E, Israel O, Keidar Z. PET/CT Imaging in Soft Tissue Infection and Inflammation-An Update. Semin Nucl Med 2020;50(1):35–49.

12. Chau CLF, Griffith JF. Musculoskeletal infections: ultrasound appearances. Clin Radiol 2005;60(2): 149–59.

13. Ellis Simonsen SM, van Orman ER, Hatch BE, et al. Cellulitis incidence in a defined population. Epidemiol Infect 2006;134(2):293–9.

14. Tong SYC, Davis JS, Eichenberger E, et al. Staphylococcus aureus infections: epidemiology, pathophysiology, clinical manifestations, and management. Clin Microbiol Rev 2015;28(3): 603–61.

15. Loyer EM, DuBrow RA, David CL, et al. Imaging of superficial soft-tissue infections: sonographic findings in cases of cellulitis and abscess. AJR Am J Roentgenol 1996;166(1):149–52.

16. Chang C-D, Wu JS. Imaging of Musculoskeletal Soft Tissue Infection. Semin Roentgenol 2017;52(1): 55–62.

17. Simpfendorfer CS. Radiologic Approach to Musculoskeletal Infections. Infect Dis Clin North Am 2017; 31(2):299–324.

18. Bonne SL, Kadri SS. Evaluation and Management of Necrotizing Soft Tissue Infections. Infect Dis Clin North Am 2017;31(3):497–511.

19. Giuliano A, Lewis F Jr, Hadley K, et al. Bacteriology of necrotizing fasciitis. Am J Surg 1977;134(1):52–7.

20. Hakkarainen TW, Kopari NM, Pham TN, et al. Necrotizing soft tissue infections: review and current concepts in treatment, systems of care, and outcomes. Curr Probl Surg 2014;51(8):344–62.

21. Fernando SM, Tran A, Cheng W, et al. Necrotizing Soft Tissue Infection: Diagnostic Accuracy of Physical Examination, Imaging, and LRINEC Score: A Systematic Review and Meta-Analysis. Ann Surg 2019;269(1):58–65.

22. Wysoki MG, Santora TA, Shah RM, et al. Necrotizing fasciitis: CT characteristics. Radiology 1997;203(3): 859–63.

23. Chaudhry AA, Baker KS, Gould ES, et al. Necrotizing fasciitis and its mimics: what radiologists

need to know. AJR Am J Roentgenol 2015;204(1): 128–39.

24. Fayad LM, Carrino JA, Fishman EK. Musculoskeletal infection: role of CT in the emergency department. Radiographics 2007;27(6):1723–36.

25. Bruls RJM, Kwee RM. CT in necrotizing soft tissue infection: diagnostic criteria and comparison with LRINEC score. Eur Radiol 2021;31(11):8536–41.

26. McGillicuddy EA, Lischuk AW, Schuster KM, et al. Development of a computed tomography-based scoring system for necrotizing soft-tissue infections. J Trauma 2011;70(4):894–9.

27. Wong C-H, Khin L-W, Heng K-S, et al. (Laboratory Risk Indicator for Necrotizing Fasciitis) score: a tool for distinguishing necrotizing fasciitis from other soft tissue infections. Crit Care Med 2004;32(7): 1535–41.

28. Levenson RB, Singh AK, Novelline RA. Fournier gangrene: role of imaging. Radiographics 2008; 28(2):519–28.

29. Parenti GC, Marri C, Calandra G, et al. Necrotizing fasciitis of soft tissues: role of diagnostic imaging and review of the literature. Radiol Med 2000; 99(5):334–9.

30. Kim K-T, Kim YJ, Won Lee J, et al. Can necrotizing infectious fasciitis be differentiated from nonnecrotizing infectious fasciitis with MR imaging? Radiology 2011;259(3):816–24.

31. Kwee RM, Kwee TC. Diagnostic performance of MRI and CT in diagnosing necrotizing soft tissue infection: a systematic review. Skeletal Radiol [Internet] 2021;51(4):727–36. https://doi.org/10.1007/s00256-021-03875-9. Available at:.

32. Sorensen MD, Krieger JN, Rivara FP, et al. Fournier's Gangrene: population based epidemiology and outcomes. J Urol 2009;181(5):2120–6.

33. Eke N. Fournier's gangrene: a review of 1726 cases. Br J Surg 2000;87(6):718–28.

34. Ballard DH, Raptis CA, Guerra J, et al. Preoperative CT Findings and Interobserver Reliability of Fournier Gangrene. AJR Am J Roentgenol 2018;211(5): 1051–7.

35. Yanar H, Taviloglu K, Ertekin C, et al. Fournier's gangrene: risk factors and strategies for management. World J Surg 2006;30(9):1750–4.

36. Voelzke BB, Hagedorn JC. Presentation and Diagnosis of Fournier Gangrene. Urology 2018;114:8–13.

37. Ballard DH, Mazaheri P, Raptis CA, et al. Fournier Gangrene in Men and Women: Appearance on CT, Ultrasound, and MRI and What the Surgeon Wants to Know. Can Assoc Radiol J 2020;71(1):30–9.

38. Tang L-M, Su Y-J, Lai Y-C. The evaluation of microbiology and prognosis of fournier's gangrene in past five years. Springerplus 2015;4:14.

39. Aridogan IA, Izol V, Abat D, et al. Epidemiological characteristics of Fournier's gangrene: a report of 71 patients. Urol Int 2012;89(4):457–61.

40. Backhaus M, Citak M, Tilkorn D-J, et al. Pressure sores significantly increase the risk of developing a Fournier's gangrene in patients with spinal cord injury. Spinal Cord 2011;49(11):1143–6.

41. El-Qushayri AE, Khalaf KM, Dahy A, et al. Fournier's gangrene mortality: A 17-year systematic review and meta-analysis. Int J Infect Dis 2020;92:218–25.

42. Auerbach J, Bornstein K, Ramzy M, et al. Fournier Gangrene in the Emergency Department: Diagnostic Dilemmas, Treatments and Current Perspectives. Open Access Emerg Med 2020;12: 353–64.

43. Goh T, Goh LG, Ang CH, et al. Early diagnosis of necrotizing fasciitis. Br J Surg 2014;101(1):e119–25.

44. Avery LL, Scheinfeld MH. Imaging of penile and scrotal emergencies. Radiographics 2013;33(3): 721–40.

45. Parker RA 3rd, Menias CO, Quazi R, et al. MR Imaging of the Penis and Scrotum. Radiographics 2015; 35(4):1033–50.

46. Crum-Cianflone NF. Bacterial, fungal, parasitic, and viral myositis. Clin Microbiol Rev 2008;21(3):473–94.

47. Maravelas R, Melgar TA, Vos D, et al. Pyomyositis in the United States 2002-2014. J Infect 2020;80(5): 497–503.

48. Chauhan S, Jain S, Varma S, et al. Tropical pyomyositis (myositis tropicans): current perspective. Postgrad Med J 2004;80(943):267–70.

49. Theodorou SJ, Theodorou DJ, Resnick D. MR imaging findings of pyogenic bacterial myositis (pyomyositis) in patients with local muscle trauma: illustrative cases. Emerg Radiol 2007;14(2):89–96.

50. Shittu A, Deinhardt-Emmer S. Vas Nunes J, Niemann S, Grobusch MP, Schaumburg F. Tropical pyomyositis: an update. Trop Med Int Health 2020;25(6): 660–5.

51. Habeych ME, Trinh T, Crum-Cianflone NF. Purulent infectious myositis (formerly tropical pyomyositis). J Neurol Sci 2020;413:116767.

52. Lovejoy JF 3rd, Alexander K, Dinan D, et al. Team Approach: Pyomyositis JBJS Rev 2017;5(6):e4.

53. Carra BJ, Bui-Mansfield LT, O'Brien SD, et al. Sonography of musculoskeletal soft-tissue masses: techniques, pearls, and pitfalls. AJR Am J Roentgenol 2014;202(6):1281–90.

54. Endo Y, Miller TT. Myositis and fasciitis: role of imaging. Semin Musculoskelet Radiol 2018;22(3): 286–98.

55. Lacout A, Jarraya M, Marcy P-Y, et al. Myositis ossificans imaging: keys to successful diagnosis. Indian J Radiol Imaging 2012;22(1):35–9.

56. Horton WB, Taylor JS, Ragland TJ, et al. Diabetic muscle infarction: a systematic review. BMJ Open Diabetes Res Care 2015;3(1):e000082.

57. Resnick D, Kang SH, Pretterklieber LM. Internal derangements of joints. Philadelphia: Saunders/Elsevier; 2007.

58. Lormeau C, Cormier G, Sigaux J, et al. Management of septic bursitis. Joint Bone Spine 2019;86(5): 583–8.

59. Truong J, Mabrouk A, Ashurst JV. Septic Bursitis. In: StatPearls. Treasure Island (FL): StatPearls Publishing; 2021.

60. Zimmermann B 3rd, Mikolich DJ, Ho G Jr. Septic bursitis. Semin Arthritis Rheum 1995;24(6):391–410.

61. Baumbach SF, Lobo CM, Badyine I, et al. Prepatellar and olecranon bursitis: literature review and development of a treatment algorithm. Arch Orthop Trauma Surg 2014;134(3):359–70.

62. Laupland KB, Davies HD. Calgary Home Parenteral Therapy Program Study Group. Olecranon septic bursitis managed in an ambulatory setting. The Calgary Home Parenteral Therapy Program Study Group. Clin Invest Med 2001;24(4):171–8.

63. Yoshida S, Shidoh M, Imai K, et al. Rice bodies in ischiogluteal bursitis. Postgrad Med J 2003;79(930): 220–1.

64. Costantino TG, Roemer B, Leber EH. Septic arthritis and bursitis: emergency ultrasound can facilitate diagnosis. J Emerg Med 2007;32(3):295–7.

65. Small LN, Ross JJ. Suppurative tenosynovitis and septic bursitis. Infect Dis Clin North Am 2005; 19(4):991–1005.

66. Patel DB, Emmanuel NB, Stevanovic MV, et al. Hand infections: anatomy, types and spread of infection, imaging findings, and treatment options. Radiographics 2014;34(7):1968–86.

67. Giladi AM, Malay S, Chung KC. A systematic review of the management of acute pyogenic flexor tenosynovitis. J Hand Surg Eur Vol 2015;40(7):720–8.

68. Chapman T, Pyogenic Flexor Tenosynovitis Ilyas AM, Evaluation, et al. J Hand Microsurg 2019;11(3): 121–6.

69. Draeger RW, Bynum DK Jr. Flexor tendon sheath infections of the hand. J Am Acad Orthop Surg 2012; 20(6):373–82.

70. Kennedy CD, Huang JI, Hanel DP. Brief: Kanavel's Signs and Pyogenic Flexor Tenosynovitis. Clin Orthop Relat Res 2016;474(1):280–4.

71. Jeffrey RB Jr, Laing FC, Schechter WP, et al. Acute suppurative tenosynovitis of the hand: diagnosis with US. Radiology 1987;162(3):741–2.

72. Bureau NJ, Chhem RK, Cardinal E. Musculoskeletal infections: US manifestations. Radiographics 1999; 19(6):1585–92.

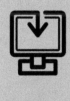

Printed and bound by CPI Group (UK) Ltd, Croydon, CR0 4YY

08/05/2025

01864723-0019